Medicine and Conflict

This book focuses on an important but neglected aspect of the Spanish Civil War, the evolution of medical and surgical care of the wounded during the conflict. Importantly, the focus is from a mainly Spanish perspective – as the Spanish are given a voice in their own story, which has not always been the case. Central to the book is General Franco's treatment of Muslim combatants, the anarchist contribution to health, and the medicalisation of propaganda – themes that come together in a medico-cultural study of the Spanish Civil War. Suffusing the narrative and the analysis is the traumatic legacy of conflict, an untreated wound that a new generation of Spaniards are struggling to heal.

Sebastian Browne is Associate Lecturer at Canterbury Christ Church, Kent and holds a PhD from the University of Kent.

Routledge/Cañada Blanch Studies on Contemporary Spain
Edited by Paul Preston and Sebastian Balfour, Cañada Blanch Centre for Contemporary Spanish Studies, London School of Economics, UK

20 Claiming the City and Contesting the State
Squatting, Community Formation and Democratization in Spain (1955–1986)
Inbal Ofer

21 Guns, Culture and Moors
Racial Perceptions, Cultural Impact and the Moroccan Participation in the Spanish Civil War (1936–1939)
Ali Al-Tuma

22 Revolution and the State
Anarchism in the Spanish Civil War, 1936–1939
Danny Evans

23 Medicine and Conflict
The Spanish Civil War and its Traumatic Legacy
Sebastian Browne

Also published in association with the Cañada Blanch Centre:

Spain and the Great Powers in the Twentieth Century
Edited by Sebastian Balfour and Paul Preston

The Politics of Contemporary Spain
Edited by Sebastian Balfour

Medicine and Conflict

The Spanish Civil War and its Traumatic Legacy

Sebastian Browne

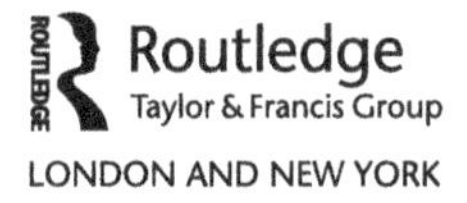

LONDON AND NEW YORK

First published 2019
by Routledge
2 Park Square, Milton Park, Abingdon, Oxon OX14 4RN

and by Routledge
52 Vanderbilt Avenue, New York, NY 10017

First issued in paperback 2020

Routledge is an imprint of the Taylor & Francis Group, an informa business

British Library Cataloguing in Publication Data
A catalogue record for this book is available from the British Library

Library of Congress Cataloging in Publication Data
A catalog record for this book has been requested

ISBN 13: 978-0-36-758764-2 (pbk)
ISBN 13: 978-0-8153-9423-5 (hbk)

Typeset in Times New Roman
by Out of House Publishing

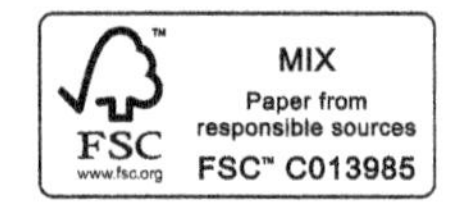

Printed in the United Kingdom
by Henry Ling Limited

To the memory of my mother Anne Browne (1932–2017).

This book is also dedicated to Andrés Barenno Pérez (1898–1936) and the villagers of La Sauceda, and to all those who died in the aerial attack and in the nearby detention centre of El Marrufo farm; but also to Ángeles Vásquez León (1922–2010), who trod the hard and difficult road from Málaga to Almería in February 1937.

Contents

Images

Acknowledgements

I have received invaluable help from numerous people, while researching and writing this book. Without this generous and patient assistance, finishing it would have been a far more arduous and difficult task. First and foremost, I have to thank my wife Jill and my sons Nathan and Adam for their unending and continued support, and also for their tolerance and forbearance. My mother, Anna Browne, also deserves special mention here, as despite a protracted illness she was unfailing in her support and even during the most difficult part of her illness had an attentive ear and helped me in keeping my eye on the target.

No book of this nature would be complete without acknowledging the enormous debt owed to Professor Paul Preston, whose enduring and ongoing scholarship on the Spanish Civil War lies at the forefront of the literature on the conflict. I was also fortunate to work at the Cañada Blanch Centre at the London School of Economics, where the support of the Centre's manager Susana Grau and of Paul Preston, the head of the Centre, was invaluable in the successful completion of this project.

I am indebted to my supervisor Ulf Schmidt for the many and incalculable ways he has helped me since I first started this project. I am also indebted to Julie Anderson from the University of Kent, and David Wilkinson, retired anaesthetist, who put me in touch with Avelino Franco Grande, a retired anaesthetist from Galicia, and who in sharing the fruits of his research carried out over a number of years, gave me access to research materials that would have been difficult to access otherwise. I am also grateful in this regard to Isabel Antón Solanas who also shared her research with me when first starting out. Avelino was just the first of the many people to help me in Spain, and special gratitude is owed to Ricardo Navarro Suay, consultant anaesthetist in the Spanish Army, and Ricardo Muro Garcia of the Museo de la Sanidad Militar for their gracious and invaluable assistance during and after my research visit to Madrid in 2014.

I am also grateful for the kind assistance of Xavier García Ferrandis, and that of Àlvar Martínez Vidal, Jon Arrizabalaga, Dolorés Martin Moruno, Richard Baxell, Jesús Majada Neila and Linda Palfreeman, all who have helped me in so many ways. It was Linda who put me in touch with Jesús

Majada Neila, who so generously provided me with much of the photographic material to be found in this study.

It is difficult to fully express the enormous gratitude due to Andrés Rebolledo Barreno for his unfailing work as president of the Asociación de Familiares y Represaliados por el Franquismo en La Sauceda y el Marrufo (Association of the Relatives of Repressed Victims of Francoism in La Sauceda and El Marrufo), work that has inspired my own efforts of addressing in this book the continuing traumatic legacy of Francoism. My brother Marcus requires special mention for helping inspire in me many years ago an interest in the Spanish Civil War, and I also owe thanks to my brother Ben and my sisters Joanna and Georgina for their understanding of my frequent absences in their lives during the writing of this book.

The acknowledgements here would not be complete without the special thanks due to Stuart Palmer for his untiring efforts in assisting me in making ready a draft suitable for submission. Aske Brock also deserves special mention for his invaluable help in this regard, as do Pip Gregory and Robert Newman who also helped me in so many ways. Alongside these towering figures of the University of Kent postgraduate world I would also like to thank Adam Rolewicz and Peter Keeling, towering figures in their own right, whose input and advice has always been gratefully received.

Special thanks are also due to Carl-Henrik Bjerström, David Bryan, Kerrie Holloway, Nick Sharman, and all those who have participated in the Cañada Blanch Centre's Discussion Group, for providing valuable and much-needed feedback and for their friendship and companionship over the past few years. I would also like to extend my gratitude to Guiomar Acevedo López, Helen Graham, Mary Vincent, Richard Cleminson and Peter Anderson, who have all helped or inspired me along the way.

I am also grateful for the kind assistance of the various personnel at the Archivo General Militar de Ávila, El Centro Documental de la Memoria Histórica de España, the British Film Institute, the Filmoteca de Catalunya, the Filmoteca Española, the Biblioteca Nacional de Catalunya, the Museo de Sanidad Militar, the Wellcome Library, the British Library, the National Archives and the Library of the University of Kent.

Special thanks are also due to my examiners Mark Connelly at the University of Kent and Sebastian Balfour at the London School of Economics. Additional thanks are owed to Sebastian Balfour, not only for challenging so many of the misconceptions concerning the participation of Moroccan troops during the Spanish Civil War, but also for his ceaseless efforts in confronting the continuing legacy of the chemical warfare inflicted upon the population of the Rif in Northern Morocco in the 1920s.

Last and by no means least, I would like to acknowledge a debt to Sir Peter Chalmers Mitchell (23 November 1864–2 July 1945), who cared enough to save the lives of not only his Francoist neighbours, but then helped local anarchists convert his neighbour's house into a hospital, as it was humanitarian efforts such as his that made the difference to so many lives during the Spanish Civil War, and inspired me throughout the writing of this book.

Abbreviations

ACMS	Archivo Casa de la Memoria de La Sauceda
ADPV	Archivo de la Diputación Provincial de Valencia
AGMAV	Archivo General Militar de Ávila
BFI	British Film Institute
BL	British Library
BLSA	British Library Sound Archive
BMJ	*British Medical Journal*
BNE	Biblioteca Nacional de España
BOE	Boletín Oficial del Estado
CASD	Canadian Committee to Aid Spanish Democracy
CCS	Casualty Clearing Station
CDMH	Centro Documental de la Memoria Histórica
CEDA	Confederación Española de Derechas Autónomas
CIG	Comité de Industrias de Guerra
CNT	Confederación Nacional del Trabajo
CSI	Central Sanitaire Internacional
CSV	Corpo Truppe Volontarie
CULA	Cardiff University Library Archive
FAI	Federación Anarquista Ibérica
FET y las JONS	Falange Española Tradicionalista y de las Juntas de Ofensiva Nacional Sindicalista
GDP	Gross Domestic Product
IHT	Institute of Haematology and Blood Transfusion at Moscow
IWMSA	Imperial War Museum Sound Archive
JSU	Las Juventudes Socialistas Unificadas
MML	Marx Memorial Library
MO	Medical Officer
MRCUW	Modern Records Centre University of Warwick
MZA	Madrid-Zaragoza-Alicante
OSO	Organización Sanitaria Obrera
PCE	Partido Comunista de España
PP	Partido Popular

POUM	Partido Obrero de Unificación Marxista
PSOE	Partido Socialista Obrero Español
PSUC	Partit Socialista Unificat de Catalunya
RTVE	Radio y Televisión Española
SERE	Servicio de Evacuación de Refugiados Españoles
SMAC	Spanish Medical Aid Committee
TPFS	Three Point Forward System
UGT	Unión General de Trabajadores
WLAM	Wellcome Library Archives and Manuscripts
WWI	World War One
WWII	World War Two

Prologue

Los Alcornacales, Spain, 2012

On 13 July 2012, *El País*, a leading Spanish newspaper reported on the recent archaeological finds from the Finca Marrufo, a deserted farm deep in the heart of Los Alcornacales, the world's largest forest of cork oak. At the farm, close to the mountain pass of Puerto Gáliz connecting Jerez, Alcalá, Ubrique, and Jimena, in a grave five metres by two, there had recently been uncovered the neatly aligned remains of twelve skeletons.[1] Victims of the Francoist repression at the beginning of Spain's savage Civil War of 1936–1939, the bones had lain hidden for seventy-six years. One of the skeletons still had a chain that held his wrists together, and in the seven other burial pits and individual graves uncovered at El Marrufo, where the victims had been interred with seemingly far less care, the remains of a further sixteen people were found. Of the total of twenty-eight skeletal remains disinterred at the farm, seven of whom were women, eleven still had bullets lodged in their bones and seven had gone to their deaths with their hands tied.[2]

For the forensic anthropologists, involved alongside archaeologists and other members of the team investigating the site, 'the presence of bound individuals, with non-life-threatening limb fractures and the manner in which they were buried, represent evidence of a moment of conflict ... with everything indicating the elimination of an undefended population'; essentially, disarmed and defenceless.[3]

It was in the nearby village of la Sauceda, on 31 October 1936, that four columns of Insurgent volunteers converged from the four points of the crossroads, and, with the support of aerial bombardment, attacked the villagers, refugees and militiamen gathered there, who were fleeing the repression that accompanied the Insurgents.[4] It is estimated that between 300 and 600 people were executed and tortured in the immediate vicinity of the Finca Marrufo, which had been converted for use as a detention centre by the Insurgents.

The bones of the remaining villagers of La Sauceda, and those who had sought refuge there that still lie beneath the soil of the forest slopes, represent but a tiny fraction of the conservative estimate of 30,000 who lie in unmarked graves across Spain.[5] It is the excavation of this site and its victims, led by the Association of the Relatives of Repressed Victims of Francoism in La

Sauceda and El Marrufo, that stand testimony to the continuing relevance of the Spanish Civil War today. Not only for those of the current generation of Spaniards seeking to recover a history repressed, but also in its wider European and world context.[6]

La Sauceda, on the eve of the conflict a thriving village with two colleges and two schools, with its own doctor based in nearby Alcalá de los Gazules, was the last centre of resistance to the insurgency in this part of southern Spain. Despite being razed to the ground, its survivors dispersed or killed, it is now one of a growing number of focal points across Spain, that speak of the traumatic legacy of the conflict, a trauma addressed in this book.[7]

A study that addresses the medical aspects of the Spanish Civil War also needs to examine the deeper wounds it left behind, and the now peaceful ruins that shelter among the oaks of the cork forest are a testament to that legacy, as are its few survivors and the descendants of those who lived there.

Notes

1 *El País* (Andalucían edition printed in Sevilla) 13.07.2012.

2 *El País*, 13.07.2012; Archivo Casa de la Memoria de La Sauceda (ACMS); Guijo Mauri, J. M., & Pecero Espín, J. C., *Estado de las investigaciones antropológicas en el cortijo de el Marrufo: Fundamentos científicos de inhumaciones clandestinas y episodios de violencia* (Jimena de la Frontera, 2012), pp. 1–24. This report also comments on the fact that for most of the burials, the evidence is for a lack of normal funerary rituals – one small pit had three bodies packed tightly together, one of which was lying on its side – and which marks out the largest grave as unusual in that despite showing unmistakeable evidence of having been executed, 'seeming' care had been taken in the arrangement of the skeletons, probably as a result of being buried by others under detention at El Marrufo.

3 Ibid.

4 Perales Pizarro, J. C., "El Marrufo. Fosa común: La Sauceda de Cortes de la Frontera, Málaga", available at: www.todoslosnombres.org/sites/default/files/investigacion131_1.pdf (last accessed 23.03.2016). The term 'Insurgent' is used throughout this study as the more commonly applied term of 'nationalist' is in most respects erroneous and was in fact a title chosen by the Insurgents to describe themselves, whereas the realities of Spanish society at the time meant that political parties that enjoyed popular support in both Catalunya and the Basque Country had nationalist agendas, which had in part been supported by the Republican Government with the grant of limited autonomy statutes. See Graham, H., *The Spanish Civil War: A Very Short Introduction* (Oxford, 2005), pp. 9–10, 22–23.

5 Graham, *Spanish Civil War*, p. 141. The figure of 30,000 may well be considerably higher as it is based upon incomplete evidence for those still missing. See Preston, P., *The Spanish Holocaust: Inquisition and Extermination in Twentieth-Century Spain* (London, 2012), pp. xi–xx.

6 Perales Pizarro, El Marrufo.

7 "Andalucía y Gobierno central firman la paz sobre la Ley de Memoria", *Publico*, 1.12.2017, available at: www.publico.es/politica/andalucia-gobierno-central-firman-paz-ley-memoria.html (last accessed 20.12.2017).

1 Introduction

The Spanish Civil War, one of the defining ideological struggles of twentieth-century Europe, has attracted the interest of writers since its inception. The majority of this literature, for much of the following four decades, originated outside Spain and favoured interpretations that reflected international participation in the conflict.[1] Before 1986, however, little had been written on the history of medicine of the Spanish Civil War.[2] Much of the writing that appeared after that date on medical aspects of the conflict maintained this international focus, that put at the forefront the foreign medical volunteers who came to Spain, predominantly in aid of the legally elected Republican Government. As a result of this, the Spanish contribution to the development of their own medical services has not always received the attention it deserves, and this book is also aimed at redressing this imbalance.[3]

The conflict, which embroiled Spain in a bloody Civil War and which was to last for nearly three years, was from its inception an international conflict. The Insurgents, who launched a coup that was to quickly fail, almost from the start benefitted from military aid from fascist Italy and Nazi Germany, with the Republican Government's main armed support coming from the Soviet Union and the thousands of international volunteers who came to aid the Republic. However, the assistance received by the Insurgents was far superior; both in terms of military hardware and manpower, and this tipped the balance decidedly in their favour.[4] This military aid to the Insurgents, coupled with a policy of non-intervention by the main European powers, which also included Germany and Italy, effectively denied the legally elected government their rights under international law to openly purchase arms for much of the war, although the Spanish gold reserve was transferred to Russia to pay for expensive shipments of arms from the Soviet Union.[5] This policy, however, also served as a convenient mask behind which Italy and Germany could hide their extensive support for Franco while flouting the terms of the agreement, and ultimately resulted in victory for the Insurgents on 1 April 1939 and the start of a dictatorship that was to last nearly forty years.[6]

A recognisably modern conflict, the Spanish Civil War was also the arena for a dress-rehearsal by Germany, Italy and, to a lesser degree, Russia for the coming World War. It was also the first European conflict that saw large-scale aerial bombardments behind the lines of civilian populations, with Republican-held areas particularly hard hit by Italian and German planes, resulting in thousands of civilian deaths.[7] In total, 200,000 soldiers died at the battlefronts and approximately 80,000 were permanently disabled during the conflict. For the disabled victims who served the Insurgency, there were reserved a number of positions as doorkeepers and receptionists, with a percentage of those unable to work granted war pensions. Disabled Republican servicemen, however, were imprisoned and denied employment, and were denied the right to claim pensions, which were only awarded to soldiers injured in action and who had fought for the 'liberation and aggrandisement of Spain and in the struggle against Marxism'.[8] As a result of this law Republican combatants did not receive pensions until after Franco's death.[9]

Despite the nature of warfare practised in Spain and the widespread destruction that ensued as a result, the conflict was also notable for a number of advances in medical practice that occurred during its course.[10] Advances in preservation and storage of blood for transfusion and in the treatment of traumatic orthopaedic injuries went on to be employed beyond Spanish borders during WWII, and within Spain medical services were organised on both sides that took forward lifesaving models for the treatment of the wounded that had begun to emerge towards the end of WWI.[11] Efforts made in this regard were particularly noteworthy in the Republican Zone. With most of the military infrastructure, including military medical facilities, under Insurgent control, and with the distinction between what constituted the frontline and the rear-guard not always clear, existing medical services were improved and new ones facilitated by a variety of organisations and political groupings and by medical volunteers from outside of Spain. Within a short period of time these helped to save lives both at the front and in the rear-guard.[12] Nevertheless, in the Insurgent Zone, the existing military medical infrastructure was not sufficient to cater for the sheer number of casualties that stemmed from the failure of the attempted coup. As such, medical advances were made, and new facilities organised that were also based on organisational models for the forward delivery of care that had evolved during WWI.[13]

The impetus for this reorganisation and evolution in surgical practice was largely the work of Spanish doctors and surgeons, but it also had the effect, at times, of limiting the further development of established practices. Spanish surgeons on both sides, who shared common backgrounds in training, often preferred the use of tried and tested existing techniques, such as the arm-to-arm direct method of blood transfusion. Likewise, anaesthesia in the opposing zones, with one or two notable exceptions, did not change significantly over the course of the war for similar reasons.[14]

British and American surgeons and nurses have garnered particular interest from historians over the past thirty years, with the role they played often portrayed as innovative and new. Their contribution was undoubtedly important in several regards. They helped save lives, collaborated with their Spanish counterparts, and contributed directly to the Republican war effort by providing medical assistance and boosting morale by being part of a transnational anti-fascist alliance of people and organisations that supported the legitimate Spanish Government.[15]

Spanish surgeons, it should be noted are not absent from these accounts. Josep Trueta, who helped popularise the closed plaster method for the treatment of fractured limbs outside Spain, a technique for reducing the number of infections that resulted in amputation or death (and frequently both), is cited in many of these works.[16] Although not necessarily the one exception that proves the rule, he is nevertheless one of the few Spanish names associated with the conflict known outside of Spain.[17]

The model that stresses the international nature of the Spanish Civil War has resulted in most historians of medicine writing in English barely scratching the surface of the contributions made by Spanish surgeons and physicians, within Spain and beyond, both before and during the Spanish Civil War. This book sets out to redress this imbalance by tracing the important role played by Spanish medical personnel, particularly surgeons, in the development and organisation of their own medical services during the conflict.

This study, therefore, is not strictly a history of medicine during the conflict, nor does it seek to further explore international efforts in this regard; rather it analyses through an examination of the medical personnel involved on both sides, the causes, treatments and long-term consequences of injury and trauma, including that of exile, on the wounded of the Spanish Civil War.

Anatomy of a conflict: Concepts and methodologies

In order to properly chart the development of changing models of care and the application of evolving techniques of surgical intervention, this study examines these developments from 1909, when Spanish troops set out on their long drawn-out journey of occupation of the northern zone of Morocco.[18] The campaigns that followed, that did not see Spanish Protectorate of Morocco subdued until 1927, was the fire in which was forged the surgical skills of so many military surgeons who later served on both sides during the Spanish Civil War, a number of whom were to make significant contributions to the evolution of surgical and medical practice during the conflict.[19] It is, also through an exploration of these different strands that chart significant medical development over a thirty-year period that the hospital and surgical care available to the significant number of North African indigenous troops who fought on behalf of Franco can be evaluated. This is important as an exploration of medical-ethical issues surrounding race, religion and differing cultural values and norms are revealing of some of the fault lines that lay at the heart of the conflict.

The surgical techniques described here were not in themselves new. The origins of the closed plaster method for the treatment of fractures can in fact be traced back to the Crimean War and the Siege of Sebastopol, where 580 fractures were treated through immobilisation and the application of plaster casts. This treatment was then further developed during WWI.[20] It was during the inter-war years that these techniques were further improved. Spanish physicians and surgeons in the 1920s and 1930s, in collaboration with other European doctors, were in the vanguard in developing new blood transfusion methods, orthopaedic and surgical treatments, including treatments for complicated fractures of bones.[21]

Spanish doctors had acted as neutral observers during WWI, and medical publications and journals published during and after WWI acted as transnational agents of change as they disseminated developing techniques in surgery and blood transfusion. As such, doctors from both opposing camps shortly after the outbreak of the Civil War in Spain were in the forefront in the development of mobile blood transfusion units that would go on to save thousands of lives during the conflict and the World War that was to follow.[22] The importance of the connecting vectors within the medical literature in this regard should not be underestimated, an exploration of which lies at the heart of the chapter on the organisation of the medical services. This analysis also examines preparations for civil defence and the protection against the possible use of chemical weapons within a medical organisational framework. The debt owed to this medical body of work written following the use of chemical toxins during WWI, is the starting point and common referent for much of the civil defence literature published during the conflict and is writ large across many of its pages. It therefore constitutes an important case study within this chapter, which is used not only to demonstrate how these services were organised, but also demonstrates how competing ideologies regarding civilian participation in civil defence were strongly influenced by anarchist medical personnel within the Republican Zone.[23]

It was through an engagement with – and by an extension of this literature through their own contribution to it – that Spanish doctors involved in treating the wounded of the Civil War were able to disseminate empirical-based observations on evolving techniques and describe changing models of care.[24] The level of dissemination of this literature is, of course, open to question, as journals, like newspapers, can pass through many hands. Therefore sales figures, even if these were available (which they are not), would not necessarily reflect their wider impact. Nevertheless, articles and references in the contemporary British medical literature to medical and surgical developments and the reports written by Spanish doctors, much of which concerned surgery, clearly demonstrate the diffusion and the transnational nature of much of the medical literature.[25]

Propaganda, broadly defined here as the dissemination of material that attempts to influence and change people's perceptions, and the press more widely, are an important concurrent historiographical strand that provide additional medical evidence in which this study is based.[26] Propaganda can be revealing on several levels. Not only is there to be found evidence for the contribution made by individuals of whom only brief glimpses are seen in the official military publications and papers, but it also provides examples of localised efforts and initiatives in the provision of surgical care, including the important contribution made by medical personnel associated with the anarchist movement, that are absent from the wider literature.[27]

Some of the propagandist material clearly originates in the medical sources cited throughout this study. A clear example of this is provided in the many articles and features aimed at the education of a much wider readership and which addressed medical aspects of civilian defence relating to the possible use of chemical weapons.[28] These 'medical articles' adapted by the journalists themselves, provide evidence not always available in other sources and form part of the foundations upon which this study is built.[29] Therefore, if good journalism is the first draft of history, then effective propaganda can also provide a provisional rough draft.[30] Articles and images selected by newspaper editors to fix meaning beyond the moment or moments captured not only constitute an invaluable resource, but the propagandist discourse in which they are placed provides an additional layer of 'evidence' that can be explored for wider social and cultural narratives.

This is clearly demonstrated in this book's second chapter, which examines the surgical and hospital care of Franco's Moroccan troops. The more traditional archival material analysed for this chapter include 400 hospital admission and discharge cards from the Military Archive in Ávila, the personal papers of the New Zealand-born anaesthetist Robert Mackintosh held by the Wellcome Library, and the diary of the British nurse Priscilla Scott-Ellis, held by Cardiff University. Together they provide complementary evidence of the type of surgery being performed on wounded combatants and provide insights into conditions in hospitals specially set up for the Moroccan troops.[31] This type of evidence is important as there has been very little written concerning medical care of Franco's Muslim combatants during the Spanish Civil War. However, it is the contemporary articles in the press, that not only provide additional evidence for the existence of mosques, ablutions halls and canteens attached to the hospitals, but the images selected to accompany the writing provide evidence beyond their desired propagandist purpose.[32] It is this wider cultural analysis that precludes a quantitative analysis of the hospital admission and discharge cards from the Military Archive in Ávila. Such an analysis would offer only limited statistical data in the absence of a full evaluation of all the hospital records for Muslim combatants held in the archive in Ávila, something outside the remit of this study, and would contribute little to the broader understanding of the social and cultural aspects of care of the Moroccan wounded explored here. It is only through an evaluation of the newspaper articles, which situate their propagandist discourse within a wider paternalist colonial rhetoric aimed at portraying the Moorish other as part of a Catholic crusade sanctioned by much of the Spanish Church against the infidel 'red', that it is possible to shed further light on the religious and cultural aspects relating to care of the Moroccan wounded.[33]

This propagandist-slanted evidence base is also a useful departure point for exploring the evolution of different models of forward surgical provision.

This provides an additional layer of interpretation in Chapter 3 on the organisation of the medical services during the conflict, which alongside the medical literature is explored in order to demonstrate similarities and differences of care provision in the opposing zones, but which also highlights the under-researched anarchist contribution to medical organisation during the conflict and provides important evidence by which their input can be assessed.

Film, despite being a kinetic medium often at the heart of Spanish Civil War propaganda, also fix moments in time, which through the recording of thousands of rapidly captured images contain details within their frames that can be interpreted separate to the message of the wider propagandist discourse. The moving image could therefore serve as an educational instructional tool, as was the case with medical films during the conflict. However, even in the most scientific films, wider propagandist discourses are not entirely absent. This is demonstrated in an analysis of the blurring of the lines between propaganda and medicine in the chapter on blood transfusion, which explores how propaganda was medicalised during the conflict.[34]

The complex relationship between propaganda and medicine not only informs the chapter on developments in the field of blood transfusion early in the conflict, it is also at the heart of its wider analysis. The history of medicine in relation to the Spanish Civil War has to a large degree been reconstructed by historians as a result of close examination of propagandist sources, and yet the role of propaganda itself is rarely discussed.[35] It is, however, the examination of the contrasting narratives constructed around blood transfusion that go a long way to explaining how those at the forefront of developments can then be overlooked, and is a theme that unites much of this book.

This study, which mines the different seams of historical evidence in charting the role played by the Spanish surgeons in the development and treatment of injuries, also examines those who sustained these wounds, not only from a physical perspective but also a psychological one. These wounds, the lesions and scars, the shattered bones and torn flesh of modern industrial warfare, represent the visible legacy of war, in other words, the visual evidence of traumatic injury. However, the unseen psychological trauma caused by the conflict, especially for the vanquished who were systematically punished for an adherence to a different set of values than those held by the Insurgents, and which for many carried long-term consequences that also affected wider family networks, are a legacy of the Spanish Civil War that still resonates in Spain today.[36] This is as a result of the fact that in Spain there were no trials for war crimes and crimes against humanity committed during the conflict as a result of the amnesty law of 1977.[37] This, despite extrajudicial killing in Francoist occupied areas during the conflict exceeding the current conservative figure of 130,199. Additionally, the execution of 20,000 Republicans following the war and the imposition by the new regime of a policy of 'redemption through sacrifice' saw many thousands more die in prisons, concentration camps and labour battalions as a result of disease and starvation.[38] The use of torture and rape as instruments of terror, which had been widespread during Insurgent occupation of territories, did not stop once Franco's forces occupied the whole of Spain, yet there have been no convictions for the crimes carried out by a number of supporters of the Insurgency and the ensuing dictatorship, despite such acts continuing long into the post-war period.[39]

Republican atrocities, which predominantly occurred during the first six months of the conflict, were responsible for the death of an estimated 50,000 people. Yet Franco's victory ensured that those responsible for such acts were, in the main, held to account for their actions, with the majority of the victims of the 'red terror' identified and 'honoured' as martyrs.[40] Therefore, in its concluding chapter, this book charts the unseen injuries caused by the trauma of this war, with an emphasis on the Republican experience of defeat, as not only were the disabled and wounded among the defeated punished for failing to have been 'adherents of the regime' (*adictos al régimen*), but collective punishment of the vanquished led to further widespread suffering through famine and disease in post-war Spain.[41] Thousands of disabled soldiers and civilians did escape direct punishment by fleeing into exile, but for the majority of those who fled, their post-war experience would not be radically different to those held in the prisons and camps in Spain, as they too were incarcerated, their wounds often left untreated, and they too experienced having to live under an army of occupation. For those in Spain this experience was also prolonged, as martial law was in place in Spain until 1948.[42] It is the impact on medical provision occasioned by the fall of Catalunya and the end of the Spanish Civil War, the flight of refugees into exile, and the impact that the defeat and loss of between fifteen to twenty per cent of the medical profession to the purges and exile that form the focus of this chapter.

A thematic exploration of different models of organisation from forward care to civil defence; the importance of propaganda as a cypher and filter; the role played by religion, race and gender in care of the sick and wounded; and the lasting legacy of trauma as examined here; all provide an analysis that projects the narrow definition of 'past' injuries caused to Spain during its brutal Civil War into an unresolved present. A present where the experiences of the suffering caused during and in the aftermath of the conflict remain injuries largely unhealed. It is only through examining both physical and psychological trauma that new insights reflecting evolving models of military and civilian care, and the longer-term consequences of the suffering caused by civil war itself, can be fully understood.

This study, in a number of important respects, then, is the study of bones, and the memories and flesh that encased them. It tells the story of shattered limbs restored to functionality by careful hands, and the evolution and improvement of techniques that contributed towards a diminution of the trauma that violent injury brings in its wake. It is also the tale of those bones, both broken and whole, that could never be mended or healed, the ossified remains that lay and continue to lie hidden in unidentified graves and burial pits across Spain. This has not only contributed to the scars of the surviving defeated, forced to endure the punishing years of the dictatorship, but also the difficult legacy bequeathed to their descendants.

If it is necessary to address ongoing issues arising out of the trauma caused by the Civil War, it is also necessary to challenge those within Spanish society who seek to deny expression and historical identity to the inert and unidentified remains in burial pits and unmarked graves across Spain. This study forms an interlocking part of a new historiographical strand examining the origins and evolution of a traumatic conflict whose repercussions continue to be felt across Spain.[43] It seeks to provide its own unique historical perspective that contributes towards this trauma being addressed, through an inclusive examination of the contribution made by Spanish medical professionals across Spain during the Spanish Civil War and its aftermath.

This study, therefore, by placing itself at the heart of the new historiography that has emerged since the turn of the millennia in Spain, also offers new interpretations and approaches to the source materials outlined above allowing for a more comprehensive analysis of what this evidence has to offer.[44] This has involved not only a re-examination of more traditional documentation such as military medical material and the official state gazettes published in the respective zones during the conflict, but also an extensive engagement with archival visual media, including film and press from the conflict, with the daily *ABC* – published in both Republican Madrid and the Insurgent controlled city of Sevilla – an important resource in this regard. It is this wider scrutiny of the image and the word in conjunction that allows for a comprehensive analysis of the role played by propaganda in shaping our medical understandings of the Spanish Civil War.

Historiography and the history of medicine of the Spanish Civil War

For the purposes of this study, which has its primary focus on how the historiography relates to the historical/medical context of the conflict, it is necessary to reflect briefly upon the wider historiography of the conflict. This is important as it helps situate this study at the centre of a new historiography, in that not only does it examine developments in surgery and medicine (for example, the treatment of fractures and the conservation of stored blood) but does this by examining the effect of propaganda and mass media as an important part of this evolution. This sets it apart from other studies as this allows for a multifaceted analysis, broader and more inclusive in its scope, as at the heart of this study, is an examination that charts these developments in both the Republican and Insurgent Zones. Although this book is concerned primarily with the medical history of the conflict, it also seeks to explore these developments within national, European and international (extra-national) contexts, which thus by definition involves an examination of the conflict itself.

Furthermore, in order to track and interpret models of organisation and development, a lens with a wide aperture that does not restrict interpretations to too narrow confines is needed to focus on how changes unfolded over time and how these in turn were applied both regionally and nationally. Major campaigns such as the Jarama Offensive of early 1937, an attempt by the Insurgents to sever the capital's connections with Valencia; the four-month Battle of the Ebro launched in July 1938 by the Republican Government to relieve pressure on Valencia; or the fall of Catalunya to the Insurgents early in 1939; were on the one hand battles that can be used to chart progression and changes in the organisation of medical provision over a period of time, but also reflected wider social and cultural issues relating to the history of medicine of the Spanish Civil War.

There is not the space here, nor is it necessarily the place, to discuss the wider historiographical trends and changes that unfolded after the death of Franco (or the thousands of publications these engendered). Those that immediately followed his death were concerned with a new approach to the causes of the Civil War itself, which included the exploration of social and economic models, with the history of medicine in relation to the conflict, a largely absent and dormant discipline.[45] Accounts of and by the wounded are of course not absent from this literature, but as these touch primarily upon the foreign combatants and volunteers who went to Spain, they, in the main, fall outside the remit of this study. Nevertheless, a brief outline of how the dominant strand in the historiography developed is required, as the writing of history within Spain was heavily censored for much of the period of the dictatorship, and this had an impact on how the conflict was interpreted by historians outside of Spain.

There are a number of studies that chart the evolution of the historiography from the Crusade-driven narrative of the early Francoist historians within Spain, through to the more rigorous international studies that both preceded and came after the death of the Spanish dictator in 1975.[46]

However, it was not until after the death of Franco in 1975 that things gradually began to change. Nevertheless, Franco's imposition of a single version of Spain's past during his long dictatorship of the nation made this a slow and difficult process, as other non-official memories of the conflict had been systematically supressed.[47]

This was, however, a fruitful period for historians thanks to the opening of certain archives shortly after the death of Franco. The year 1977 was to prove an important turning point as, with access permitted to the archives of the Spanish Ministry for Foreign Affairs, a more comprehensive analysis became possible of the Francoist regime's reactions, responses and place within an international framework, a synthesis that had been difficult to achieve before that point.[48] The year 1977 also saw the publication of the first volume of Javier Rubio's *La Emigración de la Guerra Civil de 1936–1939: Historia del éxodo que se produce con el fin de la II República española* (*Emigration during the Civil War of 1936–1939: History of the Exile Produced by the Demise of the II Spanish Republic*), a social history of the exile of nearly half a million people in France at the end of the Civil War, a work still cited by historians today. This study analyses the social and geographical composition of those who sought refuge in France, and contains statistics relating to disease and mortality rates within the internment camps in France where the Spanish refugees were concentrated.[49]

This valuable access to otherwise closed-off archival materials also saw the tentative beginnings of the history of medicine within Spain with new studies that related to the conflict. Research carried out after 1977 by military surgeons and doctors, which appeared in military journals, was a nascent discipline that nevertheless saw the slow birth of research into both national and international contributions to the wartime medical services. These studies, which benefitted from access to archival sources denied to many historians, were published as a result of their perceived non-political objectivity.[50]

For the purposes of this study, the main turning point for the historiography came in 1986, on the fiftieth anniversary of the start of the conflict. This saw an upsurge of publications on the Spanish Civil War generally, but more importantly, within Spain itself.[51] It also saw the beginning of a wider exploration of the conflict by historians of medicine, both in Spain and beyond, which marked a new direction in Spanish Civil War studies.

In 1986, *Los médicos y la medicina en la Guerra Civil Española: Monografías Beecham* (*Medical Practitioners and Medicine in the Spanish Civil War: Beecham Monographs*) was published in Spain.[52] This was also the year that saw the publication in Britain of *The Signal was Spain: The Aid Spain Movement in Britain, 1936–1939* by Jim Fyrth.[53] The importance of these books lay not just in their fresh insights into a hitherto little-explored area of the conflict, but also in that they mark a departure point in the historiography, as the first major studies from the emergent field of the history of medicine that examined the Spanish Civil War.[54]

The collection *Los médicos y la medicina en la Guerra Civil Española* attempted a not always successful synthesis of, predominantly, the military medical services offered in both the Insurgent and Republican Zones and their development during the three-year conflict. This collection of essays and accounts were almost exclusively derived from male doctors who participated on both sides during the struggle; the three notable exceptions being the accounts by the anarchist Federica Montseny – Minister of Health early in the conflict, Mercedes Milá Nolla – Inspector General of the Insurgent Nursing Services, and the study on the application and advances in treatments for the wounded by Dr Maria Herraiz Muñoz. The collection claimed to have 'revolutionised the existing historiography … by breaking with traditional works and tackling those new and original aspects by which future essayists would without doubt have to work'.[55] Although undoubtedly an important work, especially in that the accounts it contains do come from doctors who worked in both the Republican and Insurgent Zones (and occasionally in both), this monograph did not engender a wider historiographical engagement within Spain. This is, in all likelihood, because in its attempt to show a balance between the conflicting sides, its 'neutrality' and its emphasis on medicine over people failed to stimulate debate, something that a study that clearly nailed its colours to the mast might have achieved. Nevertheless, these eyewitness accounts, combining both autobiography and medical and surgical data, helped in bridging the gap between more traditional approaches of physicians writing histories of medicine with an emphasis on its medical aspects, with an emergent trend seeking to analyse history from multidisciplinary perspectives. In this new discipline, oral history was both the forerunner and a natural companion.[56]

Jim Fyrth's *The Signal was Spain* was a significant contribution to the emerging trend of utilising the history of medicine as a way of reinterpreting existing historical perspectives. It differed from *Los médicos y la medicina en la Guerra Civil Española* in that, instead of being a predominantly medically driven account by mainly male professional personnel, it engaged closely with issues of memory and gender. This was principally the result of the author's unorthodox Marxist approach to the sources. It is a book that owes much to British archival sources, but its strength lies in its judicious use of personal accounts and letters backed by other source materials to create an account that influenced later approaches, admittedly mainly within the English-speaking world, through to the present day.[57]

An important but oft-overlooked work published in 1994 is the four-volume *Historia de la sanidad militar española* (*A History of Spanish Military Health*), which examines the evolution of Spanish military medicine.[58] Written by José María Massons, a Catalan surgeon appointed chief of the surgical team of the International Brigades in March 1937, Volume II dedicates 212 pages to the military health services during the Spanish Civil War. Massons, who escaped the purges of the professional classes that followed the war, had access to a number of sources for constructing his account, including interviews with Spanish doctors and nurses who had participated in the conflict. The book has a medico-military focus, but is thorough in its research, although there is an attempt by the author, directly intruding on his own account, to portray himself as an apolitical liberal military doctor during the war; a Medical Officer (MO) rather than an idealist, an important distinction for Massons as it largely excused him from engaging in this work with the conflict's wider political dimensions.[59]

Following the seventieth anniversary of the start of the Spanish Civil War, new publications continued to proliferate. The year 2006 saw the publication of *La sanidad en las Brigadas Internacionales* (*Healthcare in the International Brigades*), which examined medical aspects of the conflict from surgery to psychiatry; and in the same year a major study of one of the key medical innovators of the Spanish Civil War, Frederic Durán-Jordà, was also published.[60]

A slow trickle of publications written in English also continued to make their mark. Nicolas Coni's *Medicine and Warfare: Spain, 1936–1939*, published in 2008, concentrated on the doctor's perspective. Although he brings his medical knowledge to bear with expertise and without recourse to obscure medical language, his analysis nevertheless lacks the scope that a more inclusive focus would have afforded.[61] It is a monograph that owes more to the 1986 study *Monografía Beecham* (and indeed to earlier generations of historians of medicine) in that its format consists of several chapters examining different topics from nursing (briefly) through to the International Brigades but lacks a strong narrative thread on which to centre its analysis. It is, nevertheless, a thoroughly researched book, rich in biographic detail, and even in its more limited scope of analysis, is a useful reference book for a modern generation of historians of medicine writing about the Spanish Civil War.[62]

Publications such as these share a common thread in that they gave voice to medical personnel involved in the Civil War, including nurses from many parts of the world. These form an important strand in the continuing understanding of the international dimensions and context of the conflict, which in turn engenders an interest from those engaged with events in the Spain of the 1930s, and has led to further research and publications creating a better and more nuanced understanding of the Spanish Civil War within national and international contexts. Nevertheless, beyond the Beecham monograph, and the studies by Masson and Coni, the role of the Spanish surgeon during the conflict was still largely unexplored in much of the literature, although with the emergence within Spain of new directions in historical study, with local and regional studies coming to the fore, this is now slowly changing.

Local and regional histories of medicine

Autonomy, which as part of the transition to democracy has been entrenched in the Spanish mainland regions since the early 1980s, has helped strengthen regional identities that had come under assault during the Francoist dictatorship. As a result of this move towards greater autonomy, local and regional historical studies of the conflict have flourished.[63] A number of these take a history of medicine approach in studying their localities.[64] Fortunately, however, these studies do not confine their conclusions to localism or regionalism, and frequently place themselves within a wider national and international context.

Ángel Beneito Lloris' book, *El Hospital Sueco-Noruego de Alcoi durante la Guerra Civil Española* (*The Swedish-Norwegian Hospital of Alcoi during the Spanish Civil War*), published in 2004, combines these approaches with its comprehensive analysis of the genesis and functioning of the hospital alongside oral testimony from surviving nurses still resident in their common locality at the time of writing.[65]

Even those studies that engage more closely with local and regional contexts have contributed to a greater understanding of social and cultural aspects of the conflict.[66] An example of this can be found in the monograph published in 2004, *Entre el frente y la retaguardia. La sanidad en la Guerra Civil: El hospital 'Alfonso Carlos', Pamplona 1936–1939* (*Between the Front and the Rearguard. Healthcare during the Civil War: The Hospital 'Alfonso*

Carlos', Pamplona, 1936–1939), by the Spanish medical doctor and historian Pablo Larraz Andía. On one level, the book's analysis of the hospital and the 'community' it serves stresses the local links between the city and within the wider region of Navarra, but equally it examines this within a wider national context of the Spanish Civil War and helps provide a regional perspective on the provision of medical care in this part of Northern Spain.[67]

Another study that threw new light on aspects of medical care during the conflict was the monograph *Hospitales en Burgos durante la Guerra Civil* by Martin de Frutos Herranz. This study of the hospitals in Burgos, a centre of government for the Insurgents throughout the Civil War, has a clearly localised focus that, nevertheless engages with wider issues of ideology, religion, race and gender. Its chapter that examines the hospital for Moroccan soldiers in the city helps to shed light on the geographic origins of combatants who died in the hospital but also highlights the difficulties faced by housing Muslim patients in a converted monastery where anti-Muslim imagery could be seen on the walls.[68]

Studies continue to be published that continue to contribute to a greater understanding of how medical provision developed and evolved during the conflict, and in turn broaden the lens through which the Spanish Civil War can be examined.[69]

Conclusion

The themes addressed in this introduction that speak of the relevance of the Spanish Civil War as an area of study within a modern contemporary context also explain why the historiography of the conflict is continually growing. The small body of literature that addresses medical aspects of the Spanish Civil War also continues to grow, and within Spain it is regional perspectives of healthcare during the conflict that predominate over more national narratives.[70] Additionally, a number of regionally funded documentaries have examined the lasting legacies of Francoism, particularly those surrounding memory and trauma. These too have contributed to a wider-ranging and multidisciplinary debate, which has further enhanced the historiography of the conflict.[71]

Monographs continue to be printed examining the role played by international medical volunteers during the Spanish Civil War, with the publishing partnership between the Sussex Academic Press and the Cañada Blanch Centre for Contemporary Spanish Studies at the London School of Economics the leading contributor in this regard.[72]

The act of remembering the Civil War in Spain, however, where the term 'regime' is more habitually applied than 'dictatorship' when referring to the Francoist period, is still a contested battlefield. It is therefore necessary to address ongoing issues arising out of the trauma caused by the Civil War and challenge those within Spanish society who seek to deny expression and historical identity to the inert and largely unidentified remains that lie in burial pits and unmarked graves across Spain. Existing excavations continue to reveal new archaeological and related data, and the creation of new archives – such as the recently opened centre in the Casa de la Memoria La Sauceda, with its small but growing collection of materials, including forensic studies – are an integral part of this ongoing challenge, as new material continues to come to light that questions existing narratives.[73]

This study, by picking over the bones of a wide body of literature and by engaging with a variety of different sources, not only forms an interlocking part of a new historiographical strand examining the origins and evolution of a traumatic conflict whose repercussions continue to be felt throughout Spain, it is also the first full-scale study to offer a comprehensive overview of medical provision on both sides of the line. Through its engagement with a diversity of sources, its analysis of the relationship between medicine and propaganda, and through an inclusive examination of the contribution made by Spanish medical professionals across Spain during the Spanish Civil War and its aftermath, this study provides its own unique historical perspective of a conflict whose living legacy of trauma and of wounds unhealed is still alive in Spain today.

Notes

1 Payne, S. G., "Historiography on the Spanish Republic and Civil War", *The Journal of Modern History*, Vol. 60, No. 3 (1988), pp. 540–556; Blanco Rodríguez, J. A., "La Historiografía de la guerra civil española", in S. Gálvez (ed.), *Dossier generaciones y memoria de la represión franquista: un balance de los movimientos por la memoria en Hispania Nova. Revista de Historia Contemporánea*, No. 7 (2007), pp. 741–775, pp. 744–748.

2 Acier, M., *From Spanish Trenches: Recent Letters from Spain; Collected and Edited by M Acier* (London, 1937); Colmegna, H., *Diario de un Médico Argentino en la Guerra de España 1936–1939* (Buenos Aires, 1941); Jolly, D. W., *Field Surgery in Total War* (London, 1940); Mira, E., *Psychiatry in War* (New York, 1943); Bastos Ansart, M., *De las guerras coloniales a la guerra civil: memorias de un cirujano* (Barcelona, 1969), are the main monographs written prior to 1986.

3 Fyrth, J., *The Signal Was Spain: The Aid Spain Movement in Britain, 1936–1939* (London, 1986); Requena Gallego, M. & Sepúlveda Losa, R. M. (eds.), *La sanidad en las Brigadas Internacionales* (Cuenca, 2006); Jackson, A., *'For Us It Was Heaven'. The Passion, Grief and Fortitude of Patience Darton: From the Spanish Civil War to Mao's China* (Brighton, 2012); Palfreeman, L., *¡Salud! British Volunteers in the Republican Medical Service during the Spanish Civil War, 1936–1939* (Brighton, 2012); Lethbridge, D., *Norman Bethune in Spain: Commitment, Crisis, and Conspiracy* (Brighton, 2013); Palfreeman, L., *Aristocrats, Adventurers and Ambulances: British Medical Units in the Spanish Civil War* (Brighton, 2014); Palfreeman, L., *Spain Bleeds: The Development of Battlefield Blood Transfusion during the Civil War* (Brighton, 2015); Derby, M., *Petals and Bullets: Dorothy Morris, New Zealand Nurse in the Spanish Civil War* (Brighton, 2015); Pretus, G., *La ayuda humanitaria en la Guerra Civil española, 1936–1939* (Granada, 2015).

4 Graham, *Spanish Civil War*, pp. 1, 41f.

5 Beevor, A., *The Battle for Spain: The Spanish Civil War 1936–1939* (London, 2006), pp. 153–154.
6 Graham, *Spanish Civil War*, p. 7.
7 Preston, *Spanish Holocaust*, p. xi; Thomas, H., *The Spanish Civil War*, revised edition (Toronto, 2001), pp. 900–901.
8 *Boletín Oficial de Estado* (*BOE*), No. 540 (Suplemento), 14.04.1938, "Reglamento Provisional del Benemérito Cuerpo de Mutilado de Guerra por la Patria (Decreto de 5 de abril de 1938.-11 Año Triunfal)", pp. 1–72, p. 4.
9 Aguilar, P., "Agents of Memory: Spanish Civil War Veterans and Disabled Soldiers", in J. Winter & E. Sivan (eds.), *War and Remembrance in the Twentieth Century* (Cambridge, 1999), pp. 84–103, pp. 87, 101.
10 Palfreeman, *¡Salud!* p. 2.
11 Ibid. World War One and World War Two are referred to throughout the text as WWI and WWII respectively.
12 Estellés Salarich, J., "La sanidad del ejército Repúblicano del centro" in *Los médicos y la medicina en la Guerra Civil Española: Monografías Beecham* (Madrid, 1986), p. 39; Guerra, F., *La medicina en el exilio republicano* (Madrid, 2003); Jackson, *For Us It Was Heaven*; Palfreeman, *¡Salud!*; Lethbridge, *Norman Bethune*; Palfreeman, *Aristocrats, Adventurers and Ambulances*; Palfreeman, *Spain Bleeds*; Derby, *Petals and Bullets*; Pretus, *La ayuda humanitaria.*
13 Massons, J. M., *Historia de la Sanidad Militar Española: Tomo II* (Barcelona, 1994), p. 415.
14 Browne, J. S., "Anaesthesia and the Spanish Civil War: The Delivery of Anaesthetic Care in a Divided Spain", *History of Anaesthesia Society Proceedings*, Vol. 46 (2013), pp. 74–80.
15 Jackson, *For Us It Was Heaven*; Palfreeman, *¡Salud!*; Lethbridge, *Norman Bethune*; Palfreeman, *Aristocrats, Adventurers and Ambulances*; Palfreeman, *Spain Bleeds*; Derby, *Petals and Bullets*; Acier, *From Spanish Trenches*; Jolly, *Field Surgery*.
16 Ibid.; Trueta, J., *El tractament de les fractures de Guerra* (Barcelona, 1938); Trueta, J., "The Organization of Hospital Services for Casualties Due to the Bombing of Cities, Based on Experience Gained in Barcelona—with Special Reference to the Classification of Casualties", *Journal of the Royal Society of Medicine*, Vol 33, No. 1 (1939), pp. 13–23; Trueta, J., *Treatment of War Wounds and Fractures: With Special Reference to the Closed Method as Used in the War in Spain* (London, 1940).
17 *Spain Bleeds* by Linda Palfreeman examines the role of four doctors involved with blood transfusion, two of whom were Spanish. However, it is the role played by the Reading GP Reginald Saxton that lies at the heart of this study.
18 Balfour, S., *Deadly Embrace: Morocco and the Road to the Spanish Civil War* (Oxford, 2002), p. 4. This resulted in 1912 in the establishment of the Spanish Protectorate of Morocco. See "The Treaty Between France and Spain Regarding Morocco", *The American Journal of International Law*, Vol. 7, No. 2 (April, 1913), Supplement: Official Documents, pp. 81–99.
19 Bastos Ansart, *De las guerras coloniales*, pp. 89–144.
20 Moral Torres, J., "El 'método español' en el tratamiento de heridas de Guerra", in *Los médicos y la medicina en la Guerra Civil Española* (Madrid, 1986), pp. 157–166, p. 161.
21 Fernández Sabaté, A., *Nuestros fundadores y maestros en 1935 y 1947: Sociedad Española de Cirugía y Traumatología* (Madrid, 2013), pp. v, 4, 15, 33, 57, 240.

22 Ibid., pp. 244–245; Schneider, W. H., "Blood Transfusion Between the Wars", *Journal of the History of Medicine and Allied Sciences*, Vol. 58, No. 2 (2003), pp. 187–224; Navarro Carballo, J. R., *Frederic Duran i Jorda: Un hito de la historia de la transfusión sanguínea* (Madrid, 2006).

23 Parrilla Hermida, M., *Los gases de combate: Síntomas, tratamiento y protección* (La Coruña, 1936); Parilla Hermida, M., "Los gases de guerra", in L. Girones (ed.), *Cuestiones médico-quirúrgicas de guerra* (Castellón de la Plana, 1938), pp. 527–553; Balmori, H., "Servicios sanitarios de antigás: Táctica y organización de estos servicios en el ejército", *Revista Española de Medicina y Cirugía de Guerra*, Vol. 2, No. 5 (1939), pp. 49–63; Consell de Sanitat de Guerra, "Instruccions sobre defensa passiva de la població civil, per al cas d'atac amb gasos", *La Medicina Catalana*, Vol. 7, No. 39–40 (1936–1937), pp. 375–383; Guindal y Calderero, J. M., "Problemas de salubridad que ha planteado la guerra", Real Academia Nacional de Medicina, Instituto de España, *Anales de la Real Academia de Medicina* – 1943 (Madrid, 1944), pp. 503–538; Morata Cantón, J., *Defensa de guerra tóxico química: En colaboración con otros compañeros y ed. por el "Sindicato Unico de Sanidad"* (Madrid, 1937); Morata Cantón, J., *Guerra química y bacteriológica* (Barcelona, 1938); Viñuales Fariñas, M., "La ciencia al servicio de la barbarie: los horrores de la guerra aeroquímica", *Revista Blanca* (Barcelona, 1936); España, Servicio de Guerra Química, *Información del servicio de guerra química* (Madrid, 1938).

24 Gordon-Taylor, S. R. A. G., & Hamilton, F. H., "Surgical Experience in the Spanish War", *BMJ*, Vol. 2, No. 4164 (1940), pp. 560–561; Martín Santos, L., "Nuestro criterio en el tratamiento de los fracturados de guerra en la zona de vanguardia", *Medicina Española*, Vol. 1 (1938), pp. 653–681; "Hospital de Sangre", *Crónica* (07.03.1937), pp. 1–3; Gómez Durán, M., "Principios fundamentales en cirugía de guerra", *Revista Española de Medicina y Cirugía de Guerra*), Vol. 3, No. 2 (1939), pp. 2–35; Gómez Durán, M., "Principios fundamentales en cirugía de guerra: Parte 2ª, hospitales de evacuacion y especialidades", *Revista Española de Medicina y Cirugía de Guerra*, Vol. 3, No. 12 (1939), pp. 81–101; Bastos Ansart, M., "Dos problemas de asistencia a los heridos en retaguardia", *Revista de Sanidad de Guerra*, No. 1 (1937), pp. 9–14; Gordon-Taylor & Hamilton, Surgical Experience in the Spanish War; "Treatments of War Wounds and Fractures", *BMJ*, Vol. 2, No. 4108 (1939), p. 694; Trueta, "The Organisation of Hospital Services for Casualties due to the Bombing of Cities, Based on Experience Gained in Barcelona – with Special Reference to the Classification of Casualties", *Proceedings of the Royal Society of Medicine*, Vol. 33, No. 13 (1939), pp. 13–23; López Cotarelo, A., "Organización de los Servicios sanitarios militares de vanguardia", in L. Girones (ed.) *Cuestiones médico-quirúrgicas de guerra* (Castellón de la Plana, 1938), pp. 527–553; Oleo Herraiz, I., "Apostillas a los servicios de sanidad militar en campaña", *Revista Española de Medicina y Cirugía de Guerra* Vol. 2, No. 9 (1939), pp. 254–261; Coller, F. A, & Valk, W. L., "The Delayed Closure of Contaminated Wounds: A Preliminary Report", *Annals of Surgery*, Vol. 112, No. 2 (1940), pp. 256–270; Moynahan, E. J., "Treatment of War Wounds and Infected Fractures", *BMJ*, Vol 1, No. 4127 (1940), p. 229; Winnett Orr, H., "Treatment of War Wounds and Infected Fractures", *BMJ*, Vol 1, No. 4135 (1940), p. 585; Ross, J. A., & Hulbert, K. F., "Treatment of 100 War Wounds and Burns", *BMJ*, Vol. 1, No. 4190 (1941), pp. 618–621; Broster, L. R., "A Survey of War Surgery", *BMJ*, Vol. 1, No. 4207 (1941), pp. 273–5; Wilson, P. D., "The Treatment of Compound Fractures Resulting from Enemy Action",

Annals of Surgery, Vol. 113, No. 6 (1941), pp. 915–924; Ponseti Vives, I., "History of Orthopaedic Surgery", *The Iowa Orthopaedic Journal* (1991), pp. 59–64.

25 Ibid.

26 Corse, E., *A Battle for Neutral Europe: British Cultural Propaganda during the Second World War* (London, 2013), p. 6; Cull, N. J., Culbert, D., & Welch, D., *Propaganda and Mass Persuasion: A Historical Encyclopaedia 1500 to the Present* (Santa Barbara, 2003), p. 318.

27 Álvarez, A., "El Cuerpo de Sanidad Militar ha organizado un tren-hospital para los heridos del Frente", *Crónica* (01.11.1936), pp. 4–5; Nombela Gallardo, D., "Nuestro Servicio Sanitario en la toma de Albarracín", *Libertad,* Vol. 1, No. 6 (1937), pp. 4–6; Rico Belestá, F., "Servicio Sanitario en Campaña", in *Libertad,* Año 1, No. 7 (1937), pp. 6–7; Sarto, J. de, "Actividades de la Cruz Roja Española: El secretario general de esta magnífica institución, señor Morata, habla para los lectores de Crónica", *Crónica* (16.01.1938).

28 *La Voz*, 05.10.1936, p.3; *ABC* (Madrid), 12.01.1937, p. 7; *ABC* (Madrid), 07.05.1937, p. 8; *ABC* (Madrid), 08.05.1937, p. 8; *ABC* (Madrid), 12.05.1937, p. 13; "La guerra química III", *Mundo Gráfico*, 02.06.1937, pp. 10–11; *ABC* (Madrid), 30.06.1937, p. 4; *ABC* (Madrid), 10.07.1937, p. 6; "La Cruz Roja y la guerra: La labor de los comités locales, los consultorios gratuitos, los puestos de socorro, las patrullas antigás", *Mundo Gráfico*, 08.09.1937, p. 10; *Mi Revista*, 19.07.1937, p. 72; Sarto, J. D., "Actividades de la Cruz Roja española: Cómo se prepara a la población civil para su defensa contra la guerra química", *Crónica* (30.01.1938), p. 5; *Crónica*, 06.03.1938, p. 3.

29 Ibid.; "Visita a un hospital: como se efectuá la transfusión de sangre en el frente", in *La Vanguardia*, 25.11.1936, pp. 2–3.

30 Zelizer, B, "Why memory's work on journalism does not reflect journalism's work on memory", in *Memory Studies*, Vol. 1, No 1 (2008), pp. 79–87, p. 80.

31 Archivo General Militar de Ávila (AGMAV): AGMAV, C. 42385, 1; AGMAV, C. 42385, 3; AGMAV, C. 42385, 5; AGMAV, C. 42386, 1; AGMAV, C. 42386, 2; & AGMAV, C. 42386, AGMAV, C. 29297, 1; AGMAV, C. 29297, 2; & AGMAV, C. 29297, 5; Scott-Ellis, P., *The Diary of Pip Scott-Ellis* (Cardiff University Library Archive (CULA): manuscript no. 3/233); Sir Robert Reynolds Mackintosh Papers, Wellcome Library, Archives and Manuscripts (WLAM): WLAM, PP/RRM/D1/76; & WLAM, PP/RRM/C/2.

32 *ABC* (Sevilla), 27.03.1938, p. 4; *ABC* (Sevilla), 22.08.1937, pp. 11–12; *ABC* (Sevilla), 26.08.1937, p. 11; *ABC* (Sevilla), 24.08.1937, p. 1.

33 Ibid.

34 *Blood Bank Service in Spain* (Laya Films, 1937).

35 Fyrth, *The Signal Was Spain*; Requena Gallego & Sepúlveda Losa, *La sanidad en las Brigadas Internacionales*; Jackson, *For Us It Was Heaven*; Palfreeman, *¡Salud!*; Lethbridge, *Norman Bethune*; Palfreeman, *Aristocrats, Adventurers and Ambulances*; Palfreeman, *Spain Bleeds*; Derby, *Petals and Bullets*; Pretus, *La ayuda humanitarian.*

36 Preston, *Spanish Holocaust*, pp. 502–503, 508–509, 514–515, 519–521; Aguilar, Agents of Memory, pp. 90–92.

37 *BOE*, 17.10.1977, Ley 46/1977, de 15 de octubre, de amnistía, pp. 22765–6.

38 Ibid.; Aguilar, P., "The Timing and the Scope of Reparation, Truth and Justice Measures: A Comparison of the Spanish, Argentinian and Chilean Cases", in K. Ambos, J. Large, & M. Wierda (eds.), *Building a Future on Peace and*

Justice: Studies on Transitional Justice, Conflict Resolution and Development: The Nuremberg Declaration on Peace and Justice (Berlin, 2009), pp. 503–532, pp. 505–509.

39 Ibid., pp. 502–503, 508–509; *BOE*, 17.10.1977, Ley 46/1977, de 15 de octubre, de amnistía, pp. 22765–6.

40 Preston, *Spanish Holocaust*, pp. xvi, 503–504; Richards, M., *After the Civil War: Making Memory and Re-Making Spain since 1936* (Cambridge, 2013), pp. 64–65.

41 Aguilar, Agents of Memory, p. 87.

42 Ibid.; Anderson, P., *Friend or Foe? Occupation, Collaboration and Selective Violence in the Spanish Civil War* (Brighton, 2016).

43 Larraz Andía, P., *Entre el frente y la retaguardia. La sanidad en la Guerra Civil: El hospital "Alfonso Carlos", Pamplona 1936–1939* (Madrid, 2004); Frutos Herranz, M. de, *Hospitales en Burgos durante la Guerra Civil, 1936–1939* (Burgos, 2009); Beneito Lloris, A., *El hospital Sueco-Noruego de Alcoi durante la Guerra Civil Española* (Alcoi, 2004); García Ferrandis, X., *L'assistència sanitària a la ciutat de València durant la Guerra Civil* (Valencia, 2015); Hervás I Puyal, C., *La xarxa hospitalária a Catalunya durant la Guerra Civil 1936–1939* (Manresa, 2014); Algarbani, J. M., *Y Jimena se vistió de negro: II República, Guerra Civil y posguerra en Jimena de la Frontera* (Cádiz, 2011), pp. 106–11; Romero Romero, F., *Alcalá del Valle. República, Guerra civil y represión 1931–1946* (Cádiz, 2009); Cabañas González, J., *La Bañeza 1936. La vorágine de julio. Golpe y represión en la comarca Bañezana*, Vol. 1, (León, 2010).

44 For a full list of archival sources see Bibliography.

45 Preston, P., *The Coming of the Spanish Civil War: Reform, Reaction, and Revolution in the Second Republic, 1931–1936* (London, 1978); Fraser, R. *Blood of Spain: An Oral History of the Spanish Civil War* (London, 1979); Carr, R., *Spain 1808–1975*, 2nd edn. (Oxford, 1982); Beevor, A., *The Spanish Civil War* (London, 1982); Bernecker, W. L., *Colectividades y Revolución social: El Anarquismo en la Guerra Civil Española, 1936–1939* (Barcelona, 1982).

46 Preston, "The Historiography of the Spanish Civil War", in *People's History and Socialist Theory*, History Workshop Series (London, 1981), pp. 193–194; Thomas, *Spanish Civil War*; Payne, Historiography; Blanco Rodríguez, Historiografía.

47 Preston, P., *The Spanish Civil War: Reaction, Revolution, and Revenge*, revised and expanded edition (London, 2006).

48 Campos, M. L., "La historiografía española y la internacionalización de la Guerra Civil (1936–1939): un estado de la cuestión", *Ab Initio*, No. 5 (2012), pp. 59–79, p. 67.

49 Rubio, J., *La emigración de la guerra civil de 1936–1939: Historia del éxodo que se produce con el fin de la II República española* (Madrid, 1977).

50 Bescós Torres, J., "Las enfermeras en la guerra de España (1936–1939)", *Revista Historia Militar*, Vol. 53 (1982), pp. 97–143; Bescós Torres, J., "La Sanidad Militar en la guerra de España (1936–1939). 1ª parte – La Sanidad en el Ejército Republicano", *Medicina Militar*, Vol. 43, No. 1 (1987), pp. 88–100; Bescós Torres, J., "La Sanidad Militar en la Guerra de España (1936–1939), 2ª parte – La Sanidad en el Ejército Nacional", *Medicina Militar*, Vol. 43, No. 4 (1987), pp. 434–447; Garate Córdoba, J. M., "Las tropas de África en la Guerra Civil Española", *Revista de Historia Militar*, No. 70, (1991), pp. 9–66; Jackson, M., *The Oxford Handbook of the History of Medicine* (Oxford, 2001), pp. 1–2.

51 Campos, La historiografía española, p. 67.
52 Beecham Research Laboratories, *Los médicos y la medicina en la Guerra Civil Española: Monografías Beecham* (Madrid, 1986).
53 Fyrth, *The Signal Was Spain.*
54 Jackson, *The Oxford Handbook of the History of Medicine*, pp. 1–2.
55 Ramiro Rivera, Dr., Presidente de la Organización Médico Colegial, "Epilogo: Soldados de la ciencia, el humanismo y la libertad", in *Los médicos y la medicina en la Guerra Civil Española* (Madrid, 1986), pp. 347–350, p. 347.
56 Fraser, *Blood of Spain.*
57 Keene, J., *The Last Mile to Huesca: An Australian Nurse in the Spanish Civil War* (Sydney, 1998); Fyrth, J. & Alexander, S. (eds.), *Women's Voices from the Spanish Civil War* (London, 1991); Mangini, S., *Memories of Resistance: Women's Voices from the Spanish Civil War* (New Haven, 1995); Scott-Ellis, *The Chances of Death: A Diary of the Spanish Civil War*, edited by Raymond Carr (Norwich, 1995); Vásquez León, A., *Un boomerang en Jimena de la Frontera: guerra, huida y exilio de una niña campogibraltareña* (Algeciras, 1998); Preston, P., *Doves of War: Four Women of Spain* (London, 2002); Jackson, A., *British Women and the Spanish Civil War* (London and New York, 2002); Hastings, M., *The Real Band of Brothers: First-Hand Accounts from the Last British Survivors of the Spanish Civil War* (London, 2009).
58 Massons, J. M., *Historia de la Sanidad Militar Española: Tomos I–IV* (Barcelona, 1994).
59 Massons, *Historia de la Sanidad Militar Española: Tomo II*, pp. 312–525.
60 Requena Gallego & Sepúlveda Losa, *La sanidad en las Brigadas Internacionales*; Navarro Carballo, *Frederic Duran i Jorda.*
61 Coni, N., *Medicine and Warfare: Spain, 1936–1939* (Abingdon, 2008), p. 8.
62 Jackson, *For Us It Was Heaven*; Palfreeman, *¡Salud!*; Lethbridge, *Norman Bethune*; Palfreeman, *Aristocrats, Adventurers and Ambulances*; Palfreeman, *Spain Bleeds*; Derby, *Petals and Bullets.*
63 Ametlla, C., *Catalunya: Paradís perdut. La guerra civil i la revolució anarco-comunista* (Barcelona, 1984); Domínguez Pérez, A., *El verano que trajo un largo invierno: La represión político-social durante el primer franquismo en Cádiz, 1936–1945*, Vol. 1 (Cádiz, 2004); Ávila Álvarez, A (ed.), *Todos los nombres. Base de datos sobre la represión franquista en Andalucía accesible a través de internet* (Sevilla, 2007); Aracil, R., & Villarroya, J., *El país valencià sota les bombes, 1936–1939* (Valencia, 2010); Rina Simón, C., *La construcción de la memoria franquista en Cáceres: Héroes, espacio y tiempo para un nuevo* estado, 1936–*1941* (Cáceres, 2012); Aguirre González, J. V., *Al fin de la batalla, y muerto el combatiente … La Rioja 1936–1939* (Logroño, 2014); Rodríguez Padilla, E., *Mujeres de Almería condenadas a muerte o reclusión perpetua tras la Guerra Civil 1939–1945* (Almería, 2014); Giner Jiménez, A., & Porcar Orihuela, J. L. (eds.), *El temps perdut: Memòrica històrica de Vistabella* (Castelló de la Plana, 2015).
64 Larraz Andía, *Entre el frente y la retaguardia*; Frutos Herranz, *Hospitales en Burgos*; Beneito Lloris, *El hospital Sueco-Noruego*; García Ferrandis, *L'assistència sanitària*; Hervás I Puyal, *La xarxa hospitalária.*
65 Beneito Lloris, *El hospital Sueco-Noruego.*
66 García Ferrandis, X., & Munayco Sánchez, A. J., "La asistencia sanitaria en el frente de Teruel durante la primera campaña repúblicana (agosto de 1936-febrero de 1937)", *Sanidad Militar*, Vol. 66, No. 4 (2010), pp. 245–249; García

Ferrandis, X., "La Asistencia sanitaria in la provincia de Valencia durante la Guerra Civil Española (1936–1939)", *Llull*, Vol. 34, No. 73 (2011), pp. 13–38; García Ferrandis, X., "La cobertura sanitaria de un ejército en retirada: la actuación de un Capitán Médico durante la Batalla del Maestrazgo (abril-julio de 1938)", *Sanidad Militar*, Vol. 68, No. 3 (2012), pp. 189–194; Larraz, P. & Barrola, C., " 'Los pies de Teruel': Asistencia y tratamiento de las heridas por congelación en los hospitales navarros durante la guerra civil", *Anales de Sistema Sanitario de Navarra*, Vol. 28, No. 2 (2005), pp. 197–212; Larraz Andía, *Entre el frente y la retaguardia.*

67 Larraz Andía, *Entre el frente y la retaguardia.*

68 Frutos Herranz, *Hospitales en Burgos*, pp. 126–127.

69 Gurriarán, R., *Fernando Alsina E O Seu: Diario de Guerra* (Santiago de Compostela, 2015).

70 Palfreeman, *Spain Bleeds*; Valls, R., et al., Infermeres catalanes a la Guerra Civil espanyola (Barcelona, 2008); Hervás I Puyal, *La xarxa hospitalária*; García Ferrandis, *L'assistència sanitària.*

71 *Las maestras de la República*, Director: Pilar Pérez Solano (FETE-UGT, Transit Producciones, 2013); *La Sauceda, de la utopía al horror*, Director: Juan Miguel León Moriche (Foro por la Memoria del Campo de Gibraltar/Asociación de Familiares de Represaliados por el Franquismo en La Sauceda y el Marrufo, 2013); *Els internat de la por*, Directors: R. Vinyes, M. Armengou, & R. Belis (Televisió de Catalunya, 2015).

72 Jackson, *For Us It Was Heaven*; Palfreeman, *¡Salud!*; Lethbridge, *Norman Bethune*; Palfreeman, *Aristocrats, Adventurers and Ambulances*; Palfreeman, *Spain Bleeds*; Derby, *Petals and Bullets.*

73 www.elplural.com/andalucia/2016/11/21/la-memoria-ya-tiene-casa-en-la-sierra; www.europapress.es/andalucia/noticia-psoe-defiende-memoria-historica-vigilara-cumpla-ley-andaluza-todos-municipios-20180114141132.html.

2 Military conflict and medical care of Moroccan wounded 1909–1939

Introduction

On the evening of 17 July 1936, the garrisons of Melilla, Ceuta, Larache and Tetuan in Northern Morocco rose up in rebellion as part of the coup orchestrated by General Mola. By the early hours of the following morning, apart from isolated pockets of resistance, the Spanish Protectorate in Morocco had been secured for the Insurgents. Key to the success of this operation was the role played by indigenous troops, the Regulares, led by Spanish officers, and units of the Foreign Legion, the units within the Spanish Army of Africa most trusted by the Insurgent leadership.[1] The first troops mobilised were the fifth Tabor of Regulares (a brigade-sized unit), who set out on the night of 16 July from the south of the Protectorate toward the Bay of al-Hoceima across the difficult terrain of the Rif Mountains.[2] On 19 July, Franco arrived in Tetuan from Gran Canaria and the Army of Africa was placed under his command.[3]

The intervention of the Army of Africa helped secure the Protectorate for the Insurgents and played a decisive role on the Spanish mainland during the first weeks of the war. The use of the Army of Africa, particularly the highly trained Regulares and the Legionnaires, helped prop up the faltering military rebellion on the mainland that would have likely failed without their intervention.[4] Between 75,000 and 85,000 Maghrebi soldiers were to see action in Spain, and it is the background to their participation in the conflict and the hospital care they received in mainland Spain that forms the central focus of this chapter.[5]

The term 'Maghrebi' is chosen here as it more accurately reflects the diverse origins of the combatants. Although the majority of troops were from the Spanish Protectorate in Morocco, there were also recruits from French Morocco, as well as a small number from Algeria and Tunisia, despite efforts by the French authorities to deter their recruitment.[6] The high levels of poverty in the Maghreb, and Spanish historical connections with Algeria and its geographical proximity to the North African coast, meant that the chance to earn a regular income as a soldier in the Insurgent army was a sufficiently attractive proposition for many who sought to enlist. Recruits from Ifni in Southern

Morocco and the Spanish Sahara also served with the Insurgent forces, as did a small number from the nomadic tribes of Mauritania. 'Maghrebi' also serves as a useful definition in that the available documents do not always stress whether the soldiers were from the French or the Spanish Zones of Morocco, or from outside these areas. The use of this term also means that the more emotive but ultimately derogatory term 'Moor' can be avoided, except in those circumstances where it is quoted directly from sources.[7]

The term 'soldiers' is also deliberately chosen here as much of the secondary literature refers to 'Moorish mercenaries', including some monographs and studies that set out to portray them in a more sympathetic light than is normally found in the historiography.[8] While technically correct as a definition, in that they fought for pay for a foreign power, the term 'mercenary' nevertheless carries a derogatory meaning. These recruits were not in the main professional soldiers, especially after the number of veterans were depleted in the opening campaigns of the Civil War. Instead, they were largely made up of civilians who were prepared to serve in the military for regular pay and the chance to acquire booty while on campaign.[9] If applied in its original meaning, then the Sikhs who fought for the British Empire during WWI and WWII were also mercenaries, or indeed the Gurkhas who serve in the British Army today, so the term soldier is preferred here as it has a more clearly defined meaning, as 'Moorish mercenaries' were effectively colonial troops.[10]

It might seem that an uprising launched by self-proclaimed 'nationalists' to wrest control of Spain from its 'legally elected' government, an insurgency that had the backing of the staunchly conservative Catholic Church in Spain, might have been indifferent to the care of Muslim soldiers under its command. This, however, was not the case. The Maghrebi troops, an integral part of the Insurgent war effort, were provided with their own hospitals, where not only were there attempts to address their medical needs, but efforts were also made to comply with their religious and cultural requirements. This engagement with Islamic precepts in relation to the combatants from the Maghreb was important to maintain recruitment and elicit support from the Moroccan elites within the Protectorate, and it was also seen as a means of ensuring the loyalty of these troops.

The use of the Regulares and the other predominantly Moroccan units, such as recruits from Ifni Sahara or the Mehal-la Khalifianas (troops who owed their loyalty to the Sultan), as the main shock troops during many of the key campaigns of the conflict meant that casualty rates among these men were often high.[11] It is for this reason that the aim of this chapter is to examine the surgical and wider healthcare that the troops from the Maghreb received during this period and the motives for their participation in a conflict on foreign soil. Part of this examination will entail a study of how attempts were made to meet the religious and cultural needs of the hospitalised patients. This analysis will also involve an enquiry into how the care provided served within the context of a wider effort by the Insurgents to portray the 'Moorish other', traditionally Catholicism's greatest foe, as part of a 'crusade' sanctioned by the

Spanish Church against the 'red' infidel who threatened the 'patria', or, fatherland. This reinvention of Christianity's 'traditional enemy' as co-defenders of religion became an important focal point of Insurgent propaganda.[12]

It was against this background that it became important to establish separate hospitals for the Muslim troops of the Insurgency. It would seem likely that it would have been possible to expand the established military hospitals, or simply create new hospitals that could treat all Insurgent casualties under one roof. For a time, the Regulares and other indigenous troops did indeed receive treatment in hospitals other than those designed specifically for their use, but it soon became desirable from a religious and cultural viewpoint to provide separate healthcare, a move that would also have helped assuage Catholic sensibilities.[13]

The treatment received in hospitals by Spanish troops on both sides of the conflict has, to a limited degree, been covered above, and is more fully explored in the following chapters, however, very little attention has been paid to the care of wounded soldiers from the Maghreb. María Rosa de Madariaga in *Los moros que trajo Franco* (2002), Francisco Sánchez Ruano in *Islam y Guerra Civil Española* (2004), and Mustapha el Merroun's *Las tropas Marroquíes en la Guerra Civil Española 1936–1939* (2003) deal briefly with the topic, with Madariaga dedicating ten pages out of 422 to the subject, and Sánchez Ruano three.[14] José Luis de Mesa in *Los moros de la Guerra Civil española* (2004), provides a more detailed nine-page study, in which the creation of individual hospitals is also examined. However, his overall analysis is on the military participation of the 'Moors', and his brief study on medical care focuses on the numbers of those hospitalised and the permits of leave granted to the wounded.[15]

The most detailed study carried out to date is to be found in the monograph by Martín de Frutos Herranz, *Hospitales en Burgos durante la Guerra Civil, 1936–1939*. The study is, however, a traditional micro-history, focussing on the hospitals in Burgos, the Muslim hospital being just one among these. Included within this work is an examination of the Hospital del Rey in Burgos, which was converted from civilian use in March 1937 to provide care for the wounded soldiers from the Maghreb. Various aspects of the care received by the hospitalised patients in the Muslim hospital of Burgos are analysed, including their religious and dietary needs. Also of interest is a chart that details the deaths of thirty-nine in-patients hospitalised between 1936 and 1939. Thirty-five of these were from the Spanish Protectorate, three from French Morocco and one from Algeria.[16] Elsewhere, Ali al Tuma, from the University of Leiden, has carried out and continues to research social and religious aspects of 'the participation of Moorish (Moroccan) troops in the Spanish Civil War'. Part of this research includes an examination into care of the wounded and, although not the main focus of his research, he is nevertheless advancing our understanding of a topic that remains sorely neglected.[17]

There are a variety of possible reasons for this neglect. Much of the focus of attention on the Spanish Civil War has traditionally been on the political and military, rather than the medical, aspects of the conflict. Studies examining participation by North African troops have tended to look predominantly at their military role, or focus on perceptions of the 'other' in order to re-evaluate the traditional stereotype of the supposed savagery of the 'Moors'.[18] The participation of the Regulares (and of the Legionnaires) in the brutal suppression of the Asturias rising of October 1934, and the terror employed in Andalucía, Extremadura and beyond during the opening months of the Civil War (and indeed throughout much of the conflict), where summary execution, mutilation and rape were frequent, has commanded the attention of some historians.[19] This combination of factors goes some way to explaining why so little has been written with regards to the healthcare on offer to soldiers from the Maghreb.

Two further considerations ought to be taken into account. The first is the role played by the perceived image of the 'savage Moor' during the conflict that still permeates much of the collective memory within Spain today.[20] The second equally important factor is the almost total lack of written records by soldiers from the Maghreb who participated in the conflict. The majority of those who fought in Spain were illiterate subsistence farmers and herdsmen (most of whom spoke little or no Spanish), primarily from the Rif, where the majority eked out a meagre living, a way of life that most returned to once the conflict was over.[21] The combination of these influences largely explains the lacuna in the historiography of the history of medicine with regards to Maghrebi participation during the Spanish Civil War.

This lacuna is even more regrettable as there is a largely untapped yet accessible source of documents in the Archivo General Militar de Ávila.[22] It is a selection of these documents, which take the form of index cards covering two of the main Muslim hospitals, El Hospital Musulman de Zaragoza and El Hospital Militar Musulman de la Vega/Hospital Militar de la Vega Salamanca, which constitute the supporting evidence for the central case study of this chapter. These index cards, often only consisting of a few lines of text, contain the admission and discharge details of Maghrebi soldiers from 1936–1940.[23]

At first appearance, these index cards seem to hold only the briefest of details.[24] Nevertheless, these index cards reward careful study. Those from the hospital in Zaragoza provide more detailed information. This material includes patients' injuries, the location where they sustained their wounds, which hospital or hospitals they had been transferred from, the unit they were serving in, which hospital they were being discharged to, and how much leave they had been granted as a result of their injuries. Together the information contained comprises a rich body of material from which it is possible to reconstruct a picture of the surgical treatment received by a number of hospitalised soldiers. It also throws additional light on their overall health, by providing information on endemic illnesses suffered by the indigenous troops of the Army of Africa. The 400 documents collected for the purpose of this study were chosen carefully from a total of 4,000 cards examined to represent a variety of conditions suffered by a number of soldiers serving in a variety of units. Nevertheless, this sample represents only a small part of the index cards regarding the inpatients of the Muslim Hospitals. This, in turn, represents an even smaller part of the overall number of files contained in this one archive in relation to the health records of the military hospitals during the Civil War.[25]

As this chapter is also concerned with religious and the cultural aspects of care examined within the context of Muslim participation in Franco's 'Catholic Crusade of Reconquest', a subversion of the original idea of the *Reconquista*, the other main primary source drawn upon is the Insurgent edition of the daily newspaper *ABC*.[26] An invaluable resource, it contains references to Muslim hospitals and visits by a variety of Spanish and Moroccan dignitaries during the years 1937 and 1938, with this frequently framed within a religious and cultural discourse that is inclusive rather than exclusive of the 'Moor'. Although this discourse is primarily concerned with the glorification of the Francoist cause and notions of empire, it nevertheless provides an insight into the construction of a paternalistic model that has at its centre the 'protector' (Insurgent Spain), and the 'protected' (the Spanish Protectorate in Morocco).[27] It is by a careful utilisation of these and other sources that it is possible, for the first time, to reconstruct a more comprehensive account of the care received by the Maghrebi wounded during the Spanish Civil War.[28]

The roots of a conflict: Regulares and the Army of Africa

If the estimated figure of 85,000 is widely accepted for the participation of troops from the Maghreb, then the vast majority of these came from the Northern Zone of the Spanish Protectorate.[29] Furthermore, if we accept the figures quoted by Sebastian Balfour of 11,500 killed and 55,468 wounded during the conflict (this figure includes those injured on more than one occasion), then the question must be asked why so many were prepared to face injury and death in a foreign war on foreign soil.[30] To understand the participation of what amounted to an estimated ten per cent of the native male population of the Northern Zone of the Spanish Protectorate (and the conservative figure of fourteen per cent of the male population of Ifni Sahara), it is necessary to first examine Spanish colonial involvement in North Africa between 1908 and 1936.[31] This is important, as the policies pursued by successive governments during this period go some way towards explaining this participation.

The role played by Franco and his fellow officers in the Protectorate during this period is also a matter of some importance in this regard. The experiences of Spanish officers serving in the Protectorate would shape how the indigenous 'colonial' troops of the Army of Africa would be used during the Spanish Civil War as the shock troops of the Insurgency, which in turn helps to explain the high casualty rates suffered by these combatants. Alongside this, the role played by the surgeons Manuel Bastos Ansart and

Fermín Palma García during the early period of the Protectorate will also be briefly examined, as they were both later to contribute in providing care during the Spanish Civil War, albeit on opposite sides.[32] Indeed, during the period under consideration here, almost all Spanish military doctors served in the Protectorate at one time or another.[33]

The Spanish Protectorate of Morocco: The birth of a military elite

Spain's early twentieth-century colonial expansion in Africa had its roots in the late Middle Ages. Ceuta, a Portuguese possession, was ceded to Spain by the Treaty of Lisbon in 1668, and has remained as a Spanish overseas possession ever since. Melilla, Spain's other enclave on Morocco's north coast, was conquered in 1497 and, like Ceuta, is now an autonomous city administered by Spain.[34] With the loss of the Philippines and Cuba in 1898, the last two vestiges of the Spanish Empire, Ceuta and Melilla were to become important bases for Spain's new imperial venture when she belatedly became involved in the tail end of the scramble for Africa in 1908. During the negotiations, which led to the Entente Cordiale between Britain and France in 1904, Spain was given a sphere of influence in Northern Morocco.[35]

Spain, which was in no position to contest French claims in North Africa, was forced to accept a sphere of influence that covered only one-fifth of Moroccan territory.[36] France and Spain were ostensibly charged with ensuring that the *Makhzen* (the Moroccan state), under the sovereignty of the Sultan, remained the governing power in Morocco. This, however, meant that they were effectively to be the new colonial powers in Morocco, as the agreement made them responsible for policing this accord.[37]

By 1908, the French had extended the area of Morocco under its control. The Spanish government saw this as a threat to their own interests in the region, which were centred round the mines of the North-Eastern Rif, rich in high-quality iron ore.[38] Part of French efforts included trying to spread her influence within and beyond her own 'territory' by opening medical dispensaries in Fez, Rabat and Marrakech, and in Larache, which fell within the Spanish sphere, even if it was not yet under direct Spanish control. French doctors were also sent to Alcazarquivir and Tetuán in the Spanish Zone, although no dispensaries were opened in these areas.[39] The Spanish military, in response to this multipronged expansion, and still smarting from the loss of empire only ten years previously, decided to directly intervene in Moroccan affairs. It was against this background that, on 14 February 1908, the Spanish military began its invasion of Morocco when a small contingent of troops set sail from Melilla and occupied a small port nineteen kilometres to the south.[40] This was to be one of the few outright victories the Spanish military were to enjoy in the next seventeen years, and it was the disasters that would follow which led to the formation of the Fuerzas Indígenas Regulares (Indigenous Regular Forces) in 1911.[41]

The Spanish soldiers who first saw service in Morocco were predominantly poor conscripts undertaking military service, and were badly equipped and poorly trained. Facing them was an elusive enemy, the tribesmen of the Rif, described by the historian Sebastian Balfour as among 'the most accomplished guerrilla fighters in the world'.[42]

It was an attack on the mines close to Melilla by Riffian tribesmen (from where so many of the Regulares were later recruited) in July 1909, that led to the Spanish government intervening more actively in Moroccan affairs.[43] The Spanish premier, Maura, under pressure from the army and Spanish investors, sent an expeditionary force to expand Spain's territorial control to include the mines whose output was threatened by continuing attacks by Riffian fighters.[44] The call up of reservists led to anti-war protests in Catalunya, Aragón and Valencia, and also served to widen the gulf between the military and the government, an increasingly fraught relationship. The subsequent disaster of El Barranco de Lobo in July 1909, when Spanish troops were heavily defeated after efforts to protect the railway connecting Melilla with the mines, had the effect in Spain of swinging public opinion in favour of military intervention. It also had the adverse effect of reinforcing racist stereotypes concerning the *Imazighen* (Berbers) and Arabs.[45] Some 42,000 troops were mobilised between July and November 1909, and occupied an area of 17,000 square kilometres, with half of these troops remaining to consolidate the territorial gains.[46]

A witness to this attack and its aftermath was Víctor Ruiz Albéniz, also known as *El Tebib Arrumi* (the Christian Doctor), as he dispensed medicine in a wide area beyond the mines. In a telling passage from his book *España en el Rif* (Madrid, 1921), his summary of the events of 1909 perfectly encapsulate the attraction for the officers who served in the Rif, who could gain promotions even when the actions they were involved in resulted in defeat:

> After six months of campaigning, of many men lost, of much money spent, and above all, after the victory obtained, the country continued to look on with indifference, if not with aversion at things (*las cosas*) in Morocco. The politicians did not worry themselves with creating an understanding of the problems that was accessible to popular opinion, and the military only saw on the ground of the Rif a chess board where the pawns could be manoeuvred either towards death or promotion.[47]

It also helps to explain the rise of the Africanistas (the Africanists), the military officers that included Mola, Franco, Millán Astray, Varela and the other chief plotters of the 1936 coup, who participated in the pacification of the Protectorate.[48] It was this ability of the officers to gain promotion in a harsh colonial environment that set them apart from their counterparts in Spain. This separate identity was later additionally reinforced by their control over indigenous soldiers, whom they not only saw as tools of 'empire', but also a means of restoring Spain to her imperial glory, through the destruction of the Republic. These factors would define how the Army of Africa was used during the Civil War.

As part of the expeditionary force despatched in 1909, a young surgeon Manuel Bastos Ansart who had recently joined the Army Medical Services, was sent to Morocco. His job as an army surgeon not only required that he attend those who fell in battle, but as an army medic he also had to tackle conditions aggravated by poor hygiene, adverse climate conditions and a poor diet. Nevertheless, during the many postings that he spent in Spanish Morocco between 1909 and 1921, he honed his skills in surgery, specialising in orthopaedics and traumatology.[49] He wrote extensively on his specialty, and in 1924 described the closed plaster method of treatment for open fractures, also known as the 'Spanish Method', helping to re-popularise its use.[50] However, it was the publication of his book just prior to the outbreak of the Spanish Civil War in 1936, *Algunos aspectos clínicos de las heridas por arma de fuego*, which ensured that many Spanish surgeons at the start of the conflict were familiar with this method.[51]

The closed plaster method was a technique that had first been used in its modern form by the US surgeon Winnett Orr during WWI.[52] It involved the careful and full debridement (cleaning) of the wound site, the application of paraffin-impregnated gauze, followed by the application of plaster of Paris so as to fully encase and immobilise the affected limb.[53] This process often meant that limbs that had previously been amputated due to the presence of gas gangrene and other infections could now be healed. Josep Trueta, an important figure in popularising this method outside of Spain, treated 605 open fractures using this method during the course of 1938 in Spain without having to amputate and without a fatality.[54]

The experience gained by surgeons within the Protectorate and in the Spanish military hospitals was to prove important during the Civil War, especially when placed in the context of public expenditure on health within Spain during the opening decades of the twentieth century, which gave little scope for a national programme for the training of doctors. In 1910, this figure was just 0.12 per cent of Gross Domestic Product (GDP), rising to 0.24 per cent by 1921. During the dictatorship of Primo de Rivera, this figure stabilised at 0.25 per cent, but with the devaluation of the peseta during this period there was a fall in real terms. The figure rose between 1930 and 1933 to 0.71 per cent of GDP, but tailed off again when the Spanish Confederation of the Autonomous Right (CEDA), under the leadership of Gil Robles, attempted to reverse many of the liberal reforms begun during the first two years of the Second Republic.[55]

With the limited opportunities offered by public employment in health, surgeons predominantly relied on private practice to gain experience. However, with large sections of Spanish society unable to afford their services, the experience gained in the Protectorate by military doctors undoubtedly proved beneficial in the treatment of an array of traumatic injuries common during the Spanish Civil War.[56]

The high casualty rates among Spanish reservists that resulted from the El Barranco de Lobo debacle and the subsequent unrest, led to reforms under the new liberal government of Canalejas (1910–1912). In 1911 the first units of the Regulares were formed from recruits drawn mainly from the Protectorate, but among these early recruits were a number of soldiers from French Morocco, Algeria and Tunisia.[57] In pushing for military reform the government had one eye on reducing Spanish casualties, and the other on addressing popular unrest that rose out of forced conscription within Spain.[58]

In 1911 the French occupied Fez, with the Spanish responding by occupying Larache.[59] It was conquests such as these that led to the creation on 27 November 1912 of the two protectorates in Morocco, when the Treaty between France and Spain Regarding Morocco was signed.[60] The Sultan was supposedly nominally in control throughout Morocco, but his authority was vested in his representative, the Khalif in the Spanish Zone, whom the Sultan selected from a shortlist of two chosen by the government in Madrid.[61]

It was in February 1912 that Franco first saw service in Morocco. In 1913, the year in which Tetuán was occupied, he applied for and received a transfer to serve with the Regulares as a lieutenant. Already in use as shock troops, Franco, along with the tabor of Regulares he was serving with, was posted initially to help defend Ceuta, which was under attack by tribesmen from the Rif.[62] This was to be the beginning of a close relationship for Franco with the Regulares that would last until the end of the Spanish Civil War and beyond.[63] It was this relationship that Franco and his fellow officers were to share with the soldiers of the Protectorate that would define many aspects of how the Civil War was to be fought. The brutal colonial war of attrition that unfolded in the Protectorate was the approach favoured by Franco during much of Spain's later internal war, as he systematically purged 'undesirable elements' in those areas that came under his control. This resulted in a high casualty rate among the Maghrebi soldiers and the Tercio, and prolonged the conflict at the cost of thousands of extra lives.[64]

In the years between 1912 and 1921 the Spanish military in the Protectorate had, to a limited degree, extended its control over the Protectorate, but consolidating their hold over the territories gained had cost many lives and incurred huge expenditure.[65] As a result, there were renewed efforts towards continued recruitment of indigenous troops. This process was accelerated by the Spanish High Commissioner in the Protectorate, General Jordana, between 1915 and 1919. A policy of patronage of *qaids* (local notables) and administrators played an important part in recruitment. These 'pensioned' (pensionados) local officials and chiefs and their successors were to play a key role in the recruitment of soldiers during the Spanish Civil War.[66]

Nevertheless, despite efforts to 'buy' support among the local population between 1913 and 1924, the Spanish Army was involved in a total of 410 military engagements in the west of the Protectorate. The reason for the number of conflicts was due to the unpopularity of what was essentially an occupying power, which did not flinch from punishing any opposition it encountered.

These campaigns were primarily against the forces of its one-time ally, Mulai Ahmed al-Raisuni.[67]

In 1921, in what became known as the Disaster at Annual, General Silvestre, intent on occupying the territory between Melilla and the Bay of al-Hoceima, was warned by the Riffian leader Abd al-Karim that if he crossed the Amekran River he would be resisted in force. Due to the fact, however, that concerted action by the tribes of the Rif was uncommon, this warning was ignored. Silvestre, confident that he could easily meet any threat, overextended his line and in what turned out to be a rout lasting three weeks, suffered the loss of over 9,000 men, considerable quantities of military hardware and 5,000 square kilometres of territory.[68] Additionally, more than 500 troops were captured, which only added to the uproar created in Spain by the news of the disaster.[69]

Carlos Puig, a doctor in the expedition was an apparent witness to the death of Silvestre at the hand of the 'Moors', although other witnesses claim that he committed suicide in his tent. Perhaps of more interest, however, was Puig's observation of the desertion of Regulares, Harkas (small bands of predominantly Riffian auxiliaries from the same village or villages, formed and disbanded at need, and led by their *qaid*) and Idalas (temporary units formed from troops owing their loyalty to the Sultan), who joined the forces of Abd al-Karim. These desertions exposed an early weakness of Spanish 'colonial' policy: the preoccupation with gaining territory instead of seeking to build ties of loyalty with local communities by investing in infrastructure within those territories gained.[70] Large numbers of indigenous troops did desert and join Abd al-Karim, nevertheless, Melilla, under attack from the forces of Abd al-Karim, was relieved by the Tercio and by Regulares from Ceuta.[71] One of the captives who was to die in captivity, on 18 July 1922, was Fernando Serrano Flores, a young doctor. From the start of his captivity he had attempted to aid the wounded prisoners. He had also been called upon to treat the wounded among his captors, and due to the heavy workload, trained fellow prisoners to aid him in this task. Some supplies from the Spanish Red Cross did get through, but with typhus and typhoid fever rampant, Flores contracted typhoid which resulted in his death.[72]

Disease, rather than injury, was the main cause of hospitalisation throughout most of this period, with the most widespread illness, venereal disease, the possible cause of more fatalities than the war itself.[73] Malaria, typhus, typhoid fever and rheumatism were also common, and these ailments, as well as gonorrhoea, were a frequent reason for the hospitalisation of Maghrebi soldiers during the Spanish Civil War.[74] Conditions in many of the hospitals, with the exception of Red Cross hospitals, were generally very poor. These establishments were put under severe strain after the disaster at Annual, and in many instances, were unable to cope with the sheer number of diseased and injured patients. Conditions did improve with more investment in infrastructure, but this improvement was modest compared to French efforts in their own area of control in Morocco.[75]

As a result of the defeat at Annual, an independent republic was established in the Rif under the leadership of Abd al-Karim. This did impact upon the recruitment of indigenous troops in the Rif by the Spanish military during its existence, but this impact was mitigated by a policy of renewed recruitment and the reintegration of deserters.[76] It was also accompanied by more repressive measures, which included a localised version of a scorched earth policy in those areas where there was resistance to recruitment and re-enlistment. Nevertheless, by 1926 there were five groups of Regulares organised into twenty tabors, all from the north of the protectorate.[77]

Professionalising the troops

Abd al-Karim, whose success in part rested on his ability to appeal to religious and nationalist sentiments, made the mistake of attacking the French Zone in 1925.[78] Despite aerial bombardment that included the extensive use of the toxic chemical agents mustard gas, phosgene and chloropicrin by the Spanish military in the Rif, Abd al-Karim had consolidated his position as the leader of the Riffian Republic between 1921 and 1925.[79] When French troops tried to occupy the no-man's-land (an important source of grain for the forces of the Rif) that defined the border between the French and Spanish Protectorates in the spring of 1925, Abd al-Karim inflicted heavy losses on the French. This was to result in a joint action by the French and Spanish when a Franco-Spanish force in a combined naval and aerial assault landed at al-Hoceima on 8 September 1925, and which included contingents of Regulares and Legionnaires.[80] This joint landing on a heavily protected area of coast was also significant in that it saw the combined use of frontline mobile hospitals that were established on a large beach in the bay of al-Hoceima, the use of three hospital ships with a total of 814 beds, and the use of three air ambulances that could carry two patients, a medic and a pilot each.[81] This military action against Abd al-Karim had in fact been suggested as early as 1921 as a response to the defeat at Annual but it took French participation for it to become a reality.[82] Abd al-Karim surrendered to the French in May 1926, but it was not to be until July 1927 that the main resistance in the Rif was finally quashed by General Sanjurjo.[83] This period of 'pacification' between May 1926 and July 1927, which saw the tribes in the Rif largely disarmed, was characterised by a brutal campaign of summary executions of prisoners, expropriation of goods and animals, destruction of villages and the detention of hostages.[84]

In a speech given in Bab Taza on 10 July 1927 to celebrate the 'occupation in its totality of our Zone of the Protectorate', Sanjurjo paid tribute to the 'loyal Muslims at the side of the protecting nation, there because they are convinced of the benefit this brings to their country and their race'.[85] The process of pacification, however, was not entirely complete, and on 17 July 1927, *ABC* reported on the 'act of submission' in the Souk of Tetuán of the last *qaid* in rebellion in the Ketama region. Also reported upon was the return of the Harka involved in the campaign who 'returned very satisfied with the economic result of the campaign; the booty gathered in raids'.[86] This right to booty continued to be a way of rewarding participation in military actions by indigenous units up to and including during the Spanish Civil War. Also reported upon was the dissolution of the Idala of Melilla involved in the operation, under the command of the *qaid* Amarusen [*sic*] and Commander Bueno, a fatality along with the unit's Dr Correa, with indigenous casualties among the Idala numbering 200 men.[87] This relationship between local leaders and the officers of the Army of Africa was to prove an important factor in recruitment during the forthcoming conflict of the Civil War.

Those injured among the Idalas and Harkas also enjoyed the same rights to medical assistance and right of admission to hospitals as the Regulares and the Mehal-la Khalifianas. This would also have acted as an incentive to serving with the occupying forces, especially as casualty rates among these units were high. There continued to be pockets of resistance in the Rif until 1932, although this did not seem to have interfered with recruitment during this period.[88] Indeed, recruitment in the years between 1934 and 1937 was further facilitated by poor crop yields as the result of drought.[89] This, in turn, made it easier for those *qaids* in the pay of Spain to promote enlistment; the incentive offered by a regular salary and the gift of food when joining up that could then be shared with families suffering extreme poverty was sufficient for many who enrolled.

The evidence, however, in relation to recruitment, and even for drought, is sketchy at best and is based largely on limited oral testimony.[90] This paucity of evidence also applies to the promotion of ideas closely tied to *jihad* as an additional means of maintaining recruitment.[91] Nevertheless, *jihad* may well have been a further motivating factor for fighting in Spain where Republicans were frequently portrayed as atheists. Another reason should also be considered, the opportunity for taking revenge on the colonial power perceived as being directly responsible for adverse conditions within the Protectorate. These factors, although difficult to quantify, do not ultimately detract from the main reason for enlistment, namely, opportunities provided by serving in the military to provide for families living in extreme poverty.[92]

A rare testimony by a Moroccan woman, Fátima Ben Enfeddal, provides a compelling reason for why so many men in the Protectorate sought to enlist. The widow of Mohammad Ben Abdelsalam Redondo, an early recruit killed in action in September 1936, recalled how she first found out about her husband's enlistment: 'He presented himself in the house with his uniform on and with a large tin of oil "La Giralda", various loafs of sugar "La Rosa", and a packet of green tea.' For Fatima Ben Enfeddal, the enlistment of her husband in the Regulares was a mixed blessing:

> Nine years have passed and I can still not decide whether it was to my liking or not seeing him cloaked in that khaki uniform. The only thing I know is that the pay-packet of two months advanced wages that he

brought with him that day was for me like manna rained from heaven, apart from it being the first time that your father had brought into the house a five-litre tin of oil and so many cakes of sugar together.[93]

It was against this background of colonisation between 1909 and 1927, which led to the Army of Africa becoming the most efficient section of the Spanish Army. By 1927, these forces had undergone a period of reconstruction. Improvements had been made to the medical services, to the diet of the troops, and the army's military equipment and hardware was similar to that found in most advanced European armies.[94] A French military delegation that visited the Spanish Protectorate in August 1928 reported that the Army of Africa had become an efficient and powerful body, officered by ambitious men; men such as Franco, Yagüe and Varela, who would rise to prominence during the Spanish Civil War.[95] These findings were confirmed by a French military attaché in the following spring after a visit to the Protectorate. He also noted that the 'troops of Morocco form something of a separate army where the mentality is quite different to that of the metropolitan Army and much more military'.[96] It was this separate mentality, an Imperial-Africanist mindset, which made these colonial troops so different from their metropolitan counterpart.

As part of the increased professionalisation of the military during this period, military surgeons who first served in Morocco were to contribute towards the development of surgery, both within Morocco and within Spain. Bastos Ansart, after a stint as director of the Civil-Military Hospital of al-Hoceima, and further service in Ceuta and Tetuán, took up a post at the Military Clinic for emergencies in Madrid in 1913.[97]

Another surgeon who had honed his surgical skills in the Protectorate was Fermín Palma García. As a result of service in Morocco between 1913 and 1916, he took up a post in the Civilian-Military Hospital in Jaén with the responsibility for surgical care of the military wounded. It was in Jaén where he was to spend most of his career, with the exception of the period of the Civil War, where he served in a number of hospitals on different fronts. In January 1939, he was transferred to the Muslim Hospital of Ronda in the province of Malaga, a hospital where seriously wounded Maghrebi troops had been evacuated to from the Granada and Córdoba fronts by hospital train during the campaigns of 1937.[98]

An early taste of the increased capacities of the Army of Africa, especially with the Regulares and the Tercio, prior to the Civil War came in the mining areas of Asturias in Northern Spain during October 1934. It was here that the Regulares were first credited with having seen action on Spanish soil, when Franco had them brought to the mainland to quash the 'October Revolution' of the miners in Asturias.[99] Two tabors of Regulares, one from Ceuta and another from Tetuán, alongside soldiers from the Tercio and forces of the Civil Guard, were used to supress the revolutionary uprising of the Asturian miners.[100] The tactics employed were the same tactics that had been employed in the Rif, with looting, rape and summary executions common.[101] This brutal style of colonial warfare, which was to be a common feature throughout much of the Spanish Civil War, was largely attributed to the Regulares, with the equally brutal role played by the Tercio and the Civil Guard somewhat overlooked. This in turn had the effect of further reinforcing the racist stereotypes surrounding the 'Savage Moors'. These prejudices were common throughout Civil War Spain, and would have added impetus to the segregation of hospital services in the Insurgent Zone.[102]

The intervention in Asturias is frequently cited as the first time in more than 400 years that Muslim troops had set foot on Spanish soil following their expulsion during the 'Reconquista' of the Catholic monarchs. Regulares had in fact previously been sent to Spain in 1932 to aid in the suppression of the Sanjurjada (the attempted coup by General Sanjurjo), but as this coup quickly came to nothing they were not deployed and returned to the Protectorate after only a few days. Those deployed were only informed that they were to be used against an extremist uprising, and upon disembarking in Cádiz were heard saluting their previous leader with the cry of 'Long live General Sanjurjo', unaware that Sanjurjo was the author of the uprising they had been sent to suppress.[103] This was indicative of the close relationship between Spanish officers of the Protectorate and the indigenous troops, which also set them apart from their counterparts in the metropolitan army.

This forging of a colonial army, with indigenous troops from the Protectorate forming an important element of its structure, had its roots in the prolonged campaigns and wars of occupation and pacification that characterised Spanish involvement in the North of Africa. It was the army that was formed there, with the Regulares and the Tercio at its core, which was to be crucial to the early success of the Insurgency. Maghrebi soldiers were used as shock troops on several fronts, from the Strait of Gibraltar to the foothills of the Pyrenees, not only for their fighting skills, but also as a psychological weapon. It was thought that their use would instil fear and terror among Republican soldiers and civilians alike, thanks to the commonly held perceptions of the innate savagery of the 'Moors'.[104]

These men, an unknown number of whom regularly employed rape, mutilation and summary execution, were themselves the victims of a colonial process of brutalisation, and collectively suffered the most casualties among the forces of the Insurgency.[105] They were, however, an important part of Franco's initial assault of the Spanish mainland, and his control of the Army of Africa also enabled him to build a power base from which he was able to establish control over the whole of the Insurgent forces.[106] They were also to form an important element in the crusade mythology that grew up around Franco. Thus, they were, on the one hand, used as a modern fighting force, but on the other, they were also used to connect to and reinforce medieval Catholic notions of reconquest and crusade (traditionally Papal-sanctioned moves against the Islamic 'infidel'), but reconfigured as part of a community of believers fighting against the atheist creed of the 'ungodly reds'.[107] Many of these soldiers were the recipient of more than one injury, but where possible they were reintegrated into the army, and the hospital care they received was an important part of this process. However, reintegration was not always possible due to the severity of a number of injuries that included penetrating abdominal wounds and complex fractures of limbs. The implications for Muslim combatants surviving serious injuries were many, and ranged from long-term stays in hospital to being discharged home, with extended periods in hospitals posing additional challenges to the medical authorities when it came to addressing longer-term cultural and religious needs.

Surgical care of the wounded: North African amputees

In a report in the *ABC* of 27 March 1938 on the Hospital de la Vega in Salamanca, reference was made to the 'wounded Moors, young African men who in fighting for the freedom of our Fatherland relive the glory and courage of their ancestors who left us a treasury of art, valour and tradition'. The newspaper columnist, Maria Matilde Belmonte, was shown around the hospital by the MO Don Pablo Heredia, 'favourite surgeon of these Moroccan warriors'. In the opening paragraph, Belmonte also reflected upon how the once good-time-girls turned dedicated nurses, 'have been uniquely reborn … and are now dedicated to the hard mission', alongside the Sisters of Charity, of 'relieving the suffering of all classes who fight for Spain'.

The main focus of the article is the surgical care of the 'wounded Moors', who, despite the physical pain of their wounds, 'have happy smiling faces and are anxious to be cured so they can return to the fight'. A young Moroccan 'barely a boy', is described as displaying his amputated feet, the result of frostbite contracted at the Teruel Front during the harsh winter of 1937–1938. He apparently exhibited his wounds with pride, expressed his gratitude to the surgeon, Pablo Heredia, and spoke of the moment when he dreamed of getting his new feet so that he could walk 'the same as he had before'. Another patient who was missing an arm, upon seeing Heredia, smiled with pride and cried 'long live Spain'. A patient being prepared for an operation asked not to be given the 'water that makes you stupid', i.e. ether – an anaesthetic containing alcohol which is thus proscribed by Qur'anic law.[108]

Heredia, in supposed deference to the patient's wishes, anaesthetised with an intravenous anaesthetic, most probably Evipan (sodium hexobarbitol), before then giving ether, regardless, to maintain anaesthesia, as Evipan was only suitable for short procedures.[109] Heredia then goes on to describe that the soldiers' 'greatest wish is a permit to pass their convalescence with their families in Morocco', with 'all the Moroccan wounded given a twenty-day permit to go to their land'. The article closes:

> and as a typical example of spirit without equal which animates these African warriors, that young Moor, who with a child's face and tears in

> his eyes, upon contemplating his amputated leg, says in a moving voice; 'what bad luck is mine! No longer will I be able to make war for Spain.'[110]

The above propagandistic article encapsulates several of the themes surrounding the hospital care of the Maghrebi wounded addressed below. Was this, however, an accurate reflection of that care? Described frequently as brothers, cousins or even twins, soldiers from the Maghreb were often portrayed as being endowed with a simplicity and strength that implied a healthy younger brother, who was nevertheless in need of the protection of his stronger Spanish sibling. Absent, however, from these commentaries were any real attempts to describe the horrific injuries suffered by some, or the endemic diseases suffered by many.

The newspaper article is nevertheless cleverly constructed, and does contain factual elements. Out of the 54,000 Insurgent casualties suffered during the Teruel campaign, there were more than 18,000 resulting from the unusually cold conditions, something neither side had fully allowed for in the outfitting of their troops. The archives in Ávila contain the details of a number of Maghrebi soldiers hospitalised with severe frostbite of their feet.[111] The description of the administration of an anaesthetic provided in the article is, similarly, accurate.[112] Soldiers were also recruited who were often no more than between fourteen and sixteen years of age.[113] Muslim soldiers were generally entitled to permits to convalesce after being injured, including those who had suffered frostbite at Teruel, but contrary to what was stated in the *ABC*, the length of the permits varied. Many of the records for the hospital in Salamanca do not state the duration of leave granted, and those for Zaragoza show permits of fifteen days being the most common, but longer periods of leave of up to two months were also allowed for those with more serious injuries.[114] This was the case for a sergeant from the third company of the fifth tabor of the Regulares of al-Hoceima, Mohamed Ben Amar, who was wounded in the abdomen in the last months of the war in Catalunya. After a life-saving laparotomy (an exploratory operation of the intestinal cavity) and a stay in hospital of nearly a month, he was granted two months leave in 'Africa'.[115]

The newspaper item on the hospital in Salamanca, however, is unusual in that it describes amputees, a subject not normally found in the Insurgent daily *ABC*. It also states that all wounded Muslim soldiers were also entitled to 'a permit to pass their convalescence with their families in Morocco'.[116] There is evidence to suggest, however, that leave was not necessarily granted to all amputees. Massons, in *Historia de la Sanidad Militar Española* (1994), simply states that 'the evacuation of the wounded and of invalids to their place of origin was prohibited, with the aim of "not causing a bad effect within their tribal groupings (*cabilas*)"'.[117] However, in an interview in 2007 for the documentary *El laberinto marroqui*, seventy years after losing his lower right leg to a mortar, Mustafa Ben Marzouk, a veteran of the Spanish Civil War who served with Group No. 3 of the Regulares of Ceuta, reflected upon his own experience of amputation:

> I was hit by a mortar and wounded – I was picked up and taken to a hospital and they cut of my leg. I was in a lot of hospitals, because I was taken from hospital to hospital. We had our suitcases with us, but they would not let us go back in case others saw us and were frightened. Those of us who had had our legs amputated were not returned to Morocco; those of us with the suitcases were not sent back. It was not until the war finished, then we were discharged.[118]

Ben Marzouk's statement reflected the need for Insurgent propaganda to encapsulate the benefits of serving in Franco's crusade, while downplaying any negative aspects associated with this service, such as the high casualty rates suffered by soldiers from the Maghreb. By apparently restricting the movement of those with visible disabilities through prolonged hospital stays, the hope was to maintain recruitment from the main area of enlistment, the Rif. Recruitment was likely to have been impeded in a largely subsistence agricultural society of difficult terrain, if returning wounded soldiers such as amputees found themselves a burden on their families and clans.

The evidence from the records in the Archive in Ávila would seem to support the testimony by Mustafa Ben Marzouk. Although more research is needed to establish whether this was indeed the 'unwritten' policy with regards to the amputees, early indications from those records studied would suggest that this was certainly a common practice. Mohamed Ben Amar (a different soldier from the one above with the same name), of the third company of the fourth tabor of the Regulares of al-Hoceima, was 'gravely' wounded during the Aragón Offensive in the spring of 1938, and was admitted to the Muslim hospital of Zaragoza on 14 March 1938.[119] Suffering from a fracture to the tibia and fibula of his left leg, he underwent a below-knee amputation on 2 May 1938.[120] Three months later, he was granted a permit for a month's leave in Africa, but this was to a hospital, either in Ceuta or Melilla, and not the place of his origin, which was normally the case for those with other categories of wounds.[121] On 18 December 1938, he was recorded as being admitted to the hospital in Zaragoza again, but this time his condition was described as 'light'. On 20 January 1939, more than ten months after he was first admitted, he was discharged, but not to al-Hoceima, instead he was described as having been 'evacuated to the Hospital of Ceuta, no longer fit to serve'.[122]

This was also the reason given for the discharge to the same hospital of Amar Ben Amar from the third company of the ninth tabor of the Regulares of al-Hoceima on 6 February 1939. He had the lower third of his left arm amputated but was one of a number of soldiers fitted with a prosthesis.[123] Kadir Ben Alal, of the first company of the fifth tabor of the Regulares of al-Hoceima, was admitted to the Muslim hospital of Zaragoza on 6 July 1937. His record does not state when or where he was wounded or when the operation took place but he was transferred from a hospital in Valladolid to have a prosthesis fitted after an amputation to remove the lower third of his right leg, and was also discharged to Ceuta.[124]

Embarek Ben Amar, of the third company of the sixth tabor of Larache whose left leg was amputated as a result of injuries received at Las Rozas near Madrid in July 1937, was transferred to the military hospital of la Vega in Salamanca in September 1937, being later transferred to Zaragoza. Mohammed Ben Mohammed, who was admitted 22 May 1938 in 'a serious condition' with a left arm radial fracture that resulted in amputation, was 'licenced to Africa to be incorporated into' the hospital there (it does not state which hospital). What is also interesting about this particular soldier is that both entries stating the unit he was serving with have been crossed out and left blank, even though these records, even where the details for wounds are scant, usually record the soldier's number and unit. This may have been because he was in a state of shock, or for a number of other reasons, including the possibility of being from an area outside of the Protectorate.[125]

These are just a few examples of amputees who were not discharged home after becoming unfit for service. The records cited above are a representative sample from the admission and discharge cards chosen for this study and would seem to back the claims made by Massons and by Mustafa Ben Marzouk that those who had undergone major amputations were not granted leave or discharged to their home villages and towns in Morocco.[126] Additionally, José Luis de Mesa cites the example of two Moroccan amputees awaiting the fitting of prostheses in a hospital in Vigo in North-Western Spain, who requested permits to return to the Protectorate before these were fitted, but were denied passes on the grounds that this would have a negative impact upon their local community.[127] Nevertheless, additional research is required to provide further supporting evidence for this claim, although early indications do seem to point towards this indeed being the case.

Further evidence for some of the traumatic orthopaedic injuries suffered by the Maghrebi shock troops of the Insurgency can be found in the diary of Esyllt Priscilla Scott-Ellis. Priscilla, or Pip as she was more commonly known, was the only British nurse known to have volunteered to work for the forces of Franco during the Spanish Civil War.[128] Her diary – in which she wrote almost daily during her time in Spain – is an important historical document, offering an extremely rare example of a record of surgical care provided in a number of Insurgent hospitals written from a nurse's perspective.[129]

Scott-Ellis first arrived in Southern Spain on 9 October 1937. On the morning of 18 October 1937, she started a short course at a hospital in Jerez in order to qualify to practice as a nurse in Spain.[130] It is not clear, however, whether this was the Muslim Hospital in Jerez, a rear-guard hospital far from the frontline.[131] This would, however, seem likely as she makes frequent references to 'Moors', and in her entry for 26 October 1937 she refers to 'about two hundred Moors all shouting and calling one'. A further indication suggesting this being the Muslim Hospital of Jerez can be found in her entry of 14 November 1937. She states that she is:

> beginning to loathe the Moors. They are so tiresome ... it makes me mad to have a lot of filthy, smelly Moors ordering me about ... the trouble is that they are doing their periodic fasting and eat nothing till dinner, so are all very irritable ... I am getting to dislike the people intensely, I still like their wounds, which is after all the main point.

Although these sentiments echo commonly held prejudices against the 'Moors', they also offer a more realistic reflection of commonly held attitudes in contrast to the paternalistic offerings to be found in the *ABC*.

Elsewhere, her description of her first experience of an operating theatre during her first day of training provides an insight into aspects of the experience of surgical care as experienced by Maghrebi soldiers. The following extract from her diary describes her reaction to seeing her first orthopaedic injuries in the operating theatre, where she, alongside other trainees, had been sent to 'watch the dressings':

> It was very interesting and quite horrible. There were five Moors to be treated. The first one had a wound in the calf of his leg which had shattered the bone and was so big one could have put both one's fists into it; the second had one in his heel and had to have his heel bone removed, and had a wound about five inches deep that went right in behind the bone; the third was almost cured, but had his whole arm blown up and only had a semi-paralysed pulpy mess left; the fourth had two awful wounds in his knee where one could see all the veins and everything on one side and the bone of the other; the last was almost cured except for a huge raw patch on his knee and a hole the size of a ping-pong ball in his thigh. It was horrible watching as the wounds were packed with gauze, and as it was pulled out and stuffed in, the poor men, who are incredibly brave, would moan and shout and struggle and sometimes even scream.[132]

The injuries described by Scott-Ellis in her diary were frequent causes for admission to the hospitals in Salamanca and Zaragoza, as they were the types of wounds common to modern warfare: predominantly caused by projectiles, most frequently shrapnel from mortars and shells.[133] Of the admission and discharge cards examined for the Hospital Militar de la Santisima Trinidad, the hospital for legionnaires in Salamanca, these types of injuries were a common reason for admission, but as they were often in the forefront of actions alongside the Regulares, this is hardly surprising.[134]

Although there are no exact figures at present for how many soldiers of the Maghreb suffered surgical or traumatic amputations, admissions for fractures caused by firearms requiring more conservative treatments were far more frequent.[135] The admission and discharge cards for the soldiers in the hospital in Salamanca do not record the treatments received for these types of injuries.[136] The hospital in Zaragoza, however, does record some of these treatments. The most common method applied was the 'reduction and immobilisation' of the fracture 'with apparatus' and plaster.[137] The records do not state whether the 'Spanish Method' was applied in any of the cases examined, but as a technique that had been in use in the Protectorate it is likely to have been employed by at least some surgeons familiar with the procedure. Possible evidence for this can be found in references to debridement and immobilisation with plaster. Haddar Ben Mohammed, from the third unit of the ninth tabor of the Regulares of al-Hoceima, was wounded and received a right radial fracture of his forearm. This was 'operated, reduced and immobilised with plaster'.[138] This was also the treatment described for the calf injury, with fracture, of Mohamed Ben Misian of the fourth unit of the fifth tabor Regulares of al-Hoceima on 28 December of 1938, before his transfer the following day to Salamanca.[139] Although no direct mention is made of this technique, there is no reason to suggest that the soldiers from the Maghreb were not the recipients of advanced techniques in wound-care that had their origins in WWI.

Further evidence regarding amputation was provided by the New Zealand-born anaesthetic pioneer Sir Robert Reynolds Macintosh, who visited the Muslim Hospital in Zaragoza in the late summer of 1937. He went to Spain from England to volunteer his services in the insurgent zone at the invitation of the American plastic surgeon Eastman Sheehan. His invitation had resulted from the fact that Sheehan, himself a volunteer, had found himself unable to operate on the facial injuries of a soldier due to the anaesthetic practitioner, a nun, insisting on keeping the anaesthetic mask tightly clamped to the patient's face. During his three-week visit, Macintosh provided the first recorded administration in Spain of general anaesthesia with an endotracheal tube (passing a tube through the trachea for the delivery of anaesthesia to safeguard the airway), at hospitals in Zaragoza and San Sebastian.[140]

While Spain had been at the forefront in the development of techniques of spinal analgesia, with Fidel Pagés (who had himself served in Morocco in 1921) being the first to practice an epidural in 1921, general anaesthesia with the use of a tube was all but unknown.[141] This was despite it being a technique that was first used in 1880, and was used by the pioneer anaesthetists Rowbotham and Magill to facilitate head and neck surgery during WWI.[142]

Macintosh did not record in any detail the cases he provided anaesthesia for, but it is likely that at least some of his patients were from the Maghreb given that he described the visit he made to the Muslim hospital in Zaragoza.[143] His observations on the 'Moors' he encountered are typical of the orientalist perceptions of the 'other' common among his contemporaries.[144] In the diary he wrote during his time in Spain he recorded that he:

> Visited a Moorish hospital where the men appeared to be very contented … One of the doctors told me that they had great difficulty in persuading the moors to submit to amputation. It appears that their religion tells them that paradise is full of houris, whose sole mission is to smile on the fortunate men who reach paradise, but unfortunately these houris

> will have nothing at all to do with a man who has not a complete body, and I am told by the doctor that dozens of moors have preferred to die without having their leg amputated, when by having it taken off, they could have saved their lives.[145]

It is difficult to ascertain whether this statement has any validity, but fear of amputation, regardless of religious beliefs, would have been common. The reluctance of Muslim patients to submit to such an operation was more likely the result of the permanent nature of such a procedure, with the absence of a limb a visible disability that proclaimed a proscribed ability to work.

Although there is no mention in the newspaper articles of Muslim soldiers being involved in *jihad*, there are frequent references to soldiers being engaged in crusade against the atheist.[146] The ninth *surat* of the Qur'an states 'fight the polytheists totally as they fight you totally'. As such, with Paradise 'guaranteed' for those fighting in what could also be interpreted as a *jihad* against the 'godless reds', it is unlikely that the reason given by the doctor in Zaragoza to Macintosh accurately reflects the reason for refusing an amputation.[147]

Sheehan invited Macintosh to the Hospital Militar General Mola to assist him further in December 1937, but Macintosh was unable to go to Spain due to commitments at the Radcliffe Royal Infirmary in Oxford.[148] He sent Kenneth Boston, a colleague from Oxford who was also skilled in intubation.[149] Boston, unlike Macintosh, kept detailed notes of the thirty-three cases he anaesthetised while in Spain in January 1938. One of the patients he anaesthetised by introducing the endotracheal tube via the nose into the trachea was a 'moor of about 35'. This patient was described as having a 'severe sunk scar on right cheek with paralysis of facial nerve fibres to the eye and mouth'. The surgery that he underwent involved 'transplantation of muscle fibres of the temporalis to the eye and mouth, and subcutaneous fat graft from the abdomen to fill out the cheek'.[150] This soldier from the Maghreb was one of only a minute number of soldiers from either side during the Spanish Civil War to have a general anaesthetic that included the use of an endotracheal tube. Unfortunately, apart from a brief description of the soldier's wound and subsequent surgery, and the fact that the intubation was unsuccessful at the first attempt, there is no record of how this thirty-five-year-old soldier from the Maghreb did following the operation.[151] This case, however, demonstrates that at least on this one occasion advanced surgical and anaesthetic care was provided to a wounded soldier of the Maghreb. Unfortunately, it would seem from the surviving evidence that this level of provision, which included an anaesthetic with an endotracheal tube, was unavailable outside of San Sebastian during the Spanish Civil War.[152]

Soft tissue injuries were also common. Ali Ben Brahim of the Tiradores of Ifni-Sahara, and Laraichi Ben Mohammed, also from Ifni, were admitted with soft tissue injuries, as was Mohammed Ben Burzan of the Regulares of Melilla. Burzan is recorded as having an injury to the muscle of his right thigh but under the section for observations it is noted that his eye came out, a detail that is also inscribed large on the back of his admission and discharge card.[153] There were also admissions for what appears to be shell-shock, described on the cards as 'cerebral commotion' or 'general commotion caused by explosions', all these injuries being typical of the wounds received by combatants during modern industrialised warfare.[154]

Medical admissions in Salamanca and Zaragoza

Although the primary focus here has been on surgical admissions, it is also worth examining what the records for the hospitals in Salamanca and Zaragoza contain in relation to admissions for endemic diseases. The majority of these soldiers came from backgrounds where a variety of diseases were widespread, and admissions to hospital as a result of these were not uncommon.[155] These conditions, which included malaria, typhus, typhoid fever and gonorrhoea, were also prevalent among the rural poor on the Spanish mainland whose subsistence existence in many respects was similar to that of the recruits from the Maghreb.[156]

The incidence of endemic disease throughout the Protectorate seems to have been fairly extensive. Bacher Ben Hadi, of the third company of the sixth tabor of the Tiradores de Ifni, was admitted on 19 December 1937 with a diagnosis of malaria. He was discharged on 26 December 1937 and given a 'twenty days permit to Cabo Juby', an area situated in the extreme south of the Protectorate on the edge of the Spanish Sahara.[157] Mimun Ben Hadu, of the second group of the fourth tabor of the Regulares of al-Hoceima recruited in the north of the Protectorate, was admitted with malaria on 5 October 1937, but was discharged four days later fit for duty and 'cured'.[158] These are just two of the numerous incidences among the records examined that mention malaria, but they are largely typical of these types of admissions.[159]

Evidence of other chronic health conditions abound. Particularly debilitating seems to have been the high incidence of tuberculosis.[160] Again, those suffering from the disease came from a wide geographical area. Mohamed Ben Mohamed, from the third company of the third tabor of the Regulares of Ceuta, was a direct admission on 13 December 1938 to the hospital in Salamanca as a result of pulmonary tuberculosis, and was declared unfit for duty.[161] Earlier in the year, Hamido Ben Ali, of the third company of the seventh tabor of the Regulares of Larache, was transferred from Zaragoza to Salamanca on 12 January with 'tuberculosis of the skin'. His stay in hospital was for nearly three weeks before being transferred to Sevilla on 31 January 1938.[162] Ali Ben Mohamed, from the Tiradores de Ifni, was also transferred from Zaragoza to Salamanca when he was admitted on 12 December 1938 with pleural and peritoneal tuberculosis, but died four days later as a result of his illness.[163]

A less straightforward case was that of Mohamed Ben Abselan, of the fifth tabor of Regulares of al-Hoceima.[164] He was admitted to the Muslim Hospital of Zaragoza on 14 March 1937 after being transferred from the Hospital of

Pamplona. His diagnosis upon admission showed that he was suffering from chronic bronchitis and gastritis, and on the 27 March, he underwent a laparotomy and a gastro-entero-anastomosis, a surgical repair of his stomach and small bowel. Three weeks later, at four in the morning on 18 April, he was recorded as having vomited up blood and sputum. He was to have a further episode three days later. The underlying problem was diagnosed the following day when an x-ray discovered a lesion on the apex of his right lung, caused by tuberculosis. A month later, on 22 May 1937, he was declared unfit and discharged to 'Africa', most likely to the town of his recruitment as his admission and discharge card does not record Mohamed Ben Absalan being transferred on to another hospital.[165]

Admissions for rheumatism were also common, and there were also a considerable number of admissions for syphilis and gonorrhoea. These involved stays in hospital of anything from a few days to several weeks, with soldiers either transferred on to another hospital, returned to duty after a short period, or given leave.[166]

The medical hospital admissions highlighted here constitute a representative sample of the total of records examined. Nevertheless, what becomes apparent from a wider examination of these records is the large number of soldiers who were admitted with conditions indicative of the wider health concerns affecting Muslim combatants.[167] Whether these conditions were pre-existing ones or had been contracted during the many campaigns in Spain, the presence of endemic disease does not seem to have been a bar to recruitment in the Protectorate. Indeed, it seems likely that recruitment would have been adversely affected if too much attention had been paid to the prevalence of disease among these soldiers.

Religion and culture

In an editorial for the *ABC* of Sevilla 26 August 1937, Antonio Olmedo, commanding inspector of operations of the Protectorate for the Army of the South, reported on a visit by the Blue Sultan of Ifni, Sidi Mohammed Mustafa, to the Muslim Hospital of Barzola in Sevilla. The occasion for his visit, in the company of several *qaids*, was the inauguration of a mosque in the grounds of the 250-bed hospital, constructed to meet the spiritual needs of its Muslim patients.[168] Several senior Spanish officials were also present, including Antonio Olmedo. Among the officials were the Colonel-in-Chief of Inspection for Moroccan Affairs of the Army of the South, Don Juan Sánchez de Pol; the Chief of Military Health, Lieutenant Coronel Bravo Ferrer; and, from the secretariat, the Head of Interpretation, Sidi Ali al Fakir.

Olmedo's editorial, under the heading 'The visit by the Blue Sultan to Sevilla', incorporates the main elements of the propaganda surrounding the use of Islamic troops by Franco. The aim of this propaganda was a reinterpretation and reinvention of a Crusade-dominated narrative against the 'infidel Moor' as a friend, rather than as a foe:

> Accompanied by his brilliant entourage, and with the assistance of the Nationalist authorities, the Mosque of the Muslim Hospital was inaugurated. This could only be in Sevilla, stronghold of the newest Reconquista, apex of the new empire, chosen by the Muslim people as the starting point for their march on the heart of the country, which invaded by the red plague had stopped beating in Spanish.
>
> Sevilla conscious of its debt to the men of the twin race who hastened without hesitation to form the vanguard of the movement of salvation, has offered a space for the erection of a mosque, where since yesterday the Muslim brothers have called with incorruptible zeal upon the almighty for the definitive triumph of the arms of Franco, Chieftain (Caudillo) and restorer of the Hispano-Moroccan Empire ... Spain reciprocates the generosity of our Moroccan brothers who have spilled their blood on the battlefields, and which also demonstrates the splendour of our national culture, which exalting in this tradition, also respects that of others. The Muslims search for God by different paths, which are maybe not that different from our own, and we offer them the means, for the practice of their cults.

The article that accompanies this editorial refers to the Sultan having made a thorough visit of the hospital where he 'eulogised' the 'cleanliness, order, good treatment and affectionate care of the wounded Moroccans'. It was important to the Insurgent portrayal of the participation of Islamic troops in Franco's 'Reconquista' to maintain a belief in the protective relationship between a paternal and imperial Spain with their 'Muslim brothers' in the Protectorate.[169]

An important element of this was served by highlighting the similarities arising from their common Abrahamic faiths. By emphasising the special care that the wounded received, and by placing this within a context of an attention to caring for their wider cultural needs, the contribution of the 'Moors' to the Insurgency could be portrayed in a more constructive and inclusive manner. This additionally served the purpose of making it easier to accept the presence of the 'traditional enemy' in the heart of Insurgent-controlled territories. Furthermore, it served the purpose of redefining, as in the case of the Salamanca article, visible disabilities in a more positive light, portraying the results of wounds as a selfless sacrifice by the 'Moors' devoted to a paternal and caring fatherland. It additionally allowed for the Blue Sultan, whose authority was limited to the extreme south of the Protectorate, to be used as a visible symbol of religious authority, as a legitimising figurehead in Insurgent propaganda for Muslim participation in 'Franco's Crusade', and for recruitment purposes in the south of the Protectorate, including from areas of French Morocco.[170] This was all the more important, as the Sultan of Morocco, Mohammed V, in a decree issued 20 February 1937, had prohibited the enlistment of all Moroccans on either side in the Spanish Civil War, although this was largely ignored by the Insurgents as it was seen as serving French interests in the region.[171]

The picture constructed in articles such as these was of the hospital as a space for the treatment of the heroic wounded 'Moorish' foot soldier, cared for by the rightful providers of care, i.e., women; namely the 'Sisters of Charity' and the 'damas enfermeras' (female nurses).[172] The reconstruction of the hospital as a space for the care of the Maghrebi wounded sometimes required the conversion of visible Catholic architecture to avoid offending the Muslim wounded. On one occasion when Franco visited a hospital for the Regulares, he was reported as having ordered that two crosses hanging on a wall be immediately removed. At the Hospital del Rey in Burgos, two images of St James the Moor Slayer, part of the architectural fabric of the building, were covered up shortly after it was converted to medical-military use. This move was prefigured by a large-scale disturbance among the Muslim patients in response to the image of the saint on horseback, trampling on the bodies of their co-religionists.[173]

As part of the attention paid to the wider cultural needs of the patients, many of the hospitals employed a variety of staff that ideally included four religious officials.[174] These were an Iman, who was the head of the religious staff; a religious teacher – the *Mudarris;* a *Katib* or scribe; and a *Munadif el Mauta*, the cleaner of the dead, who also accompanied units on the battlefield and who attended to the fallen.[175]

The Moroccan Hospital of Granada, 'created through the initiative of Dr Guirao, militarised with the grade of Commander of Military Health', and staffed with doctors from the Granada Faculty of Medicine and Surgery, was described in the propagandist *Crónica de Granada* (*Granada Chronicle*) in 1937 as 'the first of its type installed in liberated Spain at the service of Moroccans adherent to the cause'. The 300-bed hospital contained its own mosque, quarters for the Iman, an ablutions hall, a slaughterhouse for the ritual slaughter of livestock, 'a typical Moorish café' and kitchen facilities where food prepared according to 'Arab custom' could be made ready.[176].

Meeting the dietary requirements of the soldiers appears to have been relevantly straightforward, and a number of Muslim hospitals employed Moroccan cooks to prepare food according to religious strictures, and butchers to slaughter animals in accordance with the rules of halal.[177] In hospitals without slaughterhouses local facilities could be used. In Santiago de Compostela in Galicia, the municipal abattoir was used regularly by the Moroccan butcher Mohamed Belkaid, with the slaughterhouse also used to supply halal meat to Muslim patients in the Military Hospital of San Caetano.[178] These needs were not necessarily uniformly met in all of the Muslim hospitals, but efforts were made to ensure that the soldiers from the Maghreb could observe and practise their religion.

Important religious festivals were also celebrated in many of the hospitals with the observance of feast days used by the Insurgent press to reinforce ideas of Christian and Muslim co-religiosity.[179] On 11 February 1938, the Muslim hospital of Barzola in Sevilla celebrated the Festival of Sacrifice. As part of the festivities, a lamb was ritually slaughtered for the feast that was held later that day for the patients. The Iman of the hospital, Mohamed Ben Ham-mi, read an 'expressive' discourse in which he reiterated the adhesion of the Moroccan people to the 'Caudillo'. This was immediately followed by the Inspector, Commander Olmedo, conveying to the wounded and the politico-religious personnel, 'the felicitations of Generalísimo Franco', at the end of which 'a splendid meal of traditional (Moroccan) food was served'.[180] On 22 February 1938, 'by reason of the solemnities of *Aid el Kebir* (Festival of the Sacrifice), a most brilliant fiesta has been celebrated in the Muslim Hospital of Cacarés with the assistance of the notables of Ifni-Sahara who are visiting National Spain'. The festivity was described as leaving an 'indelible memory' much appreciated by, among others, 'the head of the nurses, Señorita Matilde Garcia, who has devoted all of her hours to her patriotic and Christian duty of alleviating the sufferings of those Moroccan soldiers who have spent their generous blood for Spain and its Caudillo Franco'.[181]

Although not directly related to hospital care, Franco's greatest propaganda coup in relation to providing for the needs of the troops from the Maghreb was his provision of a ship for Muslims undertaking the *hajj* (pilgrimage) to Mecca early in 1937.[182] A second ship was laid on for the *hajj* in January 1938. This included an on-board medical team, Moroccan food and a 'religious official, an Iman'.[183] By emphasising the aid provided that facilitated 'Moroccan' participation in key Islamic duties and festivals, Insurgent propaganda was keen to stress the religiosity of their brothers in 'faith', and at the same time looked to counter growing Moroccan nationalism within the protectorate.[184]

Also reported upon in the *ABC* were non-religious festivities. In Zaragoza, on 1 February 1939, 'a fiesta was organised by the señoritas enfermeras (unmarried nurses) in honour of the hospitalised wounded'.[185] In the January of the previous year, the Muslim hospital of Zaragoza was chosen as the site for the first of a series of hospital concerts by the renowned guitarist Sáinz de la Maza.[186] Reports such as these were used to reinforce the idea of a common cultural heritage and highlighted the additional role played by nurses in providing non-nursing care within the hospitals. This engagement in the *ABC* of Sevilla with the visible face of Islam was aimed at reflecting the provision made by Insurgents for the religious and cultural needs of the patients in the Muslim hospitals as part of a wider community of the faithful. This portrayal of the happy and well-looked-after Maghrebi soldier was, nevertheless, a construct, and did not allow for a description of the wounded that reflected the disabling injuries and debilitating health conditions suffered by these soldiers.

Mosques, 'cantinas', courtesans and *kif*

Throughout the period of the Spanish Civil War there were at least thirty Muslim hospitals in operation throughout Spain. Five of these are known to have had their own mosques, a number had ablutions halls, and at least five of these hospitals had cemeteries.[187] Although the Muslim hospital of Barzola was the focus of several articles in the *ABC* in relation to its mosque, there was also a mosque attached to the Muslim Hospital in Jerez.[188] The Hospital del Rey in Burgos – where, due to pressure for beds, two patients were placed in single-occupant cubicles – opened the doors of its mosque on 27 December 1937. Mosques are typically imagined as large imposing buildings complete with a tall minaret, but this was not the case in Burgos. It was a simple structure built within the grounds, which was in ruins ten years after its inauguration. Nevertheless, it was provided with running water when it first opened so that the Muslim patients could perform their ritual ablutions. In the November of the following year a café was also opened within the grounds, and canteens such as these were an important way of providing centres where patients, especially those hospitalised for long periods, could relax in a non-ward-based environment.[189]

As part of the desire to be seen to cater for the wider need of the Maghrebi troops, musicians and dancers were also imported from Morocco.[190] Prostitutes were given permission to travel to Spain, and Yubida ben Mohamed Chaui ran a brothel in Arroyomolino for Muslim soldiers early in 1937.[191] Arroyomolino's brothel was reserved for the use of Muslim troops of the South-Western Sector near Madrid, and there were between forty to fifty prostitutes in the town. The prostitutes were also active in a number of cafeterias, and Moroccan military police, under the command of a junior Spanish officer, were responsible for overseeing order. Their health was overseen by Doctor Peyrí, a Spanish medic, whose duties included checking for venereal diseases among the prostitutes, and sending those found to be infected back to Morocco.[192]

Many of the women, whether prostitutes or dancers, were also given permits to bring with them *kif*, the marijuana grown in the Rif, with permits granted to carry as much as fifty kilos at a time.[193] It is likely that *kif* would also been available to smoke in hospital canteens. According to oral testimony, alcohol was also supplied if required, despite Qur'anic proscription.[194]

The propagandist-based engagement with the cultural and religious aspects of the Maghrebi wounded under their care served to underline and delineate the paternalist relationship between Insurgent Spain and the Protectorate in Morocco. By stressing the co-religiosity of Muslim soldiers, and by being seen to cater for their cultural as well as their medical needs when hospitalised, the Insurgent authorities were able to place these combatants at the heart of their Crusader discourse. This engagement with the non-medical needs of the hospitalised patient also served to reinforce Francoist paternalist concepts and notions of empire, with Spain – as represented in the figure of Franco – seen not only as provider, but as necessary protector.[195]

Care of the dead

The provision of cemeteries for the Muslim dead was not an issue that was so easily resolved, as requirements for those to be interred required that they be buried separately from Christians.[196] Cemeteries were specifically built for the Muslim deceased, such as those in Burgos, Zaragoza and Avilés, but these were the exception rather than the rule.[197] Normally, the deceased were buried in areas set aside in municipal cemeteries.[198] There were occasions, however, when religious officials could bless a site close to a battlefield in order to consecrate it as a Muslim burial ground.[199]

Although Madariaga and Sánchez Ruano refer to cemeteries and the burial of the Muslim dead, albeit briefly, it is the manuscript from 1945 reproduced in *La actitud de los moros ante el alzamiento, Marruecos 1936* by Azzuz Hakim that offers the most detailed account of the observance of Muslim burial rites during the Spanish Civil War.[200] During the early days of the Spanish Civil War, on 3 September 1936, Mohamed ben Abdelsalam Redondo of the third company of the second tabor of the Regulares of Xauen, husband to Fatima Ben Enfeddal, was seriously wounded in action at Talavera near Madrid. He was admitted to the hospital on the outskirts of Talavera but died the following day. The ensign of the company, the *qaid* Laarbi Hihi, who received a serious wound to his right arm in the fighting, later recalled issuing Abdelsalam Redondo with his uniform and lanyard upon enlistment. He also stated that, although Abdelsalam Redondo had never previously fired a rifle, he became a good marksman during his 'brief' period of training in the Protectorate.[201] After undergoing an operation on 5 September 1936 for the removal of a bullet from the arm he was eventually to lose, Laarbi Hihi was told of the death of Abdelsalam Redondo the previous night. He was also informed that the *faqih* (Islamic jurist), Radi Lemmagui, had inculcated the *shahada* (profession of faith) and prepared his body for burial.[202] Radi Lemmagui, the only *faqih* in the campaign hospital set up by Coronel Yagüe at Talavera, recalled that the number of casualties at Talavera on that day was high, 'but only four of these … were mortal wounds'. He remembered being:

> Woken by a nurse called Isabel to tell me that one of the four gravely wounded soldiers was dying. I went immediately to his side and found him expiring whilst at the same time trying, without success, to pronounce the *shahada* … I later called in the doctor, Lieutenant Castro, who certified the death. His body was then taken to the hall of ablutions where upon the rising of the sun I washed him and placed him in a shroud … after praying for his soul, we buried him in cemetery habilitated by myself, a cemetery where we had buried the previous day one hundred and four Muslims who died that same day. I still have the logbook where I recorded the names of the fallen Muslim soldiers I assisted in washing, placing in shrouds and burying during the three months I was at Talavera, and which came to five hundred and ninety-seven.[203]

The burial of the Muslim dead was never an easy issue to resolve. By providing separate areas within municipal cemeteries, often with a separate entrance, such as was to be found at the cemetery of San José in Burgos, and by the consecration of additional sites such as the burial ground outside of Talavera, it was possible to avoid a clash between Muslim and Catholic customs in relation to burials.[204] Nevertheless, concerns arising around separate burials led to commissions being set up after the conflict composing of both Moroccan and military officials who were to ensure that Catholics and Muslims had not been buried together.[205]

Although the surviving evidence does not allow for a full reconstruction of how the Muslim dead were 'cared for' when it came to the observation of Islamic burial customs, surviving evidence indicates that care was taken in many instances to respect Islamic religious custom. It is not, however, altogether clear whether this was principally aimed at assuaging Catholic sensibilities or respecting the needs of their fellow combatants.

Conclusion

Further studies based on research in the Spanish archives is likely to reveal more on the injuries and diseases suffered by the soldiers from the Maghreb. The cases discussed here and the records that make up this study, although based on a relatively small sample of the available records, were nevertheless chosen as a representative sample of the 4,000 admission and discharge cards examined, representing a cross-section of the ailments and diseases suffered by the Maghrebi troops. However, what quickly becomes evident from an examination of the evidence, is how prevalent a wide variety of diseases were among these soldiers. What also becomes apparent is the predominance of a variety of injuries, including a large number of fractures and soft tissue injuries connected with the use of these troops in the frontline of many of the military campaigns of the conflict. The presence of these types of injuries is not in itself surprising, as it is among frontline troops where most combat casualties occur.[206] However, the absence of significant academic work on the injuries sustained by more than 54,000 Muslim combatants and the medical care they received, is less easy to understand, as this figure represents one of the highest casualty rates suffered by any one body of men fighting at the front during the Spanish Civil War.[207] There are studies that partly address the hospital care received by the non-Muslim wounded on both sides during the conflict; nevertheless, a comprehensive examination of the medical care on offer to the Maghrebi wounded provides further insights into wider cultural and religious differences evident in Spain arising from the presence of a significant number of the 'infidel' among the 'crusader' forces of the Insurgency.[208] This in turn helps to broaden our understanding of the medical care of the wounded more generally during the Spanish Civil War, as it allows for a broader exploration arising from cultural and religious differences.

By addressing in this chapter the question of why soldiers from the Maghreb participated in the Insurgent 'Reconquista' of Spain, it has been possible to step beyond the narrow but common definition that portrays the 'Moorish' combatant as an elite fighter, involved in widespread looting and sexual violence, to provide a more defined but nuanced assessment.[209] The analysis here that clearly acknowledges the brutal excesses committed by a number of Maghrebi soldiers, also questions wider assumptions that go with this model. These assumptions, in large part based around this notion of an elite fighting force, ruthless in pursuit of its military objectives, are here further challenged through an analysis of the hospital care received by these troops, as this reveals that this model is only truly representative of the North African veterans who fought in the opening campaigns of the conflict, and not of the Maghrebi participants as a whole.[210]

This chapter by focusing on the care of the Maghrebi wounded, rather than on the Insurgent forces as a whole, throws light on an area of medical care during the Spanish Civil War that has received scant academic attention. Further research is likely to reveal more on the social composition of the Muslim troops that fought for Franco in Spain, and provide additional evidence for their reasons for enlisting.

Nevertheless, this remains an area of study that is under-researched. By contrast, the organisation of surgical care within the Republican medical services, and to a lesser degree that of the Insurgents, which forms the focus of the next chapter, has received greater historical scrutiny. This scrutiny has still emphasised international participation over that of the Spanish contributions. The soldiers of the Maghreb, predominantly from the Spanish Protectorate in Morocco, have, like their Spanish counterparts, received little of this attention. This has led to a polarisation within the limited literature on the medical care of the wounded during the conflict, reflecting external efforts in the development of surgery and the role of non-Spanish medical personnel in the evolution of these services. The following chapter, therefore, sets out to redress this imbalance through an analysis of the organisation of both the Republican and Insurgent medical services. By assessing the role played by Spanish medical personnel in the development of these services, and the evolution of the medical services during the conflict, the following study will additionally explore distinct approaches to healthcare resulting from different ideological outlooks. The exploration of religious and cultural aspects of the medical care of the Maghrebi wounded reveal a number of complexities that result from an adherence to different belief systems, and these themes are further explored and developed in the following pages, by additionally examining the role played by ideology in the provision of this medical care.

Notes

1 Beevor, *Battle for Spain*, pp. 56–57.

2 Balfour, *Deadly Embrace*, p. 269. For further information on troop composition, see García Cruz, J. F., "Las fuerzas militares nativas procedentes del Protectorado de Marruecos. Transcendencia política de su aplicación en las operaciones militares durante la Guerra Civil española", *Hispania Nova. Revista de Historia Contemporánea*, No. 2 (2001–2002), pp. 1–23, p. 11.

3 Preston, P., *Franco: A Biography* (London, 1993), pp. 141–143.
4 La Porte, P., "Civil Military Relations in the Spanish Protectorate in Morocco: The Road to the Spanish Civil War, 1912–1936, *Armed Forces and Society*, Vol. 30, No. 2 (2004); pp. 203–226: Balfour, *Deadly Embrace*, p. 312.
5 Madariaga, M. R. de, *Los moros que trajo Franco: La intervención de tropas coloniales en la Guerra Civil Española* (Barcelona, 2002), pp. 172–173. Traditionally the Maghreb consisted of Morocco, Algeria, Tunisia and Eastern Libya. The modern Maghreb compromises Mauritania, Western Sahara, Morocco, Algeria, Tunisia and Libya. See also Benjelloun, A., "La Participación de los mercenarios marroquíes en la Guerra Civil Española", *Revista Internacional de Sociología*, Vol. 46, No. 4 (1988), pp. 527–541, p. 535. Interestingly, Mekki Ben Mohammad Redondo, the son of a Regulare killed in 1936, in an interview he conducted in December 1945 was shown an appendix attached to a document drawn up by the Delegation for Indigenous Affairs, 28 April 1940, of which he made a copy, and which cites the participation of 80,500 soldiers from the Spanish Protectorate in Morocco. See Azzuz Hakim, M. I., *La actitud de los moros ante el alzamiento, Marruecos 1936* (Málaga, 1997), pp. 189–191.
6 Balfour, *Deadly Embrace*, pp. 276–277; Mesa, J. L. D., *Los moros de la Guerra Civil española* (Madrid, 2004), pp. 232–242.
7 Madariaga, *Los moros que trajo Franco*, pp. 154–156, 187; Sánchez Ruano, F., *Islam y Guerra Civil Española: Moros con Franco y con la República* (Madrid, 2004), p. 49.
8 Al Tuma, A., "The Participation of Moorish Troops in the Spanish Civil War (1936–1939): Military Value, Motivations, and Religious Aspects", *War and Society,* Vol. 30, No. 2 (August, 2011), pp. 91–107; Mesa, *Los moros de la Guerra Civil española*; Madariaga, *Los moros que trajo Franco*; Sánchez Ruano, *Islam y Guerra Civil Española.*
9 Balfour, *Deadly Embrace*, p. 277.
10 Preston, *Spanish Holocaust*, p. xii; Casanova, J., *A Short History of the Spanish Civil War* (New York, 2013). See also Benjellon, La participación de los mercenarios marroquíes.
11 Balfour, *Deadly Embrace*, p. 116; Benjelloun, La participación de los mercenarios marroquíes, p. 535; Madariaga, *Los moros que trajo Franco*, pp. 173, 104; Azzuz Hakim, *La actitud de los moros*, pp. 189–191.
12 Balfour, *Deadly Embrace*, pp. 184–202; Said, E., *Orientalism: Western Conceptions of the Orient* (London, 1978).
13 Madariaga, *Los moros que trajo Franco*, pp. 277–278; Wellcome Library Archives and Manuscripts (WLAM), PP/RRM/D1/76; Frutos Herranz, *Hospitales en Burgos*, p. 126.
14 Madariaga, *Los moros que trajo Franco*, pp. 277–287; Merroun, M. E., *Las tropas marroquíes en la Guerra Civil española, 1936–1939* (Madrid, 2003), pp. 195–6; Sánchez Ruano, *Islam y Guerra Civil Española*, pp. 237–240.
15 Mesa, *Los moros de la Guerra Civil*, pp. 254–263.
16 Frutos Herranz, *Hospitales en Burgos*, pp. 101–127.
17 Al Tuma, The Participation of Moorish Troops, pp. 102–104.
18 García Cruz, Las fuerzas militares nativas, pp. 1–23; Sotomayor Blásquez, C. T., "El moro traidor, el moro engañado: variantes del estereotípico en el Romancero repúblicano", *Anaquel de Estudios Árabes*, Vol. 15 (2005), pp. 233–249; Martin Corrales, E., "Maurofobia/islamafobia y maurofilia/islamofilia en la España del siglo XXI", in *Revista CIDOB d'Afers Internacionals*, No. 66–67 (2004), pp. 39–51; Al Tuma, The Participation of Moorish Troops.

19 Balfour, *Deadly Embrace*, pp. 253–255, 292–293; Preston, *Spanish Holocaust*, p. 21; Graham, *Spanish Civil War*, pp. 32–33; Beevor, *Battle for Spain*, pp. 56, 117–121, 245, 378.
20 Algarbani, *Y Jimena se vistió de negro*, pp. 74–75; Martin Corrales, Maurofobia/islamafobia, pp. 49–50.
21 Al Tuma, The Participation of Moorish Troops, pp. 92–93.
22 The Archivo General Militar de Ávila (AGMAV) has a collection of forty-three separate files pertaining to the same number of different Insurgent hospitals, mainly in the north and central Spain. These files in turn contain a total of 355 boxes, many of which contain hundreds of index cards. Additionally, there is a file for the hospitals of the Italian Legionnaires which contains a further 176. The file for the Hospital Musulmán de Zaragoza contains the boxes for the two hospitals cited above. See www.portalcultura.mde.es/cultural/archivos/castillaLeon/archivo_42.html.
23 AGMAV, C. 42385, 1; AGMAV, C. 42385, 3; AGMAV, C. 42385, 5; AGMAV, C. 42386, 1; AGMAV, C. 42386, 2; AGMAV, C. 42386, 3. (This series pertains to the Hospital Musulmán de Zaragoza. There are a total of fourteen boxes in this collection each containing a number of sub-files.) AGMAV, C. 29297, 1; AGMAV, C. 29297, 2; AGMAV, C. 29297, 5 (pertains to the Hospital Militar Musulmán de la Vega/Hospital Militar de la Vega Salamanca).
24 This is frequently the case with regards to the hospital in Salamanca.
25 www.portalcultura.mde.es/cultural/archivos/castillaLeon/archivo_42.html.
26 There was also a loyalist *ABC* published in Madrid as the paper was split in two at the start of the conflict. For a definition and discussion of the Reconquista see Fletcher, R. A., *Moorish Spain* (London, 1992), pp. 6–7.
27 *ABC* (Sevilla), 07.12.1937, p. 13.
28 These other sources include: The Sir Robert Reynolds Mackintosh Archive held by the Wellcome Library (WLAM), namely: WLAM, PP/RRM/D1/76; WLAM, PP/RRM/C/2; the film *Defenders of the Faith* (US, 1938), directed by Russell Palmer; and the television documentary first broadcast on the Spanish state television channel RTVE2, *El Laberinto Marroquí* (2007).
29 Madariaga, *Los moros que trajo Franco*, pp. 172–173.
30 Balfour, *Deadly Embrace*, p. 312. Balfour states that these figures are ‘a reliable account based on several sources’.
31 Madariaga, *Los moros que trajo Franco*, pp. 172, 190–192.
32 Zubelzu, L. S., “Obra Quirúrgica de Fermín Palma García”, *Seminario Medico*, No. 38 (1979), pp. 59–78; Beneito Lloris, *El hospital Sueco-Noruego*, pp. 104–121.
33 Martínez Antonio, F. J., “Entre la diplomacia médica y la política sanitaria: Médicos militares en el Protectorado Español en Marruecos (1906–1927)”, *Revista de Historia Militar*, Vol. 2 (2012), pp. 203–242, p. 204.
34 Gasch-Tomás, J. L., “Spanish Empire: Vol. 2. From 1580”, in J. M. MacKenzie (ed.), *The Encyclopedia of Empire* (Hoboken, 2015), pp. 6–7.
35 Balfour, *Deadly Embrace*, pp. 5–6.
36 Ibid.; International Boundary Study, No. 84 (Revised), July 1, 1970, Algeria – Western (Spanish) Sahara Boundary, p. 2. (Produced for the Department of State of the United States of America.)
37 Balfour, *Deadly Embrace*, p. 7.
38 Preston, *Franco*, pp. 31–33; Fleming, S., “Spanish Morocco and the Alzamiento Nacional, 1936–1939: The Military, Economic and Political Mobilisation

of a Protectorate", *Journal of Contemporary History*, Vol. 18, No. 1 (1983), pp. 27–42, p. 34.
39 Martínez Antonio, Entre la diplomacia médica, p. 228.
40 Balfour, *Deadly Embrace*, p. 4.
41 Madariaga, *Los moros que trajo Franco*, p. 40.
42 Balfour, *Deadly Embrace*, p. 20.
43 Ribeiro de Meneses, F., "Popularising Africanism: The Career of Víctor Ruiz Albéniz, El Tebib Arrumi", *Journal of Iberian and Latin American Studies*, Vol. 11, No. 1 (2005), pp. 39–63.
44 Preston, *Franco*, p. 11.
45 Balfour, *Deadly Embrace*, pp. 25–26; Crawford, D., "Morocco's Invisible Imazighen", *The Journal of North African Studies*, Vol., 7, No. 1 (2002), pp. 53–70, p. 53. The term 'Berber' is a corruption of the Latin word 'barbarus', which translates as barbarian.
46 Ibid.
47 Ruiz Albéniz, V., *España en el Rif: estudios del indígena y del país, nuestra actuación de doce años, la guerra del veintiuno* (Madrid, 1921), p. 150.
48 Ribeiro de Meneses, Popularizing Africanism, pp. 39–41.
49 Beneito Lloris, *El hospital Sueco-Noruego*, pp. 108–110. Traumatology is the branch of medicine that deals with the surgical treatment of physical injuries caused by accidents or violence.
50 Fernández Sabaté, *Nuestros fundadores*, pp. 178–179.
51 Bastos Ansart, M., *Algunos aspectos clínicos de las heridas por arma de fuego* (Barcelona, 1936).
52 Ibid., p. 112; Moral Torres, El 'método español', p. 161.
53 Beneito Lloris, *El hospital Sueco-Noruego*, p. 112.
54 Moral Torres, El 'método español', p. 162.
55 Huertas, R., "Politica sanitaria: De la dictadura de Primo de Rivera a la II^a^ República", *Revista Española Salud Publica*, Vol. 74 (2000), pp. 35–43, p. 36; Preston, *The Coming of the Spanish Civil War*, pp. 47–50.
56 Martínez Antonio, Entre la diplomacia médica.
57 Madariaga, *Los moros que trajo Franco*, p. 86.
58 Ibid.
59 Balfour, *Deadly Embrace*, p. 32.
60 The Treaty Between France and Spain, pp. 81–99.
61 Preston, *Franco*, p. 15.
62 Casals Meseguer, X., "Franco 'El Africano'", *Journal of Spanish Cultural Studies*, Vol. 7, No. 3 (2006), pp. 207–224, pp. 207–208; Balfour, *Deadly Embrace*, p. 40; Beneito Lloris, *El hospital Sueco-Noruego*, p. 109.
63 Casals Meseguer, Franco 'El Africano', pp. 207–224.
64 Preston, *Spanish Holocaust*, pp. xi–xiv.
65 Preston, *Franco*, p. 31.
66 Madariaga, *Los moros que trajo Franco*, p. 77; Azzuz Hakim, *La actitud de los moros*, p. 118.
67 Azzuz Hakim, *La actitud de los moros*, p. 12.
68 Preston, *Franco*, pp. 31–32; Casals Meseguer, Franco 'El Africano', p. 210.
69 Martínez Antonio, Entre la diplomacia médica, p. 233.
70 Oteyza, L. D., *Abd-el-Krim y los prisioneros: una información periodística en el campo enemigo* (Madrid, 1925), p. 77; Madariaga, *Los moros que trajo Franco*,

pp. 104–107; Blond Álvarez Del Manzano, C., "El Protectorado. Firma del convenio hispano-francés y Guerra del Rif 1912–1927", *Revista de Historia Militar*, Vol. 2 (2012), pp. 103–135, p.129.

71 Madariaga, *Los moros que trajo Franco*, p. 81.
72 Martínez Antonio, Entre la diplomacia médica, p.233.
73 Balfour, *Deadly Embrace*, pp. 225–226.
74 Ibid.; AGMAV, C. 42385, 1; AGMAV, C. 42385, 3; AGMAV, C. 42385, 5; AGMAV, C. 42386, 1; AGMAV, C. 42386, 2; AGMAV, C. 42386, 3; AGMAV, C. 29297, 1; AGMAV, C. 29297, 2; & AGMAV, C. 29297, 5.
75 Balfour, *Deadly Embrace*, pp. 120, 226–227.
76 La Porte, Civil Military Relations, p. 219; Madariaga, *Los moros que trajo Franco*, p. 81.
77 Madariaga, *Los moros que trajo Franco*, pp. 81–82.
78 Carr, *Spain 1808–1975*, pp. 573–574.
79 Madariaga, *Los moros que trajo Franco*, pp. 51–73. See also Balfour, *Deadly Embrace*, Chapter 5: The Secret History of Chemical Warfare Against Moroccans, pp. 123–157.
80 La Porte, Civil Military Relations, p. 219; Madariaga, *Los moros que trajo Franco*, p. 82.
81 Navarro Suay, R., & Plaza Torres, J. F., "1925: Cuando volvimos a ser grandes ... el apoyo sanitario en el desembarco de Alhucemas", *Sanidad Militar*, Vol. 68, No. 4 (2012), pp. 247–256.
82 Balfour, *Deadly Embrace*, p. 70.
83 Azzuz Hakim, *La actitud de los moros*, pp. 12–13.
84 Balfour, *Deadly Embrace*, p. 115.
85 Ibid., pp. 13–14.
86 *ABC*, 17.07.1927, p. 27.
87 Balfour, *Deadly Embrace*, p. 60; Preston, *Franco*, p. 146.
88 Madariaga, *Los moros que trajo Franco*, pp. 105–106.
89 Azzuz Hakim, *La actitud de los moros*, p. 81.
90 Ibid., pp. 1–123; *El laberinto marroqui* (2007), RTVE2.
91 Asbridge, T., *The Crusades: The Authoritative History of the War for the Holy Land* (New York, 2010), pp. 24–25. *Jihād* is normally translated as 'Holy War', but its literal translation is 'striving'.
92 García Cruz, *Las fuerzas militares nativas*, pp. 15–16.
93 Azzuz Hakim, *La actitud de los moros*, p. 83. The surname Redondo would indicate Andalusi origin (p. 85). This interview was carried out by her son Mekki Ben Mohammad as part of a series of interviews he conducted in 1945 with leading Moroccan nationalists, as part of an investigation into the recruitment and enlistment of North African troops during the Spanish Civil War (pp. 67–93).
94 Balfour, *Deadly Embrace*, p. 115.
95 Ibid., p. 115; Preston, *Franco*, pp. 174, 181.
96 Balfour, *Deadly Embrace*, p. 120.
97 Beneito Lloris, *El hospital Sueco-Noruego*, p. 109.
98 Zubelzu, Obra Quirúrgica, pp. 69–75.
99 Beevor, *Battle for Spain*, pp. 31–32.
100 Ibid.; Garate Córdoba, Las tropas de África, pp. 14–15.
101 Beevor, *Battle for Spain*, pp. 31–32.
102 Sotomayor Blásquez, El moro traidor, p. 239.

103 Garate Córdoba, Las tropas de África, pp. 10–14.
104 Martin Corrales, Maurofobia/islamafobia, p. 43.
105 Madariaga, *Los moros que trajo Franco*, p. 274.
106 Preston, *Spanish Holocaust*, pp. xii–xiii.
107 Asbridge, *The Crusades*, pp. 9–13; Palmer, *Defenders of the Faith*.
108 *ABC* (Sevilla), 27.03.1938, p. 4.
109 Ibid.; Franco Grande, A., Álvarez Escudero, J., & Cortés Laiño, J., *Historia de la anestesia en España: 1847–1940* (Madrid, 2005), pp. 219–221.
110 *ABC* (Sevilla), 27.03.1938, p. 4.
111 Larraz & Barrola, Los pies de Teruel, p. 201; AGMAV, C. 42385, 1; AGMAV, C. 42385, 3; AGMAV, C. 42385, 5; AGMAV, C. 29297, 1; AGMAV, C. 29297, 2; AGMAV, C. 29297, 5.
112 Carrie, L. E. S., & Simpson, P. J., *Understanding Anaesthesia* (London, 1982).
113 Sánchez Ruano, *Islam y Guerra Civil Española*, p. 225.
114 AGMAV, C. 42385, 1; AGMAV, C. 42385, 3; AGMAV, C. 42385, 5; AGMAV, C. 42386, 1; AGMAV, C. 42386, 2; AGMAV, C. 42386, 3; AGMAV, C. 29297, 1; AGMAV, C. 29297, 2; AGMAV, C. 29297, 5.
115 AGMAV, C. 42385, 3.
116 *ABC* (Sevilla), 27.03.1938, p. 4.
117 Massons, *Historia de la Sanidad Militar Española: Tomo II*, p. 445.
118 *El Laberinto Marroqui*, Director: Julio Sánchez Veiga (2007), RTVE2.
119 AGMAV, C. 42386, 2.
120 Ibid.
121 Ibid., AGMAV, C. 42385, 1; AGMAV, C. 42385, 3; AGMAV, C. 42385, 5; AGMAV, C. 42386, 1; AGMAV, C. 42386, 3; AGMAV, C. 29297, 1; AGMAV, C. 29297, 2; AGMAV, C. 29297, 5.
122 AGMAV, C. 42386, 2. It is not clear from the admission and discharge card which hospital he was discharged to as the handwriting at this point is difficult to decipher.
123 Ibid.
124 AGMAV, C. 42385, 3.
125 AGMAV, C. 42385, 1; Sánchez Ruano, *Islam y Guerra Civil Española*, pp. 131, 224.
126 Massons, *Historia de la Sanidad Militar Española: Tomo II*, p. 445; Sánchez Veiga, *El Laberinto Marroqui*.
127 Mesa, *Los moros de la Guerra Civil española*, p. 259.
128 Scott-Ellis, *The Chances of Death*, pp. vii, 1.
129 CULA. manuscript no. 3/233: Scott-Ellis, *The Diary of Pip Scott-Ellis*.
130 Scott-Ellis, *The Chances of Death*, p. 5.
131 Ibid.; Frutos Herranz, *Hospitales en Burgos*, p. 127.
132 Scott-Ellis, *The Chances of Death*, pp. 5–11.
133 AGMAV, C. 42385, 1; AGMAV, C. 42385, 3; AGMAV, C. 42385, 5; AGMAV, C. 42386, 1; AGMAV, C. 42386, 2; AGMAV, C. 42386, 3; AGMAV, C. 29297, 1; AGMAV, C. 29297, 2; AGMAV, C. 29297, 5.
134 AGMAV, C. 29316, 1; AGMAV, C. 29316, 2.
135 AGMAV, C. 42385, 1; AGMAV, C. 42385, 3; AGMAV, C. 42385, 5; AGMAV, C. 42386, 1; AGMAV, C. 42386, 2; AGMAV, C. 42386, 3; AGMAV, C. 29297, 1; AGMAV, C. 29297, 2; AGMAV, C. 29297, 5. HAF (an abbreviation for: herida por arma de fuego – wounded by firearm) is the main cause of injury recorded on the admission and discharge cards for those wounded in battle.

136 AGMAV, C. 29297, 1; AGMAV, C. 29297, 2; AGMAV, C. 29297, 5.
137 AGMAV, C. 42385, 1; AGMAV, C. 42385, 3; AGMAV, C. 42385, 5; AGMAV, C. 42386, 1; AGMAV, C. 42386, 2; AGMAV, C. 42386, 3.
138 AGMAV, C. 42385, 1.
139 AGMAV, C. 42385, 3.
140 WLAM, PP/RRM/D1/76.
141 Herrera, A., & Las Mulas, M. de, "In Memoriam Fidel Pages Mirave (1886–1923) on the 75th Anniversary of the Publication of Anesthesia Metamerica", *Revista española de anestesiología y reanimación*, Vol. 43, No. 2 (1996), pp. 59–66.
142 Carrie & Simpson, *Understanding Anaesthesia*, pp. 2–3, 202–203.
143 WLAM, PP/RRM/D1/76.
144 Said, *Orientalism*, p. 97.
145 WLAM, PP/RRM/D1/76.
146 Asbridge, *The Crusades*, pp. 24–25; *ABC* (Sevilla), 26.07.1936, p. 4; *ABC* (Sevilla), 10.12.1937, p. 13; *ABC* (Sevilla), 26.07.938, p. 9; *ABC* (Sevilla), 01.04.1939, p. 9.
147 Ibid.
148 Ibid.; Unzueta Merino, M. C., Hervás Puyal. C., & Villar Landeira. J, "Robert R. Macintosh y España: una relación fecunda", in *Revista española de anestesiología y reanimación*, Vol. 48, No. 1 (2001). pp. 21–28.
149 WLAM, PP/RRM/C/2; Unzueta Merino et al., Robert R. Macintosh y España, pp. 21–88.
150 WLAM, PP/RRM/C/2. There is no indication as to where this soldier originated.
151 Ibid.; Unzueta Merino et al., Robert R. Macintosh y España, pp. 21–28.
152 Ibid.; Browne, J. S., "History of Anaesthesia: Anaesthetics and the Spanish Civil War: The Start of Specialisation", *European Journal of Anaesthesiology*, Vol. 31, No. 2 (2014), pp. 65–67..
153 AGMAV, C. 29297, 1.
154 Van de Ven, H., "Introduction to Part 1", in R. Chickering, D. Showalter & H. Van de Ven (eds.), *The Cambridge History of War Volume IV: War and the Modern World* (Cambridge, 2012), pp. 9–15, p. 10.
155 Balfour, *Deadly Embrace*, pp. 225–228; AGMAV, C. 42385, 1; AGMAV, C. 42385, 3; AGMAV, C. 42385, 5; AGMAV, C. 42386, 1; AGMAV, C. 42386, 2; AGMAV, C. 42386, 3; AGMAV, C. 29297, 1; AGMAV, C. 29297, 2; AGMAV, C. 29297, 5.
156 Bernabéu Mestre, J., "El papel de la Escuela Nacional de Sanidad en el desarrollo de la salud publica en España, 1924–1934", *Revista de Sanidad e Higiene Pública,* Vol. 68 (1998), pp. 65–89.
157 AGMAV, C. 29297, 1.
158 AGMAV, C. 43385, 2.
159 Ibid.; AGMAV, C. 42385, 1; AGMAV, C. 42385, 3; AGMAV, C. 42385, 5; AGMAV, C. 42386, 1; AGMAV, C. 42386, 2; AGMAV, C. 42386, 3; AGMAV, C. 29297, 1; AGMAV, C. 29297, 2; AGMAV, C. 29297, 5.
160 Ibid.
161 AGMAV, C. 29297, 2.
162 Ibid.
163 AGMAV, C. 29297, 5.
164 AGMAV, C. 42385, 3.

165 Ibid., Gastritis can have multiple causes, including injury.
166 AGMAV, C. 42385, 1; AGMAV, C. 42385, 3; AGMAV, C. 42385, 5; AGMAV, C. 42386, 1; AGMAV, C. 42386, 2; AGMAV, C. 42386, 3; AGMAV, C. 29297, 1; AGMAV, C. 29297, 2; AGMAV, C. 29297, 5.
167 Ibid.
168 *ABC* (Sevilla), 22.08.1937, pp. 11–12; *ABC* (Sevilla), 26.08.1937, p. 11; Gómez Teruel, J. M., *La hospitalización militar* en Sevilla a través de los tiempos (Sevilla, 2006), p. 155.
169 *ABC* (Sevilla), 26.08.1937, p. 11.
170 Sánchez Ruano, *Islam y Guerra Civil Española*, pp. 230–232; *ABC* (Sevilla), 27.07.1937, p. 17; *ABC* (Sevilla), 07.08.1937, p. 10; *ABC* (Sevilla), 17.09.1937, p. 6.
171 Sánchez Ruano, *Islam y Guerra Civil Española*, p. 231.
172 *ABC* (Sevilla), 26.08.1937, p. 11; *ABC* (Sevilla), 07.12.1937, p. 13; *ABC* (Sevilla), 11.04.1937, p. 6; *ABC* (Sevilla), 01.09.1937, p. 19; *ABC* (Sevilla), 28.09.1937, p. 16; *ABC* (Sevilla), 12.01.1938, p. 21; *ABC* (Sevilla), 22.01.1938, p. 26; *ABC* (Sevilla), 01.02.1938, p. 23; *ABC* (Sevilla), 12.02.1938, p. 14; *ABC* (Sevilla), 22.02.1938, p. 15; *ABC* (Sevilla), 02.06.1938, p. 17.
173 Frutos Herranz, *Hospitales en Burgos*, pp. 125–127.
174 Ibid., pp. 125–127.
175 Al Tuma, The Participation of Moorish Troops, p. 104.
176 Ortiz de Villajos, C. G., *Crónica de Granada en 1937, II Año Triunfal* (Granada, 1938), p. 45.
177 Madariaga, *Los moros que trajo Franco*, pp. 278–281; Merroun, *Las tropas marroquíes*, pp. 197–198.
178 Ayesta y Daguerre, L., "Mohamed Belkaid. El Morito Matarife", *El Compostelano* (27.04.1937), p. 1; Gurriarán, *Diario de Guerra*, p. 239.
179 *ABC* (Sevilla), 12.02.1938, p. 14; *El pueblo gallego*, 03.07.1938, p. 8; "La estancia en Vigo del Visir del Majzen", *El pueblo gallego*, 28.02.1937, p. 10; *El pueblo gallego*, 23.04.1937.
180 *ABC* (Sevilla), 12.02.1938, p. 14.
181 *ABC* (Sevilla), 22.02.1938, p. 16.
182 Al Tuma, The Participation of Moorish Troops, pp. 104–105; *ABC* (Sevilla), 14.01.1938, p. 18.
183 *ABC* (Sevilla), 22.02.1938.
184 Casals Meseguer, Franco 'El Africano', p. 214.
185 *ABC* (Sevilla), 02.02.1939, p. 19.
186 *ABC* (Sevilla), 12.01.1938, p. 21.
187 Frutos Herranz, *Hospitales en Burgos*, pp. 126–127; Gómez Teruel, *La hospitalización militar en Sevilla*, pp. 155–157; Madariaga, *Los moros que trajo Franco*, p. 277; *ABC* (Sevilla), 01.12.1936, p. 11; *ABC* (Sevilla), 16.04.1937, p. 13; *El pueblo gallego*, 02.07.1937, p. 1.
188 *ABC* (Sevilla), 28.12.1937.
189 Frutos Herranz, *Hospitales en Burgos*, pp. 108–109.
190 Madariaga, *Los moros que trajo Franco*, p. 284.
191 Ibid., p. 285; *El laberinto marroqui*.
192 Massons, *Historia de la Sanidad Militar Española: Tomo II*, pp. 499–500.
193 Ibid.
194 *El laberinto marroqui*.

195 *ABC* (Sevilla), 12.02.1938, p. 14; *El pueblo gallego*, 03.07.1938, p. 8; "La estancia en Vigo del Visir del Majzen", *El pueblo gallego*, 28.02.1937, p. 10; *El pueblo gallego*, 23.04.1937.
196 Frutos Herranz, *Hospitales en Burgos*, p. 116.
197 Madariaga, *Los moros que trajo Franco*, p. 283.
198 Frutos Herranz, *Hospitales en Burgos*, p. 116.
199 Azzuz Hakim, *La actitud de los moros ante el Alzamiento*, p. 88.
200 Madariaga, *Los moros que trajo Franco*, pp. 283–234; Sánchez Ruano, *Islam y Guerra Civil Española*, p. 252; Azzuz Hakim, *La actitud de los moros*, pp. 67–193.
201 Azzuz Hakim, *La actitud de los moros*, pp. 85–86.
202 Ibid.; Armstrong, K., *Islam: A Short History* (New York, 2002), pp. 205–206.
203 Azzuz Hakim, *La actitud de los moros*, p. 88.
204 Frutos Herranz, *Hospitales en Burgos*, pp. 116–118; Azzuz Hakim, *La actitud de los moros*, p. 88.
205 Frutos Herranz, *Hospitales en Burgos*, p. 118.
206 Thackrah, J. R., *Routledge Companion to Military Conflict Since 1945* (Oxford, 2009), pp. xxii, 89, 95, 120, 136.
207 Balfour, *Deadly Embrace*, p. 312.
208 Casals Meseguer, Franco 'El Africano', p. 214.
209 Sotomayor Blásquez, El moro traidor, pp. 233–249; Beevor, *Battle for Spain*, pp. 56, 117–121, 245, 378.
210 Balfour, *Deadly Embrace*, p. 277; Beevor, *Battle for Spain*, pp. 56, 117–121, 245, 378.

3 Organisation

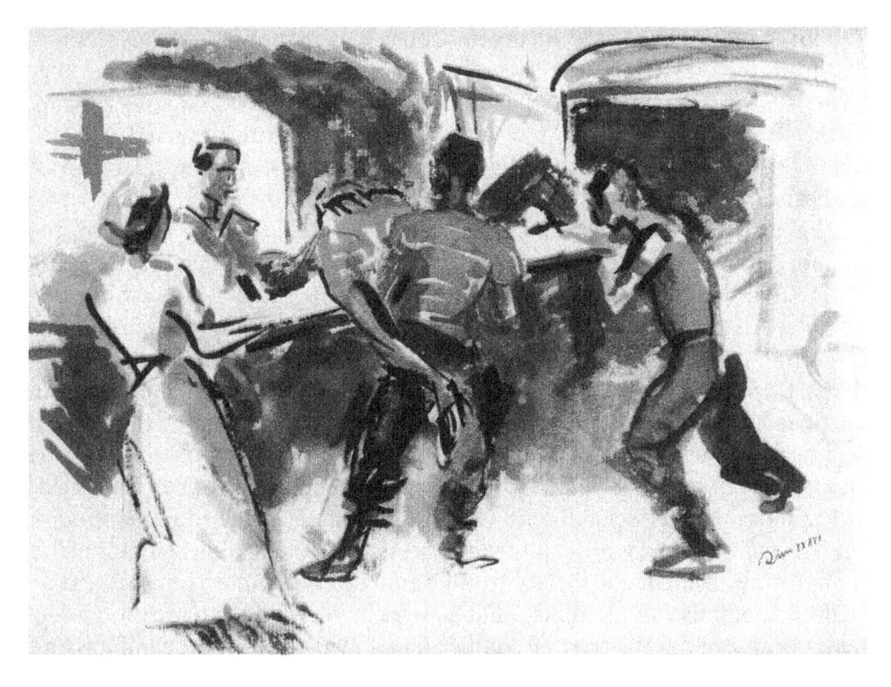

Image 1 "Final Embrace", Sim, *Estampas de la Revolución Española 19 Julio de 1936* (Barcelona, 1936).

Source: Oficinas de Propaganda C.N.T.-F.A.I. Barcelona Grafos, Colectivizada, 1936.

Introduction

The apparent chaos that characterised the provision of medical services during the opening stages of the Spanish Civil War has often been cited as being widespread across Spain, with Republican held areas described as the hardest hit.[1] The majority of the medical personnel of the Sanidad Militar (Military Health Services) sided with the Insurgents, and on the night of 17

July 1936 a number of professors from the Academy of the Sanidad Militar took advantage of the confusion accompanying the emerging news of the uprising in the Protectorate to flee Madrid and join the Insurgency.[2] However, the chaos referred to could be more accurately described as the early-stage organisation and reorganisation of new and existing medical services, which were an important step towards more regional and national models for the delivery of care.[3]

As a result of the lack of beds to treat the sick and wounded, a shortage of pharmaceutical supplies and a scarcity of ambulances, problems common to both sides, local and regional responses were to prove important and were vital in contributing towards the development of facilities and services across Spain. It is the organisation of the existing and newly created medical services in both the Republican and Insurgent Zones in response to a bloody conflict that from the very start placed severe strain on existing medical services that forms the focus of this chapter. The emphasis here is predominantly on care of the wounded combatant, but with the line increasingly blurred between what constituted the front and the rear-guard during the Spanish Civil War, medical care of the wider population is also considered.[4]

The provision of medical care, and particularly surgical care, of the wounded in both the Republican and Insurgent Zones throughout the Spain of the Civil War was notable for its similarities rather than for its differences. This is perhaps not surprising when we consider the common background and training of many of the Spanish medical staff on both sides, with the additional factor that the majority of military doctors within Spain had served in the Spanish Protectorate of Morocco.[5] However, what did mark Republican healthcare provision as different from that in the Insurgent Zone was the important contribution made by anarchist medical personnel and medical practitioners associated with, but not affiliated to the movement, with anarchists holding key posts in health throughout the Spanish Civil War.[6] It is important to highlight the contribution made by anarchists in the field of health as a number of anarchist militias were involved in the repression in the Republican Zone at the start of conflict. Their involvement in the killings and summary executions during the first months of the war in some Republican-held areas, and the failed attempt at a revolutionary uprising in Barcelona in May 1937, has overshadowed their otherwise wider contribution to the Republican war effort, with healthcare an important yet underexplored aspect of this contribution.[7]

In order to demonstrate how the delivery of care of the wounded evolved during the conflict, a number of local, regional and national responses will be explored. This will include a case study that examines how pharmaceutical provision and distribution were organised. As part of the exploration of the evolution of local and regional models of improvisation and organisation, their wider impact on national models for the provision of medical care to the wounded, and measures taken to protect both soldiers and civilians from the possible use of chemical weapons, will also be assessed as part of the wider analysis relating to the organisation of frontline medical services during the Spanish Civil War. This examination of defensive preparations taken against the possible use of chemical weapons by both the civilian and the military also allows for a wider analysis of the little-explored anarchist contribution in the area of medical organisation. Civil defence responses in the Republican Zone were led by the Spanish Red Cross, which for much of the war had an anarchist doctor, Juan Morata Cantón, as its head.[8]

The evacuation of the sick and wounded, a challenging task due to difficulties posed by geography and terrain, will also be examined with the focus here on more national models of organisation, although regional initiatives were to have an impact on the provision of these services. Finally, the chapter will demonstrate the main differences in the provision of medical care to the wounded in the opposing zones were more at an ideological and organisational level rather than in the actual medical care delivered. However, it will also demonstrate that the real differences that did exist can in part be attributed to the influence of anarchist thinking on the democratisation of medicine. There were direct parallels between anarchist approaches to the socialisation of medicine and socialist initiatives for tackling Spain's poor health services begun during the 'transformative biennial' of 1931–1933 under the leadership of the Director General for Health, Marcelino Pascua Martínez, a leading member of the Spanish Socialist Workers Party (Partido Socialista Obrero Español, PSOE). Medical reform provided a unifying platform for the disparate groups on the left in Spain and was a central tenet in their different bids to transform Spanish society. It was the desire to challenge the traditional hierarchical structure of medicine by making it free, or at least affordable, for the whole of the population, that marked the real differences between Republican and Insurgent medical services during the Spanish Civil War.[9]

Civilian and military healthcare during the Second Republic

In order to provide the wider context in which these developments took place, an examination that provide a brief background to the changes that took place in the field of military healthcare and provision during the Second Republic is required. A characteristic of the Spanish military prior to the advent of the Second Republic was the large numbers of officers that it had on its payroll, which numbered fifty-eight generals (excluding those on the reserve list) and 21,996 various chiefs and officials.[10] As a result of reforms introduced by the Minister of War, Manuel Azaña, in 1931, efforts were made to curb the disproportionate numbers of officers and petty officials within the armed services.[11] Azaña, who trained as a lawyer and was later president of the Second Republic during the Spanish Civil War, was hostile towards both the power of the army and of the church, and as part of what became known as the 'Ley

Azaña' (the Azaña Law) for military reform, the number of MOs was reduced from 900 in 1931 to 689 in 1935, before rising to 747 in January 1936.[12]

Between 1904 and 1931, increases in spending in the field of public health had been primarily directed towards preventing epidemics and infectious diseases, whereas during the liberal reformist stage of the Second Republic (1931–1933) this was expanded to promote the wider socialisation of medicine. In contrast to this, however, the Military Health Services budget as a proportion of military spending remained relatively static, although some important advances had been made in modernising the service.[13]

It was during the 'transformative biennial' that the idea of an evolved form of a national health service took root. There was no anarchist involvement in government at this stage and they had in fact encouraged voters to boycott the elections, so radical healthcare initiatives were in the hands of the socialists in government. As such, it was Marcelino Pascua, appointed as Director General of Health in April 1931, who pushed these initiatives forward. Pascua aggressively promoted the concept of public health, coordinated a programme of preventative, curative and rehabilatory action, and promoted the use of sanitary statistics for improving public hygiene and health. It was under his leadership that in 1933 a record amount was spent on health both at a national level and regionally. Unfortunately, there was still considerable resistance from elements on the right in government who had served under the dictator Primo de Rivera. As a result, the law of Sanitary Coordination of July 1934 – passed during the 'conservative biennial' phase when the right controlled parliament, and which was aimed at improving the situation of titular medics in rural areas – largely failed, as it was dependent on the limited public funds allocated to the municipalities.[14]

It was against this background of a slow but steady growth in public spending during the first half of the Second Republic before the counter-reformist phase brought in by the right in 1933, that the subsequent Republican organisation of care of the wounded at the start of the Civil War should be compared.[15]

Ideologies of care: New directions

Studies that take as their focus the provision of surgical care during the Spanish Civil War, and medical care in general during the conflict, favour analyses of the organisation of these services in the Republican Zone over those of the Insurgent Zone. While this can be a useful model in understanding how these facilities functioned in those areas controlled by the government it is, nevertheless, an imperfect model. This is because it stresses the notion, expressed in a predominantly leftist discourse on the socialisation of medicine, that the Republican approach to healthcare was as a result of an ideologically superior model of care. The realities were, of course, far more complex. The endeavours made towards creating new healthcare models during the Spanish Civil War itself were most notable during the first period of anarchist involvement in government, starting in November 1936 and which ended in May 1937 with the suppression of the anarchist uprising in Barcelona.[16] These endeavours were led at a government level by the anarchist Minister of Health, Federica Montseny, and included a failed attempt to introduce national legislation, similar to the controversial law successfully passed by the autonomous Catalan parliament, the Generalitat in December 1936, to allow planned abortions in the first three months of pregnancy.[17] Anarchist involvement at ministerial level was renewed under the premiership of Juan Negrín, when Segundo Blanco González, a former Secretary General of the Confederación Nacional del Trabajo (National Confederation of Labour or CNT), was appointed as Minister of Health and Education in April 1938, a post he held until the end of the war.[18] Félix Martí Ibañez, an anarchist doctor in charge of the General Health Office in Catalunya for ten months between 1936 and 1937, also sought the wider socialisation and democratisation of medicine with the anarchist movement, becoming a key voice in calls for healthcare to be free.[19]

The League of Nations Report on Health Organisation in Spain, while not directly referring to the influence of anarchist policies on medical issues, nevertheless noted that:

> The public health services, under the energetic guidance of Madame Montseny, are at present in process of reorganisation, considerable attention being given to hygiene, social medicine and health education. Political trade-union influence are of course not left out of the account, but – and this to us appears essential – it may be definitely asserted that the whole system is based upon the work of specialists; it is they who, at the Ministry, drew up plans whose execution depends for the most part, in the provinces, upon the co-operation of the medical profession.[20]

The specialist and trade union influence mentioned above, referred to both the anarchist CNT and the socialist Unión General de Trabajadores (General Workers Union or UGT) representatives involved in healthcare. This included the medical counsellor for social assistance, the paediatric doctor Amparo Poch y Gascon (a co-founder of the anarcho-feminist organisation Mujeres Libres), and the first sub-secretary of the Ministry of Health, Mercedes Maestre Mari, from the UGT.[21] Part of the reason for the CNT and the UGT joining forces on this occasion, was a desire to promote women candidates, but also arose from shared socialist and anarchist perspectives on the socialisation of medicine. Consequently, cooperation between these two unions in matters of health were not uncommon.[22]

Among the appointments made by Montseny was that of the anarchist Juan Morata Cantón. He held two successive government posts under her ministership, that of Counsellor of the Department of Hospitals and Sanatoria of the National Council of Health, followed by his appointment on 3 January 1937 as Secretary General of the National Council of Health, a post he held until 4 June 1937 when he resigned from government.[23] Another appointment made by Montseny was that of Francisco Trigo Dominguez, an anarchist doctor who was Delegate for Health in Madrid in 1937. Trigo Dominguez oversaw the health services in the capital but on several occasions, and at risk to his own life, protected medical personnel suspected of being Francoist sympathisers from summary execution.[24] He served throughout the conflict in a number of posts, with his last official appointment on 17 March 1939 to Sub-Secretary of Health for the Council of Public Instruction and Health.[25]

By contrast, care of the wounded and infirm in the Insurgent Zone was predicated around winning the war, and a large number of civilian doctors, providing they were not members of left-wing or Republican organisations, were assimilated into the military, with military healthcare taking precedence over that of the civilian.[26] This undoubtedly left a gap in care provision in the Insurgent rear-guard during the conflict, whereas in Republican Spain legitimising the Republic and its social and cultural agenda were key elements of its programme throughout the war. There was a record budget for educational and cultural programmes allocated to the Ministry of Public Instruction and Fine Arts in 1937 and which saw teachers' salaries increase as part of the drive towards greater literacy. This, alongside continuing the changes begun in social medicine with the advent of the Second Republic, was an important element in the policies and discourse surrounding the government's continued legitimacy throughout the Civil War.[27]

If healthcare provision for civilians and the military is examined within this context there were real differences relating to the wider issues surrounding healthcare in the opposing camps, but as will be demonstrated in this chapter, care of the wounded itself during the Spanish Civil War did not differ significantly in the Republican and Insurgent Zones. It should be noted, however, that in both zones the provision of medical care was geared towards needs dictated by the war, but that, nevertheless, in the Republican Zone martial law was not officially declared until 23 January 1939, and this allowed for more varied responses during the conflict, driven by a number of different political groupings, providing a lifeline to civilian and combatant alike.[28]

Medical services at the start of the conflict: Local and regional responses

On 17 July 1936 as the finishing touches were being put in place in readiness for the insurrection in the Spanish Protectorate in Morocco, Ignacio Ponseti Vives – a young civilian surgeon later famous for his non-surgical treatment for the correction of club foot – took and passed his final exam with the medical faculty at the University of Barcelona.[29] Within a few short days he was helping to treat the wounded at the Republican Hospital Pere Mata in nearby Reus in the team of a pre-eminent Spanish orthopaedic surgeon Francisco Jimeno Vidal.[30] The following day, on 18 July 1936, when the

Insurgency on the Spanish mainland broke out, Manuel Bastos Ansart was on his way from Madrid to Barcelona to attend the First Congress of the Spanish Society of Orthopaedic Surgery, which was due to be held in the Catalan capital the next day.[31] He returned to Madrid, but cognisant of the deteriorating situation he fled alongside his wife Consuelo to San Sebastian where their children were holidaying. During his brief stay in San Sebastian, alongside Consuelo, an experienced if unqualified theatre nurse, he attended the wounded in the military hospital there. After a brief stay in San Sebastian, Bastos Ansart returned to his own hospital in Madrid, which he achieved by first crossing into France before travelling to Barcelona and then onto Madrid.[32] His desire to return to his own hospital, likely dictated by a desire to continue his career as an army surgeon uninterrupted rather than for obvious Republican sympathies, was to have dire consequences in that he became a victim of the post-war purges.[33] Bastos Ansart helped organise orthopaedic services in the capital, before then going on to take up post as head of surgery at the Swedish/Norwegian Hospital at Alcoi in August 1937, which had been paid for through public subscription in Scandinavia.[34]

On 21 July 1936, a civilian doctor, Luis Mazo Buron, after offering his services in the provincial hospital in León, which had fallen to the Insurgents, operated on his first patient, an assault guard with a 'clean' femoral fracture caused by a rifle bullet. Within a few days the Red Cross in León requested his help in establishing a frontline hospital in León in a nursing home for the elderly (it is not stated what happened to the residents). With equipment from his own practice, which included surgical instruments and an x-ray machine, he installed an operating theatre in what was originally a fifty-bed hospital. As time went on, however, the facility had to be continually expanded with its initial installation totally 'improvised with haste and very few means'.[35]

This ability to access existing facilities or to improvise in creating new ones exemplified by the doctor's accounts was an important factor when the conflict broke out. The Republicans in the major cities of Madrid, Barcelona, Bilbao and Valencia were able immediately following the uprising to quickly access and start the work of reorganising the existing hospital systems and the wider medical infrastructure. However, with street-fighting a major factor, especially in Barcelona, and the high number of casualties this occasioned, the need arose for further surgical facilities to be made available.[36] Not only were new hospitals organised in Madrid, Barcelona and beyond by the different political Republican factions so as to provide surgical services for those injured in the street-fighting, but the rapidly organised militias also formed their own surgical units that accompanied them to the front.[37] In Barcelona due to the presence of the anarchist mutual society Organización Sanitaria Obrera (Workers Health Organisation or OSO) in several working class districts, frontline hospitals and emergency clinics were also rapidly organised to cope with the influx of civic casualties resulting from the heavy street-fighting. Medical practitioners from OSO also accompanied a variety

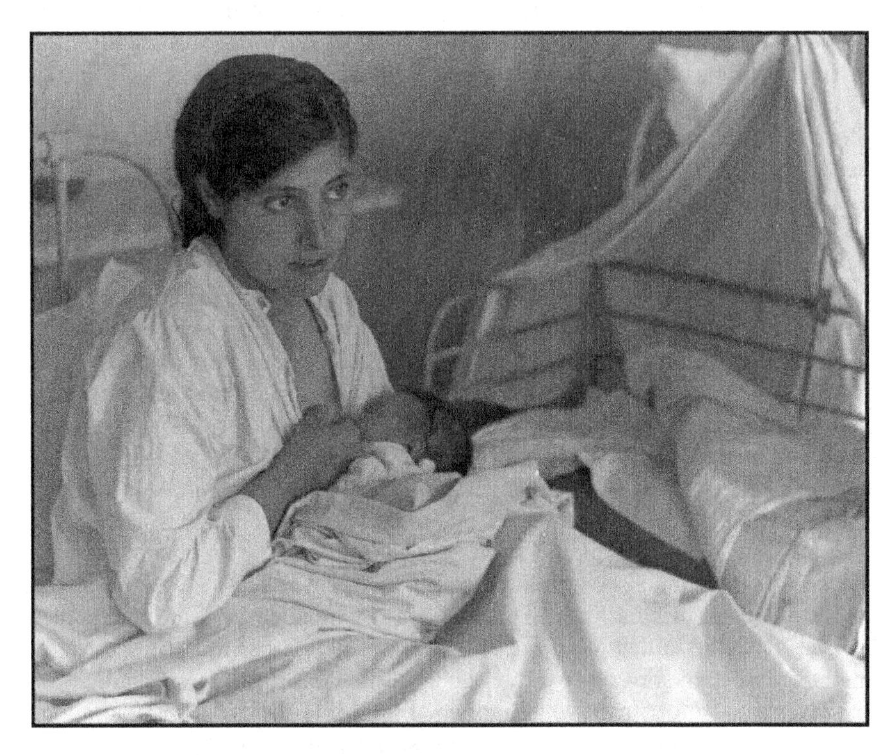

Image 2 Maternity ward by David Seymour 1936: Spain. Barcelona.
Source: Magnum.

of CNT and Federación Anarquista Ibérica (Iberian Anarchist Federation or FAI) units to the front.[38]

The CNT in Valencia set up a small frontline hospital of twenty-five beds with an operating theatre and x-ray facilities. This was funded along similar lines to that of the mutual society in Barcelona, and was where wounded or sick militiamen from the anarchist militia, the Iron Column (Columna de Hierro) were treated. Towards the end of 1936, the same organisation also set up a small maternity hospital in Valencia where treatment was free as a result of anarchist policy that promoted and advanced women's rights. It was initiatives such as these (which were used as an important visual component of Republican propaganda, see Images 2 and 3), that proved a lifeline to civilian and combatant alike early in the conflict.[39] This was despite the fact that the facilities on offer varied considerably.

The Insurgents, although not immediately in control of any of the major industrial cities, many of which benefitted from more modern surgical facilities, were nevertheless quickly able to control important sectors of the military health network of hospitals, or as in the case of provincial capitals such

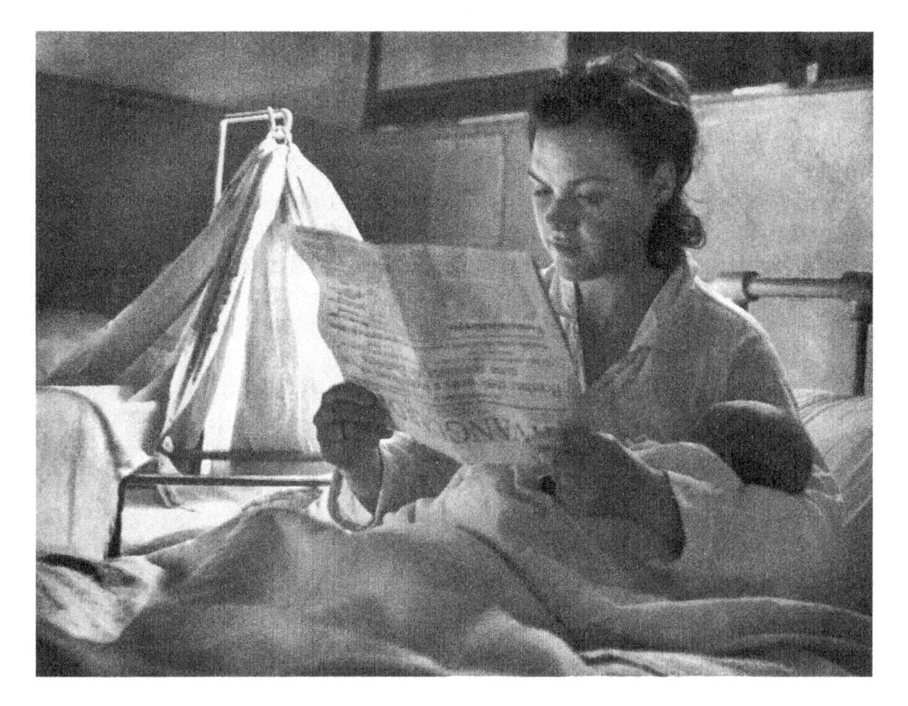

Image 3 Barcelona: Maternity ward. July 1936, by David Seymour.
Source: Magnum.

as León, organise further facilities as required.[40] The importance of controlling such facilities was soon to become evident. After the brutal uprising in the Andalusian capital Sevilla lasting several days, a city which was to become the bridgehead for the troops arriving from the Protectorate, the existing medical services were quickly placed at the disposal of the Insurgents. This included the military hospital in Sevilla whose services were to provide important medical support during the rapid Insurgent advance on Madrid in the early weeks of the war.[41]

Also important was the ability to access hospital facilities as a result of early military gains in the naval cities of Cádiz and San Fernando in the southwest, the military hospital of El Ferrol in Galicia in the northwest, and one of Spain's most prestigious military hospitals, the Hospital Militar in Valladolid in the conservative heartland of Castile.[42] The importance of controlling these establishments lay in the fact that they had benefitted from the professionalisation of the army, especially the Army of Africa, and been extensively modernised. The Insurgent medical services also benefitted from the experience gained by surgical staff who had served in the Protectorate; surgeons such as Mariano Gómez Ulla, the creator of a mobile surgical hospital based on French models from the Great War in which he participated as a neutral observer; Fernando Alsina, a Galician surgeon from Santiago de Compostela; and Fermín Palma García; who brought advanced surgical skills with them back to Spain.[43]

This initial lack of coordinated responses in both the Republican and Insurgent zones also meant that more localised initiatives outside of the provincial capitals by a variety of political bodies towards organising surgical services took place. Localised responses were not only varied and diverse, but also contributed towards the surgical care of the wounded in differing and difficult circumstances. For example, many small 'frontline' hospitals with single operating theatres were created. In the hills behind Málaga, anarchists with assistance from the retired British zoologist Peter Chalmers Mitchell, set up a hospital in the 'appropriated' house of Tomas Bolin, uncle of Franco's press agent and staff officer Luis Bolin.[44] Chalmers Mitchell in a letter to *The Times* in October 1936, commented that the CNT 'specialised in arranging new hospitals for wounded soldiers', although these did vary considerably in the services they were able to offer.[45] Forward first aid posts were also created independently, and included a Falangist unit set up in the Basque country and headed by an Argentinian volunteer doctor, Hector Colmegna.[46]

Many of these independent units soon disappeared or were swallowed up by the respective military health establishments as a result of the ongoing process of reorganisation of the health services in both zones that followed the early stage of the conflict. This reflected on the one hand efforts to centralise control in the name of greater efficiency, but on the other hand was dictated by, in the case of the Insurgents, Franco's consolidation of power over the disparate forces under his control, with the Republican Government efforts having a similar objective.[47]

The ability to rapidly organise, driven by a need for extra hospital beds, was in part dependant on an availability of suitable spaces for conversion, coupled with the ability to access surgical equipment or make new equipment in small workshops and factories.[48] Within days of the uprising the Insurgent hospital of San Carlos in San Fernando exceeded its capacity of 300 beds, even after a second surgical team was created to deal with the increased number of wounded. As a result, a second hospital with 180 beds was set up, Nuestra Señora de Carmen, sited in the ancient Academy of Marine Infantry. When it reached capacity, local infirmaries were able to provide additional beds.[49]

In Republican Gijón on Spain's northern coast, Dr Benigno Moran Cifuentes, a traumatologist and former pupil of Bastos Ansart, presented himself on the outbreak of the conflict at the Hospital de la Caridad, the town's only hospital. There was an almost complete lack of materials for the treatment of fractures, but the Popular Front Committee for the hospital placed at his disposal engineers, mechanics, soldiers, and carpenters who set about the rapid construction of a variety of orthopaedic equipment in the local School of Industry and its workshops.[50] Throughout the Civil War, Cifuentes continued to provide traumatology services at this hospital, despite the conquest of Gijón by the Insurgents in October 1937. A possible explanation for his ability to continue at the hospital after its takeover by the Insurgents was the likelihood that he had belonged to no political party or trade union and therefore could not be condemned for obvious political sympathies.[51]

These responses towards reorganisation and the establishment of new facilities to treat the ever-increasing number of wounded across Spain, whether large or small, defined the early-stage organisational structure and how medical and surgical care was delivered in the first six months of the war. With fighting taking place in in numerous locations across Spain, the necessity of being able to respond quickly in the treatment of the wounded meant that improvisation was an important factor in the delivery of medical care. That these responses varied was as much dictated by circumstances as location, and it is the organisational characteristics and how facilities were distributed in the respective zones that form the focus of the following case study that examines the evolution of pharmaceutical services during the conflict.

Pharmaceutical provision – manufacture and supply: A case study

The capacity to respond to differing circumstances through improvisation, whether through the manufacture of surgical instrumentation or the habilitation of hospital beds, could not be matched in all areas of medical provision and depended on access to the appropriate materials. The first problems faced by the respective health services whether military or civilian was that the unequal division of Spain created particular problems for organisation due to the location of key health-related industries being accessible to one side or the other, but never to both.

The following examination of how the provision of pharmaceutical materials was organised during the conflict is a case in point. With the government of the Republic in control of key industrial areas including Madrid, the Basque Country and Catalunya, where much of the pharmaceutical industry was based, access to pharmaceuticals for the Insurgents was problematic from the start.[52] Effectively, the Insurgents had to start from scratch although they did receive medical aid from Germany in the form of help to laboratories and the supply of pharmaceuticals, including the anaesthetic agent evipan not otherwise available in Spain.[53] Both sides benefitted from the ability to access supplies held in local pharmacies, and also received help from the International Red Cross who, from September 1936, supplied anaesthetics (including evipan), sera, vaccines, narcotics, insulin and a variety of other pharmaceutical materials.[54]

The Spanish system for the distribution of pharmaceuticals for the Sanidad Militar was based on a national model whereby the five administrative divisions – Sevilla, Zaragoza, A Coruña, Valladolid and Burgos – registered their requests for materials each trimester starting in January. However, with the rebellion taking place at the start of the third trimester, the distribution centres in Madrid had not yet distributed the new supplies of materials it held.[55] It is worth noting that it was precisely these depleted regional centres that the Insurgents were able to seize in the opening days of the conflict, posing problems of supply right from the start that needed to be rapidly addressed. Some of these early problems were overcome by supplies sent from abroad, with Spanish doctors sympathetic to the Insurgent cause sending medicines. The Spanish millionaire Juan March, a major financial backer of the Insurgency, also arranged for supplies to be sent from Italy.[56]

On the surface at least, supply was not a problem for the government of the Republic who were in control of Madrid and also Barcelona, an important centre for the manufacture of pharmaceuticals. Additionally they could, from early on in the conflict, rely on considerable supplies from abroad, either by directly purchasing them, or through the auspices of the Central Sanitaire Internacional (CSI), the central coordinating committee in Paris, the main distributor of outside medical aid to the Republican Zone.[57] The Republican medical services nevertheless faced their own difficulties, in part as a result of the pharmaceutical industry in 1936 being primarily geared towards the preparation and transformation of raw materials originating, in the main, from outside Spain.[58] As a result of difficulties in supply, in December 1936, Federica Montseny, a key figure in promoting anarchist and socialist cooperation in the field of health, appointed Juan Antonio Azcón Cornell, a Valencian pharmacist and a member of the UGT, to the position of Councillor for the Department of Pharmacy and Supply of the National Health Council.[59] The appointment was made with the intention of centralising pharmaceutical supply for both civilian and military use, and which, according to a speech Montseny gave at a conference in June 1937 resulted in a fully stocked central warehouse. Such statements, however, need treating with caution, as regardless of whether true or not, distribution and supply continued to pose problems throughout the conflict.[60]

By contrast, Román Casares López, a pharmacist from Málaga assimilated into the military in August 1937, in an address that he made on the occasion of his elevation to a professorial chair with the Royal Pharmaceutical Academy in Madrid in 1940, describes how the Insurgent military organised pharmaceutical provision during the Spanish Civil War. He described how, with the rapid depletion of the few remaining regional pharmacy supplies, the Insurgent Sanidad Militar was left with no other option than to organise from the ground up. This involved the construction of industrial parks in Burgos, Sevilla, Valladolid and Zaragoza, and the extensive development of laboratories in the universities of Santiago de Compostela and Granada. He also stated that it was during this period, early on in the conflict, that foreign aid in the form of supplies of pharmaceuticals not available in either military or civic pharmacies was of particular importance, with the 'production houses of friendly nations helping with their donations'.[61]

Casares López also described the importance of being able to access supplies available in pharmacies in towns and cities. Hector Colmegna, an Argentinian doctor and volunteer with a Falangist militia, shortly after his arrival in Spain early in August 1936 was taken to a local pharmacy near Ibarra in the Basque Country by the ensign detailed to take him to his battalion, so that he could stock up on materials for his first aid kit. It was access such as this to local pharmacies at the start of the war that helped alleviate shortfalls in supply.[62]

Both Republican and Insurgent hospitals in the north of Spain were able to take advantage of the proximity of France to buy supplies difficult to acquire in Spain. Cifuentes was supplied by the War Committee sent by the Republicans to facilitate the purchasing of medical materials in France, and the Carlist Hospital de Alfonso Carlos in Pamplona was provisioned by the supply service set up by the Central Carlist War Junta of Navarra headed by the hospital's head of services, Antonio Aznarés.[63]

With the war fought on several fronts in a large geographically diverse and mountainous country, whose national infrastructure had been affected by the division of the country into different zones at the conflict's outset, the routine use of national networks for the distribution of goods was not possible. Therefore, regional organisation became even more important for the transport and supply of pharmaceuticals.[64] Since the most important factory for the production of glass ampoules in Spain in July 1936 was in Republican Valencia, the Insurgents were faced with the additional problem of how to manufacture their own supplies. In Sevilla, the pharmaceutical division for the Army of the South was able to overcome early difficulties in the manufacture and supply of glass ampoules when it took over a workshop in the Trinidad factory and where subsequently 8,380,670 glass ampoules and 31,400 test tubes were produced. The factory was able to deliver the surplus from this production to the army in the north thanks to road access to the north via the territories it controlled in the west of Spain. Sevilla, due to its proximity to Portugal and Gibraltar, was also well placed geographically for accessing additional supplies in these locations.[65] Distribution, however, could be and was problematic, but this was largely mitigated by a regional model of distribution.

In the Republican Zone similar difficulties in distribution were faced in locations isolated from the centre with local initiatives taken to remedy shortfalls in supply an important response. It was through Gibraltar, although in this case from England, that Sir Peter Chalmers Mitchell brought a supply of syringes and 'a large quantity of morphia' to supplement the supplies for the hospital adjoining his house in Malaga in the last week of December 1936. To get to Malaga from Gibraltar he had to wait several days before he could board a British destroyer bound for Malaga, as by this stage, apart from the narrow coastal road to Almeria, Malaga was largely cut off, isolated and poorly supplied.[66]

Sectors of the Southern Front north of Córdoba, due to their more remote locations, also faced similar problems of supply and sought solutions to their problems at a local level. During the summer of 1937, the American Hospital at Belalcázar was able to meet many of their needs after being equipped 'by the cooperative efforts of the mayor of the town, the townspeople, the army and the American mechanics'. They were also the beneficiaries of materials, also supplied courtesy of the mayor, who turned over the equipment of 'a rich fascist doctor' and which included a centrifuge, incubator, steriliser, and other sundry materials.[67]

It was regional production centres, however, that predominantly supplied the local needs of their locales. The pharmaceutical laboratories of Granada, based at the University of Granada and headed by Professor Juan Casas Fernández, became the military pharmacy for the Insurgent Army of the South. The pharmacy produced 2,841 kilograms of anaesthetic ether during the conflict, although this quantity paled into insignificance compared with the sixteen tons produced by the pharmaceutical park of the Army of the North, after the fortunate discovery of eighteen barrels of an unknown liquid discovered in a mine in Asturias turned out to be sulphuric ether. The case of Granada is also of interest in that faced with a scarcity of materials, the pharmacy turned its attention to the collection and cultivation of the biologically diverse local flora.[68] According to the *Crónica de Granada*, plants were collected in the Sierra Nevada, with herbalists gathering their wares close to the frontline under fire from the 'reds', and the 'medicinal plants' collected included foxglove (digitalis), deadly nightshade (belladonna) and monkshood (aconite). These were used to produce cardiac drugs such as atropine from belladonna (a heart drug also used to reduce secretion of mucus during anaesthesia) and digitalis from foxglove to treat irregular heart rhythms.[69]

Elsewhere, in order for the pharmacy to be able to increase its production of silver-based medicines, a number of which were used for the treatment of venereal diseases, General Queipo de Llano in January 1938 called for the people of Sevilla and all of 'liberated Spain to hand in to the military pharmacies … objects of silver that can be sent to the chemical laboratory for the Army of the South in Granada where it can be transformed'.[70] By June 1938, 200 kilograms of silver had been donated 'from the whole of national Spain, from Spanish Morocco … and the distant lands of Spanish America', with a further fifty to sixty kilos of silver 'donated' by the end of the war.[71] The silver collected was used in the production of argirol (a topical antiseptic), protargol (a bactericidal used for the treatment of gonorrhoea), and 229 kilograms of silver nitrate, a caustic agent used widely in surgery.[72]

The role of insurgent women in pharmacy: Gendered propaganda

Female participation was to prove an important element in the early organisation of pharmaceutical provision for the Insurgents. Not only were female volunteers an integral part of the workforce, but their participation was used to reinforce traditional gender roles in newspaper articles that praised their selfless Catholic devotion in the cause of the fatherland.[73] The laboratories in Granada were staffed by a number of different personnel, with the assistance offered by women promoted in the press, with 'seven young "señoritas alumnas" (unmarried young female pupils) who every day go about their labours in a free and spontaneous manner', singled out for mention in an article in the *ABC* of Sevilla on 1 June 1938.[74]

Evidence for the important role played by women in the pharmaceutical industry can be seen by examining the contribution made by female volunteers in the Faculty of Pharmacy at the University of Santiago de Compostela in Galicia. The faculty, which was headed by Luís Maiz Eleizegui, after its incorporation into the Sanidad Militar in April 1937, functioned as a laboratory for the military pharmacy for most of the war.[75] The role played by non-professional female volunteers was to be of particular importance in Santiago, in that there was widespread distrust of teachers and professors in schools and universities by those in authority. This led to many losing employment as it was commonly believed that many within the profession held democratic, masonic or left-wing views, and female workers and volunteers with no political or professional affiliation were frequently employed to make up for this shortfall.[76] The professoriate of the faculty was also known for its liberalism and sympathetic attitudes towards Galicianism, a peculiar blend of nationalism based on a separate language and culture common to most Galicians, and was also heavily sanctioned for this reason, and this also led to a shortfall in staff and a need for their replacement.[77]

The *ABC* of Sevilla for 5 November 1937, in a five-page article above the title 'Santiago: The Fecund Rear-Guard', dedicated the whole of its front page to an image of twenty-three of the 150 women workers of the pharmacy in Santiago next to the mobile pharmacy vehicle that had been built by the faculty. The article described 'the vitally important functions' carried out by 'the selfless and admirable women of Galicia'. They are described as providing comprehensive assistance within the laboratory, with the work portrayed as being 'carried out with the utmost selflessness, and discharged with pride and exceptional competence'. It goes on to describe how the female workforce was made up of staff from the 'normal' university, some students from the faculty itself, with the majority volunteer 'señoritas from Santiago, admirable young ladies motivated by a desire to serve the fatherland'.[78]

Whereas the *ABC*, to a certain extent stressed their professional contribution, articles in the Galician newspaper *El Compostelano* of August 1937 and August 1938 phrased this contribution in a more obviously gendered fashion.[79] In the article of August 1937, Maiz Eleizegui stated that, 'the female element, which since the first moment placed their youthful strength and enthusiasm at the disposal of the laboratory services, showed their true ardour and patriotic selflessness, voluntarily renouncing all pleasure and distraction to dedicate themselves' completely to the work of the laboratory.[80] This propagandistic discourse that portrayed the selfless devotion of the female volunteers, and in the case of the *ABC*, acknowledged certain professional aspects of their work, was quickly forgotten at the end of the war. In 1940 General Peña Torrea, the chief pharmacist of the General Staff of the Army relegated the role of the female volunteers in Santiago to that of 'the proverbial femininity of the Spanish woman', with no equivalent mention of the 'exceptional competence' referred to earlier in the *ABC*.[81]

Although the pharmaceutical laboratories of Santiago were unable to produce pharmaceuticals on a scale equal to that of Granada or Valladolid, it was nevertheless the first laboratory complex to copy and then produce French medicines unavailable in Spain. In 1938 it produced Septicemina, a drug used in urinary tract infections including gonorrhoea, a common condition suffered by many soldiers across Spain; and women played an important part in the success of the laboratory.[82] The Faculty of Pharmacy in Santiago also built and supplied a fully equipped mobile laboratory with both facilities for analysis and the dispensation of medicines aboard. The mobile pharmacy, fabricated by the faculty, a nine-metre-long fully equipped dispensary, was largely financed by music and dance events put on throughout Galicia by the female volunteers. It was used on a number of fronts to dispense pharmaceuticals, including at Teruel in January 1938, during the Battle of the Ebro later that year, and also during the Levante campaign towards the end of the war. It, therefore, provided an important service to sectors of the front whose access to supplies in the rear-guard was complicated by the difficulties of the geographically diverse terrain.[83]

Ultimately, despite the important role played by women behind the lines in the Insurgent Zone, with the women's section of the Falange under the leadership of Pilar Primo de Rivera, one of the main organisations supporting the Francoist war effort during the conflict, Insurgent propaganda portrayed their contribution within a strictly gendered Catholic feminine tradition.[84] As a result of the emphasis on the subordinate role of women in Falangist and Francoist propaganda, the contribution made by women in the Insurgent Zone has largely been obscured; nevertheless, their contribution to the Francoist war effort should not be underestimated.

The focus of this examination has been primarily on pharmaceutical provision as an organisational model in the Insurgent Zone. Although there were scarcities of pharmaceutical materials in the Republican Zone, the control of major industrial centres where pharmaceuticals were produced ensured that these shortages could frequently be made good by increased production, and this was especially true of Catalunya. It was in Barcelona towards the end of the war that a pharmacist, Dr Esteve, was able to synthesise the first sulphonamides available in the Republican Zone, effective anti-bacterial drugs, with seventy-five per cent destined for military use with the remainder made available to the civilian population. The continued existence of laboratory facilities that predated the war in and around Barcelona made this production possible.[85]

Additionally, in Catalunya, as in other areas of Republican Spain, medicines donated from abroad were directly distributed from the warehouses of the Generalitat to hospitals and town halls in those areas affected by bombardments. Massons, in the *Historia de Sanidad Militar*, emphasises in relation to what he describes as the well organised pharmaceutic provision in the Republican Zone that it was only on one occasion that his unit briefly ran out of surgical alcohol. His narrative does not, however, take into account the at times serious local shortfalls that on occasion did occur. Nevertheless, the organisation of pharmaceutical provision throughout Spain, despite early difficulties in manufacture and supply, evolved during the conflict to meet the growing demands of an increasing number of the sick and the wounded.[86]

Frontline medical services

As the above case study demonstrates, the initial problem of the provision and manufacture of pharmaceutical supply in both the Insurgent and to a lesser degree in the Republican Zones was overcome through a mixture of local, regional, 'national' and international efforts. Similar problems were faced when it came to the organisation of surgical provision at or near the front, which, despite existing facilities, had to be 'created from the bottom to the top'.[87] As part of this process, forward systems of care for the wounded in both Republican and Insurgent Zones developed. These models, which shared common characteristics in their evolution, were in part based upon earlier models of forward care that emerged towards the end of WWI (but that also in the early stages of the war included more spontaneous variants). Spanish doctors during WWI, acting as neutral observers, had observed the workings of both French and British hospitals, both near the front and in the rearguard, and this was to have a direct influence on developments within military health in the Protectorate and in turn fed into changes that took place later in Spain.[88]

Building on the experiences of the First World War

The Spanish system for the provision of forward care was structured around the royal decree of 1896, 'The Regulation of Sanitary Services during Campaigns'. Despite the evolution and developments that occurred within the Sanidad Militar, this was still in force at the start of the Spanish Civil War.[89] The developments that did occur resulted from changes that took place during the period of Spain's consolidation of power in the Protectorate, when adapting to the difficulties of fighting a prolonged series of conflicts in the north of Morocco, a more mobile model of forward care evolved after the 'disaster at Annual'.[90] Gómez Ulla, who worked in Madrid before joining the Insurgents in November 1938, designed a mobile hospital with an operating theatre based upon his observations of Alpine ambulance services and forward treatment centres in the Vosges region in France during WWI. It had slatted wooden floors, Persian-blind-type wooden walls designed for easy transport that could be dismantled and carried on lorries (or on mule-back if the terrain was difficult), and was used extensively during the Moroccan campaigns of the 1920s.[91]

However, as a result of the division of Spain and the fracturing of any centralised form of organisational control over the Sanidad Militar at the start of the Spanish Civil War, the ground-up approach that characterised the early phase of the conflict led to the evolution of different approaches to the provision of forward care. It is this organisation, and the influence of models of care that evolved towards the end of WWI, that forms the focus of the following section. This connection to the lessons learnt from WWI is perhaps no more evident than in an article of 26 October 1940, in the *British Medical Journal* (*BMJ*), titled 'Surgical Experience in the Spanish War'. The article states that:

> at the present time the treatment of wounds is in the forefront of the minds of a large section of the medical profession, and the principles which guide us in this work are in the main based on extensive experience gained in the four-years [*sic*] war of 1914–1918.

It goes on, however, to make the argument that this experience had to a degree been put to the test in France earlier in the year, nevertheless, no 'systematic study' had yet been possible of 'problems that await solution' and it was for this reason that he advocated learning from the recent experience of the Spanish Civil War. It was with this in mind that the unnamed reviewer recommended that attention should be paid to the recently published work by Douglas W. Jolly, late Major of the Spanish Republican Medical Service, *Field Surgery in Total War*.[92]

Jolly, a New Zealand-born surgeon, served with a mobile surgical unit of the Sanidad Militar on a number of fronts in Spain from December 1936 to November 1938. He was well placed during this period to record first-hand how surgical care was organised and delivered during much of the conflict in the Republican Zone. In his influential monograph, he describes how the Three Point Forward System (TPFS) for the early treatment of serious casualties at or near the front evolved in Spain, with the aim of treating urgent casualties within five hours. The TPFS, 'based on the self-sufficient mobile surgical unit' as described by Jolly, evolved from pre-existing models for the treatment of casualties that began to emerge at the end of WWI.[93]

The system that evolved in Spain in the Republican Zone consisted of (1) the Casualty Classification Post; (2) the No. 1 Hospital (also known as Hospitales de Vanguardia and Hospitales de Sangre) where those cases requiring immediate surgical intervention were dealt with; and (3) the No. 2 Hospital, also known as the rear-guard hospital, for the less urgent cases.[94] The Spanish Civil War differed from WWI in that it was, for the most part, a far more mobile conflict.[95] It also differed from WWI in that major cities, such as Madrid and Barcelona were besieged, and also suffered from mass aerial bombardments that occasioned thousands of fatalities throughout the conflict.[96] Despite the fatalities that resulted from these air raids, surviving casualties were often able to access hospital facilities within a short a period of time in frontline hospitals such as in the converted hospital in the Casino in Madrid the Hotel Ritz, or the model hospital of Montjuich in Barcelona. This rapid access to treatment helped alleviate the suffering of thousands of civilians and soldiers alike.[97]

The TPFS was in part based on the forward model for the treatment of the wounded during WWI, specifically the Casualty Clearing Station (CCS), but reorganised into its 'functional elements'.[98] The CCS, however, did not begin to function properly as a surgical unit prior to July 1916 due to opposition from surgeons in base hospitals and, unfortunately, it was not until the late autumn of 1916 that casualty clearing stations, 'on the Somme front at least, adopted the policy of the "early operation" on all the seriously wounded'.[99] Despite the large distances often involved in the treatment of such casualties, adapting to the needs of a prolonged conflict with appallingly high casualty rates meant that, by 1918, some subdivision of the function of the CCS had taken place and abdominal cases that in 1914 had been deemed inoperable, were being operated upon 'at certain field ambulances'. It was primarily upon this subdivision that the TPFS was based. In Spain during the Spanish Civil War, as on the Western Front during WWI, it was adapting to the changing nature of warfare and the challenging of outdated models of forward organisation that was to prove important in the evolution of care of the wounded. However, it was in Spain, Jolly argues, where the line between the frontline and rear-guard, the military and the civilian, was increasingly blurred, that this system was most effectively deployed for the first time[100]

A point of departure from the previous experience of care of the wounded during WWI were the genuine efforts to cut down on the period between being wounded and receiving treatment, and efforts that were largely facilitated by the major battle fronts being accessible by road or rail.[101] It was the restructuring of the CCS during the Spanish Civil War, placing a greater emphasis on its role as a classification post, which marked the main point of departure from previous models, in that no longer did the wounded have to pass through numerous treatment posts to receive the appropriate care. Instead, patients were, where possible, sent directly to an appropriate hospital after having received first aid.[102] Although the early treatment of casualties was not always possible, such as during the retreat in Catalunya during the closing phase of the war, significant improvements were made in dealing with the issue of the 'time lag' in treatment.[103]

The consensus among surgeons was that the optimal time for intervention to be successful and thus avoid infection and serious post-operative complications, was within five hours to seven hours, although Jolly argued for the shorter five-hour period.[104] This time limit was important because, by the time of the Spanish Civil War, 'clean wounds', of the sort described by Mazo Buron in León at the start of the conflict, were a thing of the past, as modern weaponry meant that wounds were often contaminated with soil and other debris.[105] As a result of the overall reduction of time between being wounded and receiving treatment, mortality rates resulting from major abdominal wounds were considerably reduced. There was a reduction in the incidents of death from haemorrhagic shock (caused by the loss of blood), and amputation of limbs as a result of gas gangrene and other infections due to delayed treatment fell significantly during the conflict in both Republican and Insurgent Zones.[106] However, despite improvements in mortality rates that can in part be attributed to the TPFS, many thousands of the wounded died as a result of lengthy transfers, due to Spain's challenging geography, and the often poor state of the roads. Nevertheless, significant improvements were made in bringing down transfer times, but in a conflict with numerous fronts and in one of Europe's most mountainous countries, ideal models of evacuation could not always be uniformly and universally applied.[107]

Evidence for the evolution of the Three Point Forward System

Tracking the evolution of the TPFS in Spain is not without its difficulties; however, sufficient evidence for how the system developed during the conflict can be found in a number of sources. Nevertheless, as Jolly states in the preface to *Field Surgery in Total War*:

> unfortunately, most of the surgeons with the best right to record the experience of the Republican Medical Service, are, in present circumstances unable to do so … Many of those most concerned with this organisation are in prison, others are in exile.[108]

Many of those who served in the Republican Medical Services during the conflict who were unable to flee were either barred from public office or faced prison, and this was to have a devastating effect on public health following the war. Bastos Ansart was expelled from the army after thirty-two years of service in 1939, was briefly incarcerated after the Insurgent victory, his titles were annulled and he was barred from public practice.[109]

Bastos Ansart, did, however, leave an imprint on the literature through a number of articles he wrote during the conflict on how surgical care should be delivered, which make reference to a similar model of forward care as that described by Jolly.[110] These articles, while maintaining a focus on forward organisation, tend to in the main concentrate on surgical technique. They are all in one way or another concerned with a matter-of-fact, 'common sense' approach to surgical matters, and were aimed at the optimisation of surgical time, which he saw as being all too frequently wasted by surgeons over-concerned with either practising their own specialties or spending hours operating on patients with no hope of survival.[111] It is these articles that Bastos Ansart wrote on the organisation of surgery of the Republican Medical Services, alongside Jolly's monograph and articles written by other doctors, that provide the evidence for how medical services were organised from the frontline to the rear in the Republican Zone.[112]

The evidence for the TPFS is more difficult to reconstruct when it comes to how widely it was deployed in the Insurgent Zone, but Massons, in *Historia de la Sanidad Militar*, argues that the provision for the early surgical treatment of those seriously wounded in the Insurgent Zone evolved along similar lines.[113] This argument is given added weight by a leading Insurgent surgeon, Manuel Gómez Durán, who worked on a number of fronts including Madrid during the conflict, in articles he wrote for the medical journal *Galicia Clinica*, and in two articles he wrote for the *Revista Española de Medicina y Cirugía de Guerra* in August 1939. Further evidence for the same or a similar system being in operation is provided by Dr A. López Cotarelo in an article he wrote for *Cuestiones médico-quirúrgicas de guerra*, an edited collection of articles published in Galicia in 1938, that examined medical-surgical questions.[114] Gómez Durán and Cotarelo both describe a system that was similar in its features to that described by Jolly. Both also stressed the importance of rapid surgical treatment to prevent infection taking hold, which was important for the prevention of gas gangrene and other wound infections.[115]

Although there is no direct reference to the system as described by Jolly with reference to the Insurgent Zone, this is largely due to the term being an English one that was therefore not in use in either zone. In his monograph, Massons describes a similar system in operation in the Republican Zone, but refers to the evacuation of the wounded and the 'puestos de classificacion' (classification posts). Insurgent journals use similar language to describe this system, with Gómez Durán referring to classification posts, classification halls and 'puesto quirúrgico' (surgical post) for the same unit.[116] The journal articles examined here provide evidence for similar models of forward care in operation in both the Republican and Insurgent Zones. What is now considered is an analysis of how this organisation worked in practice in a number of settings, from small-scale offensives to larger battles and campaigns.

The July/August edition of the *Libertad*, an anarchist 'fortnightly for the front', carried an article titled 'Health on Campaign', written by the MO of the 59th Mixed Brigade, Francisco Rico Belestá.[117] Belestá describes in detail how the 'health service' at the front had evolved in the Sector of the Centre since the start of the war, with the use of this term indicative of an anarchist approach to health that saw care of the wounded combatant as an integral part of its drive for the wider socialisation of medicine.[118] *Libertad*, a periodical that contained doctrinal and propagandistic articles and was additionally aimed at encouraging a greater level of literacy among the troops, also contained articles that were accurate in their description of how the provision of military health worked.[119]

Belestá, in his description of the Sanidad Militar of the brigade also directly addressed issues surrounding the supposed disorganisation and chaos of the medical services, in order to counter what he saw as a false narrative. He states that health provision for war, in spite of claims to the contrary, was present from the start, and although he describes this as 'scarce and without direction', and despite there being no military order, that there was nevertheless a level of organisation 'through appropriate and spontaneous will'. He further emphasises this point by stating that the surgical and first aid teams were 'truly autonomous' and that it was these rudimentary structures, whether those that were in existence or those that sprung up, which was an important factor in how these services evolved.[120]

In an article he wrote for a later edition of *Libertad*, Belestá included two of his own diagrams outlining how forward care was organised in his sector.[121] The first of the diagrams is similar to the diagrammatic representation contained in *Field Surgery in Total War*, and shows that by August 1937 the TPFS as later described by Jolly was already the established model for the Republican Army of the Centre.[122] This article, apart from its anti-fascist preamble, is similar in composition to those found in journals and is matter-of-fact in its content. It is possible, however, that the diagrams, if not the article itself, had appeared in a different publication or a journal as he refers to the diagrams being numbers one and two, whereas on the diagrams themselves they are numbered differently.[123] A similar schematic appeared in the Insurgent medical journal *Revista Española de Medicina y Cirugía de Guerra* of March 1939 shortly before the end of the conflict.[124] The article by the Chief of Military Health for the Army Corps of Castilla, Medical Lieutenant Colonel Ignacio Oleo Herraiz, outlines a system of forward care similar to that described by Jolly and Rico Belestá, and a similar system is described by Gómez Durán, in the August 1939 edition of the *Revista Española de Medicina y Cirugía de Guerra*.[125] These articles, when examined alongside those previously cited, provide further evidence for the argument that forward surgical care did not differ significantly in either zone.

The anarchist-driven discourse on more spontaneous models of organisation as expressed by Belestá is usually dismissed as a reason for the disorganisation of the Republican military health services in the early stages of the conflict. However, the proliferation of local services that sprung up at the start of the conflict also meant that it was possible to assimilate numerous medical units into a bourgeoning military health service and thus provide care in a wide variety of locations.[126] Localised models for organisation took a number of forms. On 24 July 1936, a 'hospital de sangre' was created by the Partido Obrero de Unificación Marxista (Workers' Party of Marxist Unification or POUM) in Barcelona after it seized the Hotel Falcón and the Cabaret Monaco. A twenty-five-bed frontline hospital in the small town of Requena in the Province of Valencia was founded by a local 'revolutionary' committee in August 1936. During the same month, the expropriated private palace of the millionaire Juan March was converted into a hospital by the Unified Socialist Youth (Las Juventudes Socialistas Unificadas or JSU). The creation of such hospitals facilitated the work of the Sanidad Militar of the Republic in building a modern service for the delivery of medical care across those areas of Spain it controlled, as the existence of a wide array of medical units, both large and small, meant that these could be assimilated into a more centralised organised structure.[127]

The article that Belestá wrote for the July/August edition of *Libertad* is also of interest in that it explores how the system for forward care evolved within a more localised context. It makes the claim that on the Toledo Front, in the Olías del Teniente Castillo y Vargas Sector, of the 500 wounded on 28 September 1936, all passed through the forward classification post, with urgent cases sent to nearby Madrid and non-urgent cases sent on to other hospitals. Belestá describes how in October of that year the team he headed withdrew to reorganise, and that it was from that point on that the true military health began to organise itself. To support this claim, he explains how forward care was organised when the unit were sent to a new sector in the Sierra de Albarracín the following year with the aim of disrupting communication between Teruel and Zaragoza. Each battalion, he claims, had its own medical team, which were under the control of a head of service centrally located under the leadership of a Medical Commander.[128] Belestá describes how the militiamen and soldiers who passed through the first aid and classification posts were then sent further back to the No. 1 Hospital in Cuenca. Once they had reached the convalescence state in their treatment they were then sent on to the hospital of Cañizar. This hospital had been set up by Pedro Vallina Martínez, a militant anarchist doctor, and the model for the evacuation of the wounded described by Belestá, closely resembles the system described by Jolly.[129]

Further evidence for how forward care developed in this sector can be found in a separate article in *Libertad* concerning the capture of Albarracín the previous month, written by the Senior Commander for Health of the 59th Mixed Brigade, Donato Nombela Gallardo in August 1937. In an illustrated three-page article, the installation of health facilities at Albarracín and their functioning is described by the author.[130] It was in Albarracín that the mobile 'Vanguard Hospital' (of which there are two photographs in the article) was placed. This consisted of a wooden barracks hospital, similar in design to the one designed by Gómez Ulla, that could be dismantled and transported to a new location as required.[131]

Gallardo, of whom little is known, had served as an MO in the Protectorate, and it is likely that this would have had an influence on how the sanitary health services were organised in Albarracín.[132] Pedro Vallina, who apart from his role as a doctor was also an active revolutionary, and who had been in prison on several occasions and exiled or expelled from Spain many times, dismissed Gallardo as a Jesuit and a fascist spy in his memoir *Mis Memorias*.[133] This, however, would seem unlikely given that Gallardo had previously been involved in helping organise a hospital train for an anarchist militia, and *Libertad* on more than one occasion praises him.[134] Gallardo went on to serve in the Levante sector as he was transferred to the XIX Division in December 1937, but after that there is no further mention of him in official state papers, which would also suggest that he did not go over to the Francoist forces.[135]

In the Central Sector, as in other sectors on both sides of the lines, the often prompt treatment received by the wounded was not only important in reducing mortality rates but, as argued by Jolly and Belestá, was also an important factor in maintaining the morale of the troops.[136] Rapid treatment, however, was not always possible. Those wounded in night-time attacks were often not recovered before the following day, and aerial attacks on ambulances and the disruption and destruction of communication networks also impacted upon the surgical team's ability to treat patients within the five-to-seven-hour optimal period of treatment.[137] During the Battle of the Ebro, one of the largest campaigns of the Spanish Civil War, which was primarily aimed at protecting Valencia and re-establishing contact with Catalunya so as to reunite the Republican Zone, troops on both sides suffered as a result of a breakdown in organisation.[138] During a Republican retreat across the river Ebro in late July 1938, the Insurgents opened the 'flood-gates of the great hydro-electric dams on the Segre river system', which washed away the pontoon bridges and barges that were being used to facilitate troop movements and evacuate the wounded. During the rapid retreat it was impossible to establish forward hospitals and many of the wounded could not be retrieved, and problems associated with their evacuation were exacerbated by the loss of ambulances and an autochir (a mobile operating theatre) due to aerial attacks. These problems, however, were to a degree mitigated by the establishment of a tent hospital by retreating troops between Batea and Gandesa, and by the fact that the small mobile surgical units were more easily redeployed.[139]

Troops from the Moroccan Army Corps also suffered problems during the Battle of the Ebro due to delays in treatment, which actually led to a brief dispute between two Insurgent medical chiefs over whether in this instance the seven-hour period of treatment was indeed proven to reduce infection and sepsis. Shortly before the end of the Battle of the Ebro, the Chief MO of the Moroccan Army Corps wrote to his counterpart for the Army of the North expressing his concern that a large number of wounded had arrived at hospitals outside of the optimal time period. He proposed that the number of surgical teams in the frontline hospitals should be increased so that the wounded could receive forward care more promptly. In response the Head of Health for the Army of the North stated that, 'the classification that is made of the wounded is more theory than fact' when it came to whether the seven-hour rule was relevant or not, and that this also held true for the findings on the treatment of wounds within this timeframe. He also stressed that under the system proposed by his colleague 5,000 beds would have been needed, and highlighted the considerable difficulties that had been involved in organising the 2,000 beds available for that sector. He then went on to argue that in the quieter periods forward surgery had been carried out, that fracture patients were best transferred to Zaragoza, and that if the work carried out by the Classification Posts was properly applied, that his Command 'considered the health elements gathered in this sector sufficient' to meet the needs of the Moroccan Army Corps. He did, however, acknowledge that the 'sanitary organisation for this period of operations, may not have been the model to follow'. He did, however, stress that it was a model to be held up and admired when functioning properly, and that there had never been 'a lack of beds or surgical teams, more than twelve kilometres from the front'.[140]

The articles written by Belestá and Gallardo although only concerned with one front of many during the Spanish Civil War, when placed alongside the works cited above point towards the TPFS being a model for forward care that was widely deployed during the Spanish Civil War. It would appear, however, that despite the publication of a number of journals on both sides during the conflict, these were not always widely available. The North American surgeon Leo Eloesser who served with a Spanish mobile surgical unit, highlighted the need for journals and wrote to colleagues in America requesting that these be sent to him. He also pointed out that 'many doctors read theirs and discard them', which might also explain why relatively few survive.[141] Additionally, many Republican medical personnel would have destroyed written material at the end of the conflict that was in any way connected with non-Francoist publications, as possession of such materials could, and did, lead to persecution and prosecution.[142]

The scarcity of journals, also presents a problem when it comes to examining and analysing how other frontline services worked, such as the precautions taken against the use of chemical weapons, and it is for this reason that a number of different sources need to be examined when looking at different aspects of forward care. It is an examination of how the Republicans and Insurgents organised in preparation for the possible use of chemical warfare, something that many people across Spain feared might be used both at the front and at the rear, which forms the focus of the following section on forward care. This allows for an exploration of the further input by anarchist medical personnel in seeking to further their own revolutionary agenda of political and social aims within the Republican Zone, which further demonstrates that the differences that existed in how the medical services were organised during the conflict in the Republican and Insurgent Zones were as a result of opposing autonomous and centrist ideological models.

Preparing for chemical warfare: Realities and propaganda

On 8 August 1936, three weeks after the outbreak of the uprising on the Spanish mainland the besieged garrison in the Alcázar of Toledo came under attack from incapacitating agents.[143] At 7.45 am, the fortress was the target of sixteen 'conventional' bombs dropped from a large three-engine aeroplane. This was followed shortly after by another plane that 'dropped tear-gas bombs ... but as a drill had been evolved to deal with such eventualities the inconvenience caused was not great'.[144] A few months later, on 3 December 1936, Indalecio Prieto, the Republican Minister for the Navy and Aviation sent the following telegram to Josep Tarradellas, the Minister of Economics: 'I request with the utmost insistence, that if there are any masks in storage, that you send them with all urgency to Madrid where the enemy has started employing the use of gases.'[145]

There were other unconfirmed reports of the use of chemical agents during the conflict that appeared in the press and official despatches in both Spain and abroad, but there seems to be little evidence for their wider use beyond a few instances when tear gas was used.[146] There were also accusations of the use of more aggressive chemicals. The *Times* on 4 December 1936 carried a brief article in which it was alleged that a new unspecified 'gas' had been used by 'the Red Army against General Franco's forces'. The 'gas' was reported as having penetrated all masks rendering them ineffective, resulting in more than 500 casualties. The article reported that test quantities of the substance were 'taken in the ordinary way' for analysis by chemists from Germany, Italy, Spain and France; but unless these test results were suppressed (a possibility that should not be ruled out), there appeared no further reports in the *Times* that refer to the alleged attack.[147]

In the *Annals of the Royal Academy of Medicine – 1943*, Joaquín Mas Guindal y Calderero makes the claim that there was sporadic use of 'gases' (in all likelihood tear gas), that caused irritation of the nasal passages, used in the North of Spain in the locality of Cilleruelo de Bricia.[148] He also stated that fortunately for the Spanish, chemical warfare (with the above exception) did not make an 'appearance in the tragic fratricidal conflict', but that nevertheless it had still been necessary for each side to take precautions in case of its use.[149]

The precautions taken on each side in case chemical warfare operations commenced seem to have been extensive. The organisation involved in this level of preparation reflected not just the fear that chemical warfare might be deployed by either side, but that this fear was based on the knowledge that the practical deployment of such weapons was possible, if the necessary investment were made to enable their production.[150] Senior army officers on both sides who had served in the Protectorate between 1925 and 1927 would have known of their use in the Rif and therefore preparation against their possible use was seen as a necessary step in civil and military defence. Furthermore, Franco as early as August 1936 had asked Mussolini to supply him with chemical weapons and gas masks but the Italian leader had ignored this request. However, his second request in January 1937 was more successful and included the delivery of fifty tons of mustard gas bombs, and the despatch of Italian troops trained in chemical warfare. Germany too supplied similar quantities of these weapons to Franco.[151] For Republican-held Madrid, the control of the chemical weapons factory at La Marañosa close to the capital – where chemical agents, including mustard gas, had been produced for use in the Protectorate as early as June 1923 – meant that they would have had access to the residual stocks of certain chemical weapons. This is possibly where the tear gas that was used on the Alcázar originated. Nevertheless, at the start of the conflict there is no available evidence to suggest that chemical agents were being produced.[152] There were plans, however, made by the Republican Government, to produce chemical weapons, and contacts were established with the War Industries Committee (Comité de Industrias de

Guerra or CIG) of the Generalitat in Barcelona, but despite the construction of two factories in Catalunya for this purpose, chemical weapons were never produced at these sites.[153]

As part of the propaganda war, both the Republicans and the Insurgents accused each other on occasion of deploying chemical armaments, as the use of chemical munitions were banned under international law.[154] General Millán Astray, in response to the charge made by the Spanish minister Julio Álvarez del Vayo at the League of Nations that the Insurgents had used and were using chemical weapons on Madrid, accused the Republicans of attempting to produce chemical weapons at La Marañosa, albeit unsuccessfully.[155] Although La Marañosa had been the main factory involved in chemical weapons production, the Insurgents too had access to similar facilities in Melilla. In 1922, the factory in Melilla had begun the production of shells filled with phosgene (or collangite), a choking agent, and chloropicrin, an irritant with the characteristics of tear gas, and later went on to produce mustard gas for use in the Rif. However, like La Marañosa, it never resumed production.[156] La Marañosa eventually fell to the Insurgents in February 1937 during the Battle of Jarama, but by this stage the facilities of the complex had already been dismantled and transferred to the Concentaina Factory in Alcoi, in case it fell into enemy hands.[157]

Despite the presence of two factories, that, in theory at least, were able to produce chemical weapons, Spain's chemical industries were still largely subordinate to foreign interests. The French firm Cros dominated not only Spain's main chemical industrial sector in Catalunya, but the industry across Spain. Therefore, the chemical industry in Spain was not in the position of countries such as France or Germany, with large industrial chemical industries that could easily supply materials for rapid conversion into chemical weapons, as they were dependent upon supplies from abroad. La Marañosa had additionally suffered from underinvestment and neglect and it was for this reason that the CIG in Catalunya had been approached as the investment required in La Marañosa would have been costly, with its location making it particularly vulnerable to enemy attack.[158]

Despite the fact that the ability to produce chemical weapons in Spain was severely circumscribed, the fears on the Republican side that Germany or Italy – the nation that was alleged to have used chemical weapons in Ethiopia – might supply these to the Insurgents, and the additional strain this would put on existing medical services, prompted widespread measures for the protection of civilians and soldiers alike.[159] For the Insurgents, predominantly led by a military elite who had served with the Army of Africa in the Protectorate and who were familiar with the use of chemical weapons in the Rif, the fear that the Republican Government might resort to the use of chemical warfare also led to preparations to protect against their use.[160] This concern, for Franco at least, would have been exacerbated by the knowledge that, given the right opportunity, he himself would have deployed the chemical munitions he had received from both Italy and Germany in

January 1937. The likely determining factor in staying Franco's hand was the international scrutiny Spain was under, and his familiarity with their use in the Protectorate, where every effort had been made to keep their use secret, would also have meant that he was familiar with the controversy surrounding their potential use.[161]

Republican civil defence measures

The evidence for how services were organised for defence against chemical weapons in the Republican Zone is more abundant; therefore, it is these that are examined first. Military preparations on both sides were similar in organisation but, as previously stated, it was in the civilian sphere that there were noticeable differences.[162]

Francisco Trigo Dominguez was the first medical practitioner to organise an 'antigás' battalion in Spain, being both a member of its political committee as well as its captain; and Pedro Vallina was also active in this area.[163] There was a hospital set up in Madrid for the potential victims of chemical warfare, which had at its disposal designated ambulances equipped with oxygen cylinders, a commodity otherwise unavailable, even in operating theatres, except in very rare circumstances.[164] These ambulances had space for four stretchers and facilities for washing potential victims and additionally carried three artificial respirators and were fully equipped with instruments and medicines.[165] There were many shelters created as refuges against attacks, generally in basements that could be sealed against the infiltration of chemical agents by sealing doorways, windows and openings with paper tape.[166] Additionally, literature aimed at civilians provided advice both written and pictorial on how to protect homes in the same manner as the refuges.[167]

Newspapers and periodicals with a wide circulation in towns and at the front contained articles and features that followed preparations being made in Britain, where extensive measures were taking place in a nation where it was widely feared that a new world war was imminent, and that when it came, chemical weapons would be used against the civilian population. These articles, which frequently reference the use of chemical weapons during WWI, would have contributed to concerns among both the civilian population and the military. These were aimed both at preparing the population for such an eventuality, but also as propaganda aimed at maintaining a preparedness for war throughout Republican-controlled areas.[168]

The Republican popular press was the main means for the dissemination of information concerning civilian defence. Apart from carrying announcements for courses run by the National Committee for the Prevention of Chemical Warfare (Comité Nacional Antigás) established soon after the outbreak of the conflict by the Ministry of Health, or reporting on a well-attended gathering in a square in Valencia where the rapid placing of a gas mask was being demonstrated, it also carried articles warning against the purchase of fake gas masks from war profiteers.[169] There are no figures for how many gas masks were issued for civilian or indeed military use, but indications pointing towards problems of supply can be found in various references in the press to the capture of various quantities of enemy gas masks. On 7 January 1938, *La Vanguardia* carried a brief notice advising all those who worked in the port in Valencia that the gas masks they had been issued with were to be returned upon leaving employment, and that these should be disinfected for the use of new employees.[170] Valencia, in many ways exemplified an important rear-guard city that could also be described as being in the frontline, as it had suffered attacks from aerial and naval bombardments. As such, fear of chemical weapons attack on the city led to calls for a much stronger organisation within the city against such an eventuality.[171]

An article that is of particular interest in relation to a key figure in chemical warfare defence preparations appeared in *Crónica*, a Madrid weekly periodical with high circulation, on 16 January 1938.[172] The article in question was a special feature on the anarcho-syndicalist doctor Juan Morata Cantón, an important figure in the Spanish Red Cross who was first appointed as its vice-secretary on 29 July 1936, later becoming its secretary general in September 1936, a post he held throughout the war.[173] On 15 May 1937, Morata Cantón, who during the course of the war wrote and published works on chemical warfare, founded the Sanitary Brigade for the Prevention of Chemical Warfare (Brigada Sanitaria Antigás), taking up the role of inspector general.[174] This organisation, however, was suppressed later that year by decree on 30 September. This was likely due to government fear of anarchist influence within the brigade, with Morata Cantón a member of the CNT, during a period when the centrist socialist left was consolidating its hold on the reins of power during the premiership of Juan Negrín.[175]

Morata Cantón who was also president of the National Syndicate for Health and Hygiene, was also affiliated to the more militant FAI. He had worked for the Mutual Health Society for Workers (Mutua Obrera Sanitaria) in Madrid in the 1920s, was a distinguished member of the Unified Syndicate of Health and Hygiene in the capital and was an active campaigner for the socialisation of medicine.[176] In the interview that formed the basis for the special feature that appeared in *Crónica* in January 1938, he talked to the journalist Juan del Sarto about his recently published book *Defensa de guerra tóxico química* (*Defence against Toxic Chemical Warfare*).[177]

In the article, in which Morata Cantón sought to promote an anarchist discourse on health, he stated that he had written the book alongside colleagues who assisted him in the task to ensure that 'the civilian population acquire the knowledge for their own defence against the possibility of attack by chemical and bacteriological toxins during this drawn out and painful conflict'. This point was taken up by the article's author, Juan del Sarto, who stressed that the aim of the publication was to empower people through being informed of how to avoid the dangers of exposure to chemical weapons, so that 'they can liberate themselves from the terrible gases of war'. Sarto also highlighted concerns expressed by Morata regarding false information contained in the numerous pamphlets that were circulating. Many of these were stating in relation to chemical weapons that 'nothing will happen, they will not be employed', a position that was described as 'stupid optimism'. Morata Cantón concluded his interview by stating that if people were equipped to avoid 'this peril', then the job that he and his colleagues (whose 'equal' contribution he highlights) had set out to do in writing the book would have been achieved.[178]

There is a certain amount of polemic involved in such articles, but this article is nevertheless of interest as not only does it provide evidence for a relatively unknown but important medical figure, it also provides further evidence for the influence of anarchist doctors in the field of public health and civil defence. Aside from the posts described above, Morata Cantón was also the president of the Board of Directors of the College of Medicine in Madrid, secretary for public relations for the Committee of Liaison CNT/UGT, a permanent member of the National Federation of Health and Hygiene and MO of the Health Service of the Frontier Guards.[179]

Insurgent civil defence measures

The surviving evidence for how the Insurgents organised to protect against the possible use of chemical warfare is less abundant than that available for the Republicans, with only a few references outside of articles in journals and monographs which refer to how these services were organised. This scarcity of materials also extended to the Official State Bulletin (Boletín Oficial del Estado or BOE) published in Burgos, where there is no reference made to 'antigás' personnel. However, there are several references in the bulletin to sergeant practitioners, although it does not provide details of their duties, but it was these medics who were charged with providing first aid to potential chemical warfare victims.[180] Additionally MOs charged with the care of the wounded in the event of an attack with chemical weapons were appointed according to military title and rank, and therefore it is not possible to distinguish within the BOE which MO or other medical personnel was appointed to which specific task.[181] However, an article written by the MO Hermenegildo Balmori titled 'Anti-Gas Sanitary Services: Tactics and Organisation of Army Services', in the *Revista Española de Medicina y Cirugía de Guerra* in 1938, and the chapter 'Chemical Warfare' by Guindal y Calderero, in the *Annals of the Royal Academy of Medicine – 1943*, provide evidence for how these services were organised.[182]

In the *Annals* for 1943, Calderero describes how in the Insurgent Zone a school for the study of chemical warfare (Escuela de Guerra Química) was established in Salamanca. After attending the course run by the school, officials from the army, navy and air force were then qualified to join their squads. Calderero also describes how these squads always accompanied the distinct units of the army in all their operations. They were, however, referred to ironically by the author as the units of non-intervention, as their services were never called upon.[183] Balmori's article, by contrast, offers a far more detailed account of how the services were organised in the Insurgent Zone, providing photographic evidence of a drill exercise showing various personnel in masks and rubber suits, some of whom are standing next to baths and other washing facilities for the treatment of victims.[184] The article describes a system of care that in its outline is similar to the TPFS as described by Jolly and thus provides additional evidence for the TPFS being the model in use, or being aspired to, in the conflicting zones.[185] In his preamble, the author does take exception to the use of the term 'Sanitary Anti-Gas Services' for not being scientific, given that many of the chemicals in questions were not actually gases but liquids. Nevertheless, as it was the 'sanctioned' term, he uses it throughout.

Balmori describes the mission of the service as being the collection and evacuation of the affected soldiers to the forward 'antigás' posts and then on to specialist hospitals where they could receive the appropriate treatment. If treatment was necessary in these forward posts, this should be administered there, and if necessary the affected soldiers should be kept in situ until they were stable enough to be moved. He goes on to describe how each evacuation team was made up of sixteen sanitarios (sanitary assistants), eight stretcher-bearers, eight auxiliaries and a sergeant practitioner. This article goes into considerable detail, and includes information on the equipment carried by the sanitary assistants, the personal protection available to both them and the victims of chemical warfare, the procedures for treating the different types of injuries depending on the 'toxic agent' used, and a full description of the agents that might be used and their effects. The chemical agents described included phosgene, chloropicrin and mustard gas; with the treatments described ranging from ocular lavage with bicarbonate of soda for those exposed to irritant agents, through to rest, oxygen and cardiac tonics, for those exposed to phosgene.[186]

The details of the chemicals likely to be encountered and the treatments required are the same as described by Parrilla Hermida in the article titled 'Gases of War', in *Cuestiones médico-quirúrgicas de guerra*, which are also described in the *Annals of the Royal Academy of Medicine*.[187]

What is lacking in the literature on chemical warfare examined for this study, with regards to provision made against chemical warfare in the Insurgent Zone, is information relating to how defences were put into practice, particularly in the civilian sphere. During June 1938, the *ABC* of Sevilla carried an advert promoting the factory in Segovia where 'material of all classes for the protection against gases and airborne toxins of war and industry' could be procured. It also provided a contact address in Sevilla for those wanting 'details and information in the Andalusian region', but this is the only information in the *ABC* of Sevilla relating to defence against chemical warfare.[188] There are references made in the *ABC* of Sevilla regarding the capture of enemy gas masks, with reference to the capture of 12,500 masks at Teruel early in 1938, but it is likely that these were destined for reuse by the military, as references regarding the supply of gas masks for civilian use are absent from the sources examined for this study.[189] A likely reason for this absence is that the top military command, the majority of whom had seen service in the Protectorate and were familiar with the use of chemical weapons there, would have known of the efficacy of these weapons in relation to the topography of the Rif. They would have been familiar with the patterns of exposure of army personnel to chemical warfare in WWI, and thus their primary focus was the protection of battlefield troops in the open and in trenches, as it was these who were perceived to be most at risk.[190]

With regards to military preparations in the Insurgent Zone, Massons makes reference to the pharmaceutical faculty in Granada producing absorbent carbon from olive pips and almond shells for use in gas masks. There is also reference to the pharmaceutical laboratory in Valladolid producing equipment that included 100 rubberised bags for the storage of 'materials for curing' victims, and other equipment. Massons also states that the Insurgents adopted all measures required in case their troops were victims of chemical attack, but makes no mention of preparations in defence for civilians.[191] The *ABC* of Sevilla makes no reference to courses for civil defence against chemical weapons, whereas the *ABC* de Madrid and other Republican newspapers make frequent reference to courses for civilians and for the preparations necessary in case of attack.[192] The likely reason for such omissions in the Insurgent press is that the Insurgents, with a highly centralised military command, addressed their military needs first, and would have then issued commands to civilian governors if and when needed.

Government in the Republican Zone by contrast was far more diversified. Local initiatives were not subject to the same centralised control as was to be found in the Insurgent Zone, and with aerial bombardment of towns and cities far more common in the Republican Zone, civilian civil defence measures, regardless of whether chemical weapons were deployed or not, were a reality that could not be ignored.[193] Preparations made on the opposing sides differed in that, in the Insurgent Zone the emphasis was on military preparation against chemical warfare with the military in charge of civil defence, whereas in the Republican Zone the onus was also put on the civilian population to prepare. Fortunately for both sides during the Spanish Civil War, the widespread and realistic fear that chemical weapons might be deployed did not materialise. Nevertheless, this fear persisted, particularly among the military and medico-military command familiar with the extensive use of chemical weapons in the Rif in the 1920s. As late as January 1939, the Insurgents were concerned that the retreating Republican Army might, in a last-ditch attempt, deploy chemical weapons; in response to these fears, officials distributed a booklet for its Northern Army describing the correct use of a gas mask.[194]

Evacuation of the wounded

The effective provision of forward care during the Spanish Civil War ultimately rested upon the ability of getting the wounded away from the battlefield, or wherever the injury occurred, to the appropriate hospital or treatment centre as quickly as possible. Key to this was motorised transport, whether ambulance, train or ship; but in those areas where this was not possible due to difficulties caused by the terrain, the wounded could be evacuated on cacolets carried on mule-back, although this could involve journeys of several hours.[195] Mules were more widely used for the transport of the wounded in the Insurgent Zone, where the welfare of the animals was overseen by the Veterinary Services of the Sanidad Militar. On the Madrid Front in the autumn of 1937, a military doctor, José Monteys Porta, was placed in charge of a medical unit for the evacuation of the wounded in the Sierra de Guadarrama that included sixty to eighty soldiers and sixty mules.[196]

Airlifts of the wounded also took place on both sides during the conflict, but these were small in number.[197] The system for the airlifting of patients that took place during the Spanish Civil War, was based on the service first established in the Spanish Protectorate in 1925.[198] It was the service for the transport of the wounded established by the Condor Legion for the transfer of the wounded back to Germany, however, that involved the largest number of evacuation by air. These were, similarly, not large in number, and therefore the focus here is on what at the time were the more conventional forms for the evacuation of the wounded: ambulance, train and ship.[199]

Ambulances

At the start of the Spanish Civil War, the distribution of existing ambulance services across Spain was uneven. The slow but steady improvements in public health provision during the 'transformative biennial' of 1931–1933 had resulted in some changes taking place; nevertheless, shortfalls in municipal funding meant that there were large inequalities between the facilities available.[200] As a result of the budgetary constraints this imposed upon the municipalities, major cities were in a better position to respond to the sudden demand for services due to access to better facilities that included a greater concentration of Red Cross and other ambulances of different sizes. Madrid had a number of ambulances belonging to the Red Cross, which were painted white with a red cross on the roof, but many of these were large cumbersome vehicles that lacked mobility and were, on occasion, due to their visibility, the target of enemy planes.[201] In response to an increased need for ambulances that were smaller, faster and more mobile, workshops in Madrid recovered broken-down and abandoned vehicles and converted them into ambulances by either restoring them or by building new chassis.[202] Ambulances were also built in the workshops in Valencia, and this pattern of converting cars and lorries, and, where possible, building new ones, was replicated across Spain in those areas with access to the necessary materials.[203]

The distribution of ambulances across a number of fronts at the start of the conflict also varied, and local and regional initiatives in helping meet the shortfalls found in many locations were important in redressing this balance. On the Alava Front in the north of Spain in July 1936, Insurgent forces possessed seventeen ambulances, but these consisted of seven different models that had been provided by the Municipal Laboratory, the Military Governor, the Red Cross and the local Carlist Requetés. On the Aragón Front in the summer of 1936, Miguel Parrilla, an MO serving with the Insurgent forces, describes how he started out with a company of less than 100 'sanitarios', two assimilated MOs, 'a handful of stretchers, and half a dozen lorries' that had been turned into ambulances. During this early stage, these converted lorries sometimes had to make journeys lasting several hours and hundreds of kilometres to evacuate the wounded.[204]

The shortage of ambulances on both sides of the divide at the start of the conflict meant that difficulties in evacuating the wounded was a problem in need of a rapid solution. The Republicans, initially at least, had greater access to ambulances due to their control of the major urban and industrial centres where services were more concentrated. However, despite difficulties for the Insurgents caused by the inability to access similar facilities, the fact that during the uprising they were able to seize the majority of military bases, and could build upon the existing military infrastructure, would have gone some way in mitigating this shortfall.

The Insurgent medical services addressed their growing need for greater numbers of ambulances when, on 15 October 1936, the Military Command in Burgos issued a circular instructing that the Central Park for Military Health in Burgos be replaced by a new centre for the warehousing of medical material including stretchers and ambulances. This centralisation of materials in Burgos away from the frontlines would have facilitated regional distribution across those fronts in the north most in need of these materials.[205]

The Insurgents were also able to meet some of their early shortages of ambulances through donations from abroad. The Catholic weekly *Universe*, a British newspaper whose editorial stance supported Franco as well as Mussolini, launched an appeal in September 1936 for funds, as 'anti-red forces' were short of medical supplies.[206] As a result of this appeal, eight ambulances were sent to Spain, with the first a fully equipped Austin 20, despatched on 7 November 1936.[207] The British Bishops' Fund for the Relief of Spanish Distress, sent at least two ambulances to Burgos, with the first accompanied by Gabriel Herbert, sister-in-law of the writer Evelyn Waugh, and which also included a lorry with supplies.[208] This early external help, alongside the control of much of the medical military infrastructure and the large quantity of military aid that the Insurgents received from their fascist allies throughout the war, gave the Insurgents an advantage during the conflict as they were largely freed from the need to concentrate their efforts on the acquisition of military materials.[209]

The historiography, apart from the works cited here, is largely silent on the Insurgent need for ambulances from outside of Spain, although this may reflect the contradictory Insurgent discourse surrounding its own self-sufficiency in the production of military equipment. It is likely, however, that any shortfalls not met by the military or in aid from its allies were met by local initiatives, an example of which was the provision of the mobile laboratory by the faculty in Santiago, which could have been converted for use as an ambulance.[210]

Shortage of ambulances, however, quickly became a problem in the Republican Zone, with several factors contributing to this shortfall. With the Insurgents in control of much of the military apparatus at the start of the conflict and with the backing of Italian and German aviation and military technology, the Insurgents enjoyed the advantage of superior weaponry throughout much of the conflict, which made Republican ambulances more vulnerable to attack.[211] Additionally, the non-intervention policy and the presence of Italian and German ships, which for much of the war provided an effective blockade, made it difficult for the Republic to arm itself through the purchase of arms and equipment from abroad. Following the fall of Bilbao in June 1937, a centre of Spanish iron ore production, access to this important resource was also lost. It was a combination of these factors that made it so difficult for the Republic to manufacture sufficient numbers of ambulances to keep up with demand.[212]

The United Nations Report of the Health Mission to Spain of January 1937, stated that Madrid was cut off from the rest of the country by train, a statement that was in fact inaccurate as Madrid did enjoy rail connections to cities outside the capital. However, there were problems of supply in the besieged capital, with the numbers of lorries available for this work described as inadequate, providing an additional difficulty in supplying sufficient numbers of ambulances for evacuating the wounded from nearby fronts.[213]

It was within the above context that international aid became so important. On 1 September 1936, the supplement of the Barcelona daily *La Vanguardia*, under the title 'An English Ambulance for the Front', dedicated its third page to photographs of the arrival in Barcelona of some of the medical personnel that were to serve with the first foreign ambulance to reach Spanish shores.[214] The ambulance, which had been provided by the Spanish Medical Aid Committee (SMAC), left Victoria Station in London on 23 August 1936.[215] On 2 November, four ambulances were despatched by SMAC with equipment 'sufficient to enable the Spanish Red Cross to make provision for a first-class hospital and fully equipped Casualty Clearing Station or small hospital'.[216] Later that month, the first Scottish ambulances arrived, and a further four ambulances were ordered the following month from SMAC, one of which was described as a 'gas ambulance' to treat the potential victims of chemical warfare.[217] By the summer of the following year, the International Medical Services under the control of the Sanidad Militar in the Republican Zone possessed 130 ambulances of which 82 were British, and the donation of ambulances was made a focal point of the Spanish Medical Aid Committee propaganda in Britain.[218]

Hospital trains

This international aid, the majority of which was funnelled through the CSI in Paris, with funds raised in countries as far apart as Australia and Sweden, was an important element in the evacuation of the wounded in the Republican Zone.[219] Ambulances alone, however, were not sufficient in numbers for meeting the need of the evacuation of all of the wounded during a conflict with such high casualty figures. As such, hospital trains were used extensively throughout the conflict, not only for the transfer of the wounded, but several were equipped with operating theatres, pharmacies, restaurants and bars.[220] Hospital trains not only enjoyed the advantage of being able to transfer large numbers of patients in a single journey but were also useful for economies in fuel.[221]

A major offensive that has received considerable attention from historians was the Republican capture and subsequent loss of Teruel during the harsh winter of 1937–1938.[222] The first unsuccessful offensive that took place between August 1936 and February 1937, however, has received far less attention. In all, 10,430 militiamen from Valencia, including the anarchist Columna de Hierro (Iron Column), alongside 20,000 soldiers of the old Republican Army, and the 13th International Brigade, all loosely under the command of the Comité Ejecutivo Popular de Valencia (Popular Executive Committee of Valencia) attempted to take the un-garrisoned town of Teruel, which was strategically important due to its proximity to Valencia. There were a number of frontline and rear-guard hospitals available to the assailants, but the main hospitals for the evacuation of the sick and the wounded were the Municipal Hospital of Segorbe and the Provincial Hospital in Valencia. Due to a combination of factors involving difficulties of terrain, the nature of the roads, and that during this early stage improvisation was still the order of the day, the evacuation of the wounded and sick by ambulance could not be readily achieved by road alone, and from the start of the offensive the use of a hospital train belonging to the Sanidad Militar was of particular importance.[223]

During this first assault on Teruel, fierce fighting on 27 and 28 December 1936 led to local Republican forces suffering numerous casualties and losing fifty per cent of their equipment. Fatalities during this campaign would have been considerably higher if it were not for the use of the hospital trains.[224] At this early stage of the conflict, the Sanidad Militar in the Republican Zone had at its disposal a total of six hospital trains, and in the sector of the Levant throughout the war had greater access than the Insurgents to the railway network for the evacuation of wounded by train, with control of 2,565 kilometres of the 3,788 kilometres of track.[225]

The train in use on the Teruel front was the Hospital Train No. 1, which first went into service on 1 September 1936. It was responsible for transferring patients from the hospital close to the railway track at Sarrión at a distance of forty-five kilometres from Teruel, to Valencia. On its return journey it was predominantly used for transporting medical supplies to the frontline medical units. At Sarrión, the three surgical teams that were attached to the hospital train were also the teams that worked at the forward hospital in the town, and in a two-month period leading up to 2 October 1936, 156 wounded of the Iron Column who had been evacuated by train from the front were treated in the hospital there.[226] The train was still in action in July 1938, but, due to the greater proximity of Insurgent troops to Valencia, it was parked in a tunnel near Segorbe further down the line towards Valencia, being brought out as required to evacuate the wounded to Valencia.[227]

Crónica, in November 1936, carried an article on the train.[228] This article is of interest as it provides photographic evidence for the train and a description of its function, but also provides evidence for the military doctor with whom the idea for the construction of this train originated. The doctor instrumental in its construction was Donato Nombela Gallardo.[229] In common with other articles in the Republican popular press relating to medical provision, the propagandist element is evident to varying degrees throughout. However, the Spanish historian Xavier Ferrandis García who studies the evolution of the medical services in Valencia during the Spanish Civil War and who uses municipal and regional archival documentation rather than newspaper sources for the train, provides evidence in two journal articles that supports the information contained in *Crónica*.[230]

The article was written on the occasion of the train being in Madrid for cleaning and provisioning, with the author of the article, Angel Álvarez, being shown around the train by three of its doctors. One of the photographs show a wagon containing tiered beds, and visible are the system of poles with built-in suspension to which each bed is attached to reduce jolting during the transfer of the wounded. The train had an operating theatre in which on-board surgery could be carried out during transfers; two wagons or 'wards' for the lightly wounded, provisions and 'sanitary materials'; and a kitchen, restaurant and bar, with the operating theatre and the bar also shown in the photographs.

A close analysis of the article provides further evidence for a more broadly sympathetic view of an improvisational model of organisation, which was effective in providing invaluable medical services in a variety of settings and locations. Alvarez describes how, despite the enthusiasm for the project proposed by Gallardo at the Department of War, getting the train off the ground was hampered by delays and the bureaucracy of various ministries. Alvarez goes on to state that it was at this point that Gallardo directly approached the workers council in control of the railway company MZA (Madrid-Zaragoza-Alicante), who controlled all the train services of the central sector, and outlined his plans concerning the fitting out of the train.[231]

Alvarez also states that this process of outfitting the train was facilitated by Gallardo's encounter with a member of the council who had served under his command in the Protectorate, and that the train was made ready in a matter of days.[232]

By the time of the second battle of Teruel, there were a number of hospital trains operational on the Republican railway network and Joaquín d'Harcourt Got, head of the Republican Surgical Services, was in command of Train No. 12, where he carried out surgery that included abdominal operations and amputation of tissue from frostbitten feet.[233] As a result of the large numbers of casualties suffered during this campaign, those wounded not treated at the front and those not in need of immediate treatment were evacuated back down the line to hospitals in Valencia. From Valencia, those who needed further treatment could then be transferred onto Alcoi and Ontenyent, thus avoiding the conglomeration of the wounded in Valencia.[234]

In Zaragoza, in the Insurgent Zone, there were a total of twelve trains for the evacuation of casualties during the second Teruel Campaign, with six trains used for the evacuation of the wounded from Teruel to Zaragoza, and another six used for evacuating the casualties to hospitals in Pamplona, Logroño and Vitoria. The normal number for those evacuated by train to these cities in Navarra was 350, but there were occasions when the trains carried up to 400 wounded due to the numerous casualties, with a third of the Insurgent casualties bearing wounds that had resulted from frostbite. There were a large number of partial amputations of feet, and treatments that were common in WWI for frostbite of the extremities were used also in Spain. However, newer treatments were also tried, including the use of diathermy (an electrical cutting and coagulation device), meaning that amputations for frostbite were proportionally lower than during WWI.[235]

Evacuation by train was used on all fronts by both sides during the Spanish Civil War. Although the trains used were generally steam and diesel trains, electric trains were used for the transport of the wounded in and around Barcelona, where the Hospital Train No. 20 was in operation from soon after the start of the conflict, which enjoyed the same facilities as the Hospital Train No. 1.[236] Early in 1938, Republicans started using a hand railway in a disused lateral mine shaft in the side of a mountain overlooking the river Ebro for evacuating the wounded. The continued use of this tunnel for several months meant that it was no longer necessary to transfer the sick and wounded over the mountain on mules or on stretchers carried by bearers.[237]

There are no exact figures for how many of the sick and wounded were transferred by hospital train on either side during the conflict, or what percentage this figure constituted of the overall transfers, but due to the extent to which train transport was used it is likely that this figure was in excess of 100,000. It is possible to postulate such a figure based on the evacuation of the Insurgent sick and wounded during the second assault on Teruel and the Ebro campaign. During the latter, six trains evacuated 31,318 out of 48,854 wounded between July and September 1938.[238] With the Republicans in control of an extensive network of railways during the conflict and, during the

Ebro campaign able to evacuate a number of wounded by train to Barcelona, the figure postulated above may well have been higher.

Hospital ships

The articles examined above in relation to hospital trains provide evidence for the importance of regional responses in the provision of facilities during the early stages of the war. Additionally, they add support to the argument that it was the existence of a multiplicity of small organisations at the start of the conflict that were involved in the provision of care for the wounded that facilitated the process whereby the Sanidad Militar was able to build itself up from the ground up.

A more national model for the evacuation of casualties existed in the form of hospital ships. The Insurgents, however, were better able to evacuate their casualties by sea as, after the fall of Bilbao in June 1937, the Insurgents controlled the Atlantic seaboard from the French frontier to Portugal in the north-west, and from Huelva in the south-west through to Malaga on Spain's south-eastern Mediterranean coast.[239] Additionally, with the Mediterranean coastline patrolled by German and Italian shipping, and given that the Republican government were only able to retain one naval base at Cartagena and the secondary naval base of Mahon on Menorca, the transport of the wounded by sea for the Republicans was always going to be a problem.[240]

The use of Republican hospital ships appears to have been short-lived. The *Artabro*, a converted fifty-seven-metre electrical vessel (the first of its kind constructed in Spain) built in 1935, had a surgical team on-board headed by Francisco Pérez Cuadrado, who, prior to the outbreak of the conflict, had been a surgeon at the naval base at Cartagena.[241] This ship, however, only saw limited service between Malaga and the Strait of Gibraltar, as it was deliberately scuppered alongside the small battleship *Xauen* when Malaga fell in February 1937 so as to block the harbour.[242] The other Republican hospital ship of note was the *Marqués de Comillas*, but this equally only saw limited service when it was sent in support of the FAI-led amphibious Republican attempt to recapture Mallorca between August and September 1936. It was the last ship to retreat after the failure to capture the island, evacuating hundreds of the wounded.[243]

There appear to be no further references to other hospital ships in service of the Republic in the literature examined for this study. A possible reason for this is that this was a result of the Mediterranean coast being where the main Republican-held cities outside of Madrid were located. With a naval blockade effectively in place in the Mediterranean against Republican-owned shipping, the risks were too great for establishing hospitals ships in the Mediterranean. However, the need for such vessels on Spain's Levantine coast until the fall of Catalunya early in 1939 was offset by the presence of the well organised regional facilities in the Republican Mediterranean port towns of Alicante, Valencia and Barcelona.[244]

The Insurgents – who, with the exception of Cartagena and the lesser naval base of Mahon, controlled the main naval bases – were better placed to take advantage of evacuation of casualties by sea during the Spanish Civil War. This ability to move patients in large numbers over long distances was important in maintaining evolved models of forward care, as it helped maintain the movement of those treated or awaiting treatments for their wounds away from the frontline. The evidence points towards there having been only one designated hospital ship owned by the Insurgent Sanidad Militar, the *Cuidad de Palma*, a converted cruise ship that entered service in January 1938, although the battleship cruisers *Canarias* and *Baleares* were outfitted in September 1937 with operating theatres and x-ray facilities.

The *Cuidad de Palma* evacuated casualties along Spain's northern and north-western coast for treatment in rear-guard specialist centres, starting in February 1938, but also on two separate occasions evacuated casualties from Bilbao to Sevilla in August 1938, and a month later from Bilbao to Malaga, a sea journey of more than 1,000 miles. There were a total of 502 litters on board, with the lounges at the prow occupied by the walking infirm and wounded, and the second-class stern lounges reserved for the lightly wounded sub-officials. First-class lounges in the stern were reserved for the most gravely wounded, with the first-class cabins reserved for officers and officials, with the remainder of the first-class cabins given over to serious traumatology patients as there was room to accommodate orthopaedic traction equipment.[245]

In Gijón, towards the end of 1938, Moran Cifuentes received 123 fracture patients who had been evacuated 600 kilometres from the relatively quiet Ebro Front.[246] The fracture patients in question, a number of whom had been injured within the previous twenty-four hours, after receiving preliminary treatments, had all been evacuated by specially organised trains, which within a few hours had transferred them at the dockside in Bilbao to the waiting *Cuidad de Palma*. This then took them overnight to Gijón.[247] At Gijón the wounded were disembarked and transferred to the trauma hospital in nearby Granda by ambulance, where they were treated by Cifuentes and his team.[248] The hospital at Granada received numerous patients in this manner, from fronts that included Teruel, Gandesa, Castellón and Tarragona, and the wounded after receiving forward treatment in hospitals in Zaragoza and Bilbao were then transferred onto this specialist centre.[249] The *Cuidad de Palma* carried out a total of sixty-one journeys between 4 February 1938 and 21 March 1939, transporting 20,667 wounded and 7,640 sick or infirm, a total of 28,307 casualties.[250]

As far as it can be established, the Italian Corps of Volunteer Troops (Corpo Truppe Volontarie, or CSV) had at their disposal four hospital ships. These were the *SS Arquileia*, the *SS Grandisca*, the *SS Atulleia* – a large hospital ship based out of Cádiz – and, according to a report by the American Consul in Gibraltar, there was a 'large hospital ship, the SS Heluan' anchored in Gibraltar during the Insurgent assault on Malaga.[251]

The *ABC* of Madrid reported on 5 July 1938, that the *SS Atulleia*, had anchored at Gibraltar two days previously, taking aboard 1,000 wounded who were returning to Italy. In the same report it also mentioned that the *SS Grandisca* had been at anchor in Gibraltar but was now on its way to Cádiz transporting medical personnel and supplies.[252] Additionally, four steamers carried out thirty-two journeys between Cádiz and Italy, with sixteen of these journeys for the transportation of casualties returning to Italy.[253] Among this number, or possibly additional to it, were four Italian transports – *Cardeña*, *Calabria*, *Piamonte* and *Liguria* – which departed Cádiz for Italy on 14 October 1938 carrying primarily soldiers 'disfigured by war', many of whom had to be helped to embark with the aid of sanitarios.[254] This ability to free up hospital beds in Spanish hospitals, through the transfer back to Italy of the CSV sick and wounded, would have gone some way to help in avoiding the loss of bed spaces occasioned by longer-term occupancy.

Although the use of hospital ships during the conflict was limited to a small number of vessels, these nevertheless were able to evacuate a considerable number of wounded to rear-guard hospitals, or in the case of the troops of the CSV, transport the sick and wounded to Italy for further treatment, and those invalided out of the war.[255]

The evacuation of the sick and the wounded, and where possible their early treatment, during the Spanish Civil War ultimately depended upon many factors. Regional efforts were important in this regard, especially early on in the conflict and continued to contribute throughout the conflict towards the transport of casualties. Hospital trains played an important role in that large numbers of the wounded and infirm were able to be evacuated in this way, and although organised at a regional level, local efforts also proved important, as was to prove the case with the construction of the Hospital Train No. 1.[256]

It would appear that CSV casualties were the main beneficiaries of transport by hospital ships, although the Insurgent *Cuidad de Palma* transferred more than 28,000 sick and wounded during the thirteen months it was in operation, freeing up hospital beds near the frontline. These services, when combined with the more conventional service offered by road ambulance, were a significant factor in the functioning of the TPFS across Spain. The services provided also contributed to reducing the numbers of deaths caused by delays in treatment, additionally helping to reduce the number of infections caused by these delays, and freeing up beds for the newly sick and wounded in need of treatment. This not only reduced the number of amputations carried out, but also helped save numerous lives of those who otherwise might have died of their infections.

Conclusion

From the very start of the conflict the challenges faced by the opposing sides in organising their respective medical services were considerable. A country that had been slowly modernising its medical infrastructure, and had made slow but steady improvements in the field of healthcare provision, was forced into improvising and setting up services due to the unequal provision, both military and civilian, across the country. In the larger cities, but especially in the capitals of Madrid and Barcelona held by the Republicans, this was made somewhat easier by access to existing modern facilities. Although the Insurgents at the start of the conflict enjoyed access to much of the medical military infrastructure, the control of predominantly agricultural areas and the growing size of their army and the need to cater for 75,000 Italian troops and 85,000 troops from the Maghreb during the conflict, meant that they too were faced with the need to improvise and set up new medical facilities.

It was for this reason that local and regional models of organisation were important from the start, as in a divided Spain the centralised provision of medical services was not possible in a conventional sense, irrespective of which zone this applied to. These local and regional efforts also led to improvements in medical provision at a national level in both zones, and resulted in significant improvements in mortality rates among the wounded. This was largely due to the overall reduction in time between being wounded and receiving treatment due to the application of more effective models of forward care.

If the Insurgents were able to build upon the existing military infrastructure and benefit from local and regional initiatives, then initiatives on the Republican side in building upon existing civilian services were to prove equally important. What marked out the opposing camps as different was not the level of medical care provided, rather, it was the contribution made by anarchists regarding the socialisation of medicine and ideas that predated the Spanish Civil War, which in turn resulted from anarcho-syndicalist models that saw social revolution and fighting a war against the insurgents as mutually compatible goals.

This important contribution by anarchist medical personnel and thinkers, predominantly Spanish, has largely been consigned to the margins of history. This has been as result of historical models, and propaganda that originated in the Spanish Civil War, which have traditionally emphasised the role played by international medical personnel in the delivery of care during the conflict over that of their Spanish counterparts. It is this domination of the historiography by more internationally known figures that has led to the exclusion of lesser-known Spanish medical personnel, anarchist or otherwise.

It is the role played by propaganda in the distortion of the historiography that is examined in the next chapter, with blood transfusion and the advances that occurred during the conflict the theme of this investigation. The common misconception that the Insurgent model of care was inferior to that provided by the Republicans, echoed in the contemporary as well as the later literature, also has its roots in this distorted historiography. Propaganda here too has played its part. In the following chapter it will be demonstrated that the Insurgent contribution to advances in blood transfusion during the Spanish Civil War was equally important, with the provision of medical care during the conflict significant for its similarities in the opposing camps, and closer in its models of delivery than was and is generally thought.

Notes

1 Massons, *Historia de la Sanidad Militar Española: Tomo II*, p. 320; Estellés Salarich, La sanidad del ejército, pp. 40–41; Jolly, *Field Surgery*, pp. xi–xii.
2 Bescós Torres, J., "La Sanidad Militar en la guerra de España (1936–1939). 1ª Parte", pp. 88–89.
3 Jolly, *Field Surgery*, pp. xi–xii.
4 Trueta, *Treatment of War Wounds*, pp. xi–xii.
5 Massons, *Historia de la Sanidad Militar Española: Tomo II*, pp. 312–325; Estellés Salarich, La sanidad del ejército, pp. 40–41.
6 Martí Boscà, J. V., "Federica Montseny y Pedro Vallina", *Revista de Salud Ambiental*, Vol. 13, No. 1 (2013), pp. 95–102
7 Preston, *Spanish Holocaust*, pp. 221–303; Beevor, *Battle for Spain*, pp. 260–271.
8 *Gaceta de la República: Diario Oficial*, No. 213 (31.7.1936), p. 923; Sarto, Actividades de la Cruz Roja Española, p. 3; www.todoslosnombres.org/content/biografias/juan-morata-canton (last accessed 12.11.2014).
9 Bernabéu Mestre, J., "La utopía reformadora de la Segunda República: la labor de Marcelino Pascua al frente de la Dirección General de Sanidad, 1931–1933", *Revista Española de Salud Pública*, No. 74 (2000), pp. 1–13, pp. 3–4.
10 Massons, *Historia de la Sanidad Militar Española: Tomo II*, pp. 312–313.
11 Ibid.; Thomas, *Spanish Civil War*, pp. 89–90.
12 Massons, *Historia de la Sanidad Militar Española: Tomo II*, pp. 312–313.
13 Ibid., pp. 312–317; Barona, J. L., & Bernabéu Mestre, J. (eds.), *Ciencia y sanidad en la Valencia capital de la República* (Valencia, 2007), pp. 20–33; *Gaceta de Madrid*, No. 194 (15.06.1934), pp. 538–544; Espuelas Barroso, S., "La evolución del gasto social público en España, 1850–2005", *Estudios de Historia Económica*, Vol. 63 (2013), pp. 1–122, pp. 84–104.
14 González Calleja, F., Cobo Romero, F., Martínez Rus, A., & Sánchez Pérez, F., *La Segunda República Española* (Barcelona, 2015), pp. 141, 936.
15 Massons, *Historia de la Sanidad Militar Española: Tomo II*, pp. 312–313; Barona & Bernabéu Mestre, *Ciencia y sanidad*, pp. 20–33; *Gaceta de Madrid*, No. 194 (15.06.1934), pp. 538–544, "Ley de coordinación sanitaria de 11 de junio de 1934"; Espuelas Barroso, La evolución del gasto social público en España, pp. 84–104.
16 Martí Boscà, Montseny y Vallina, pp. 96–97; Pagès i Blanch, P., *War and Revolution in Catalonia, 1936–1939*, translated by Patrick L. Gallagher (Boston, 2013), pp. 150–151.
17 Ibid., p. 98; Barona, J. L., & Perdiguero-Gil, E., "Health and the War: Changing Schemes and Health Conditions During the Spanish Civil War", *Dynamis*, Vol. 28 (2008), pp. 103–126; Conselleria de Sanitat i Assistència Social, *La Reforma Eugénica del Aborto*, Generalitat de Catalunya, Ediciones de la Consejería de Sanidad y Asistencia Social, Sección de Propaganda (Barcelona, 1937).
18 Pagès i Blanch, *War and Revolution in Catalonia*, pp. 150–151; *Gaceta de la República: Diario Oficial*, No. 96 (06.04.1938), p. 111.

19 Llavona, R., & Bandrés, J., "Psicología y anarquismo en la Guerra Civil Española: La Obra de Félix Martí Ibañez", *Psicothema* (1998), Vol. 10, No. 3, pp. 669–678, pp. 669–670.
20 Modern Records Centre University of Warwick (MRCUW), 292.946.15b. 11, Laslet, A., "Report on the Health Mission in Spain: 28th December, 1936, to 15th January, 1937" (Geneva, 1937), p. 2.
21 Martí Boscà, Montseny y Vallina, p. 97.
22 Ibid.
23 *Gaceta de la República*, No. 347 (12.12.1936), p. 969; *Gaceta de la República*, No. 3 (03.01.1937), p. 45; *Gaceta de la República*, No. 155 (04.06.1937), p. 1059.
24 Martí Boscà, J. V., "Algunos hombres buenos: Francisco Trigo Domínguez", *Revista de Salud Ambiental*, Vol. 14, No. 2 (2014), pp. 151–157, pp. 152–153. The anarchists appointed by Montseny to the National Council for Health preferred the title of counsellor as this was felt to be a more appropriate title than the official government one of director general.
25 Ibid., p. 153; *Gaceta de la República: Diario Oficial*, No. 69 (17.03.1939), p. 522.
26 Serrallonga i Urquidi, J., "El cuento de la regularización sanitaria y asistencial en el régimen franquista: Una primera etapa convulsa, 1936–1944", *Historia social*, No. 59 (2007), pp. 77–98, pp. 78–79.
27 Bjerström, C. H., *Josep Renau and the Politics of Culture in Republican Spain, 1931–1939: Re-imagining the Nation* (Brighton, 2015), pp. 127–128.
28 Graham, *Spanish Civil War*, p. 165.
29 Ponseti Vives, I., "Treatment of Congenital Club Foot", *The Journal of Bone and Joint Surgery*, Vol. 74, No. 3 (1992), pp. 448–454; Fernández Sabaté, *Nuestros fundadores*, pp. 507–509.
30 Fernández Sabaté, *Nuestros fundadores*, pp. 507–509.
31 Beneito Lloris, A., "El Dr Manuel Bastos, profesor y militar represaliado", in J. L. Barona (ed.), *El exilio científico Repúblicano* (Valencia, 2010), pp. 315–333, p. 320.
32 Ibid.; Bastos Ansart, *De las guerras coloniales*, pp. 143–149.
33 Ibid.; Centro Documental de la Memoria Histórica (CDMH), *Comisión Liquidadora de Responsabilidades Políticas*, C. 75.49, 31–81, no. 1, 476.
34 Beneito Lloris, *El hospital Sueco-Noruego*, pp. 70, 114–115.
35 Burón, L., "Hospital de sangre de retaguardia: Actuación de un médico durante la guerra civil española. 1936–1939", in *Los médicos y la medicina en la Guerra Civil Española: Monografías Beecham* (Madrid, 1986), pp. 245–258, pp. 247–248.
36 Preston, P., *A Concise History of the Spanish Civil War* (London, 1996), p. 84; Carr, E. H., *The Comintern and the Spanish Civil* War (New York, 1984), p. 11; Estellés Salarich, La sanidad del ejército, p. 41; Massons, *Historia de la Sanidad Militar Española: Tomo II*, p. 321.
37 Estellés Salarich, La sanidad del ejército, pp. 43–8; & Massons, *Historia de la Sanidad Militar Española: Tomo II*, p. 322.
38 Molero-Mesa, J., "'Salud, actuación y actividad'. La Organización Sanitaria Obrera de la CNT y la colectivización de los servicios médico-sanitarios en la Guerra Civil Española', in R. Campos, A. González, M. I. Porras, & L. Montiel (eds.), *XVI Congreso de la Sociedad Española de Historia de la Medicina. Medicina y poder político* (Madrid, 2014), pp. 103–107. The FAI were the dominant militant force of Spanish anarchism.

39 García Ferrandis, X., "Anarcosindicalismo y sanidad en la retaguardia y en el frente: Los casos de Valencia y de la Columna de Hierro en la Guerra Civil Española (1936–1937)", *Asclepio*, Vol. 66, No. 2 (2012), pp. 63–76, pp. 67–68.
40 Burón, Hospital de sangre, pp. 247–248.
41 Massons, *Historia de la Sanidad Militar Española: Tomo II*, p. 365.
42 Gracia Rivas, M., "La sanidad de la armada en la Zona Nacional durante la guerra de 1936–1939", in *Los médicos y la medicina en la Guerra Civil Española: Monografías Beecham* (Madrid, 1986), pp. 103–126, p. 109; Massons, *Historia de la Sanidad Militar Española: Tomo II*, p. 446.
43 Balfour, *Deadly Embrace*, p. 115; Beneito Lloris, *El hospital Sueco-Noruego*, p. 109; Montserrat, S., "Gómez Ulla y su hospital quirúrgico de montaña", *Revista Española de Medicina y Cirugía de Guerra*, Vol. 7, No. 2 (1945), pp. 600–604; Gurriarán, *Diario de Guerra*, p. 239; Zubelzu, Obra Quirúrgica, pp. 59–78.
44 Chalmers Mitchell, P., *My House in Málaga* (London, 1938), pp. 100 & 279.
45 Chalmers Mitchell, P., "The Civil War in Málaga", *The Times* (London, England), 20.10.1936, p. 12.
46 Colmegna, *Diario*, p. 17.
47 Estellés Salarich, La sanidad del ejército, p. 41.
48 Ibid., p. 45.
49 Gracia Rivas, La sanidad de la armada, p. 108
50 Moran Cifuentes, B., "Equipo quirúrgico de Traumatología", in *Los médicos y la medicina en la Guerra Civil Española: Monografías Beecham* (Madrid, 1986), pp. 167–176, pp. 170–171; & Sabaté, *Nuestros fundadores,* p. 491.
51 Cifuentes, Equipo quirúrgico, p. 169.
52 Ibid.; Massons, *Historia de la Sanidad Militar Española: Tomo II*, pp. 415–417; Brasa Arias, B., & Landín Pérez M., "El trabajo de las mujeres voluntarias en el laboratorio de Farmacia Militar de Santiago de Compostela (1936–1939)", *Sanidad Militar*, Vol. 67, No. 1 (2011), pp. 177–192, p. 177.
53 Barona & Perdiguero-Gil, Health and the War, p. 126; Casares López, R., "La Farmacia Militar Española en la pasada guerra", *Discursos* (Madrid, 1940).
54 Brasa Arias & Landín Pérez, El trabajo de las mujeres voluntarias, p. 179.
55 Massons, *Historia de la Sanidad Militar Española: Tomo II*, p.415; Casares López, Farmacia Militar, p. 2.
56 Casares López, Farmacia Militar, p. 2.
57 Palfreeman, *¡Salud!*, pp. 55–56.
58 Massons, *Historia de la Sanidad Militar Española: Tomo II*, pp. 428–429.
59 *Gaceta de la República*, No. 347 (12.12.1936), p. 939.
60 Montseny, F., "Mi experiencia en el Ministerio de Sanidad y Asistencia Social", in J. L. Barona & J. Bernabéu Mestre (eds.), *Ciencia y sanidad en la Valencia capital de la República* (Valencia, 2007), pp. 119–125, pp. 124–125. Transcript of a speech given by Federica Montseny at a conference in Valencia at the Apollo Theatre, 6 June 1937.
61 Casares López, Farmacia Militar, p. 2; *BOE*, 28.08.1937, No. 312, pp. 3075, 3078–3079.
62 Ibid., p. 2; Colmegna, *Diario*, p. 17.
63 Moran Cifuentes, Equipo quirúrgico, p. 171; Larraz Andía, *Entre el frente y la retaguardia*, pp. 65, 279–280.
64 Herranz-Loncán, A., "Infrastructure Investment and Spanish Economic Growth, 1850–1935", *Explorations in Economic History*, Vol. 44, No. 3 (2007), pp. 452–468.
65 Massons, *Historia de la Sanidad Militar Española: Tomo II*, pp. 416–417.

66 Chalmers Mitchell, *My House in Málaga*, p. 217.
67 *AMI Periódico de la Ayuda Médica Extranjera*, No. 9, 1.02.1938 (Barcelona, 1938), unpaginated.
68 Massons, *Historia de la Sanidad Militar Española: Tomo II*, pp. 417, 424.
69 Ibid.; Ortiz de Villajos, *Crónica de Granada en 1937*, p. 36.
70 *ABC* (Sevilla), 26.01.1938, p. 12.
71 Massons, *Historia de la Sanidad Militar Española: Tomo II*, p. 416; *ABC* (Sevilla), 01.06.1938, p. 15.
72 Massons, *Historia de la Sanidad Militar Española: Tomo II*, p. 417.
73 *ABC* (Sevilla), 1.06.1938, p. 15; *El Compostelano*, 21.08.1937, p. 2; *ABC* (Sevilla), 5.11.1937, pp. 1–5; *El Compostelano*, 20.08.1938, p. 2.
74 Massons, *Historia de la Sanidad Militar Española: Tomo II*, p. 416; *ABC* (Sevilla), 01.06.1938, p. 15.
75 Brasa Arias, B., "La Facultad de Farmacia de Santiago de Compostela (1900–1971)" (Universidad de Santiago de Compostela, 2011), p, 103.
76 Maiz Eleizegui, L., "Labor realizada en el primer año por el Laboratorio Militar de Santiago", *El Compostelano*, 21.08.1937; Lloret Pastor, J. "La depuración de científicos tras la guerra civil", in J. Luis Barona (ed.), *Ciencia, salud pública y exilio (España, 1875–1939)* (Valencia, 2003), pp. 131–168, pp. 131–132.
77 Guerra, *La medicina en el exilio*, p. 112.
78 *ABC* (Sevilla), 5.11.1937, pp. 1–5.
79 *El Compostelano*, 21.08.1937, p. 2; *El Compostelano*, 20.08.1938, p. 2.
80 *El Compostelano*, 21.08.1937, p. 2.
81 Brasa Arias & Landín Pérez, El trabajo de las mujeres voluntarias, pp. 179, 183; *ABC* (Sevilla), 5.11.1937, pp. 3–4.
82 Ibid.; Brasa Arias, La Facultad, pp. 142–143; AGMAV, C. 42385, 1; AGMAV, C. 42385, 3; AGMAV, C. 42385, 5; AGMAV, C. 42386, 1; AGMAV, C. 42386, 2; AGMAV, C. 42386, 3; AGMAV, C. 29297, 1; AGMAV, C. 29297, 2; AGMAV, C. 29297, 5; AGMAV, C. 29316, 1; & AGMAV, C. 29316, 2.
83 Brasa Arias & Landín Pérez, El trabajo de las mujeres voluntarias, pp. 184–186.
84 Cenarro, Á., *La sonrisa de Falange: Auxilio Social en la guerra civil y la posguerra* (Barcelona, 2006), pp. xi–xxvi.
85 Massons, *Historia de la Sanidad Militar Española: Tomo II*, pp. 428–429.
86 Ibid., p. 430.
87 "El Ejército Popular de la República: La labor en la Guerra actual", *Mi Revista* (Barcelona), 15.07.1938, pp. 102–103.
88 Navarro Suay, R., & Plaza Torres, J. F., "Una 'hazaña prácticamente desconocida': la participación de médicos militares españoles en la Primera Guerra Mundial", *Sanidad Militar*, Vol. 70, No. 1 (2004), pp. 51–57.
89 *Reglamento para el servicio sanitario en campaña: Aprobado por real orden el 1º de Julio 1896* (Madrid, 1896); Palfreeman, *¡Salud!*, p. 65.
90 Navarro Suay & Plaza Torres, Cuando volvimos a ser grandes, pp. 247–256.
91 Torre Fernández, J. M., *Gómez Ulla, Hospital Militar Central, cien años de historia* (Madrid, 1996), pp. 35–38; *ABC* (Sevilla), 25.11.1938, p. 13; Gómez Ulla, M., "Impresiones de una visita al frente francés de los Vosgos", *La Guerra y su preparación*, Vol. 5, No. 7 (1917), pp. 152–183; Gómez Ulla, M., "Una visita a las instalaciones sanitarias de los frentes francés e inglés", *La Guerra y su preparación*, Vol. 8, No. 1 (1920), pp. 207–235; Montserrat, Gómez Ulla; Martin Sierra, F., "Hospital quirúrgico de montaña 'Gómez Ulla'", *Medicina Militar*, Vol. 56, No. 2 (2000), pp. 117–121.

92 Gordon-Taylor & Hamilton, Surgical Experience in the Spanish War.
93 Jolly, *Field Surgery*, p. xii.
94 Ibid.; Gordon-Taylor & Hamilton, Surgical Experience in the Spanish War; Martín Santos, Nuestro criterio; "Hospital de Sangre", *Crónica* (07.03.1937), pp. 1–3; Gómez Durán, Principios fundamentales: Parte 2ª; Bastos Ansart, Dos problemas de asistencia a los heridos.
95 Bescós Torres, La Sanidad Militar en la guerra de España (1936–1939). 1ª Parte, p. 91.
96 Casanova, *Spanish Civil War*, p. 159.
97 *Crónica*, 9.08.1936, pp. 1–3, pp. 10–11; *Crónica*, 7 .03.1937, pp. 1–3; *Crónica*, 21.02.1937, pp. 1–4; Treatments of War Wounds and Fractures, p. 694; Trueta, The Organisation of Hospital Services, pp. 13–23.
98 Gómez Ulla, Una visita a las instalaciones sanitarias; Jolly, *Field Surgery*, pp. 6–7.
99 Lockwood, A. D., "Some Experiences in the Last War", *BMJ*, Vol.1, No. 4130 (1940), pp. 436–438.
100 Jolly, *Field Surgery*, pp. xii, 6–7, 166.
101 Ibid.; Massons, *Historia de la Sanidad Militar Española: Tomo II*, p. 434.
102 Massons, *Historia de la Sanidad Militar Española: Tomo II*, p. 435.
103 Moral Torres, El 'método español', p. 163; Jolly, *Field Surgery*, pp. 7, 166.
104 Jolly, *Field Surgery*, p. 4; Zumel, M. F., "Cirugía de guerra", in *Los médicos y la medicina en la Guerra Civil Española: Monografías Beecham* (Madrid, 1986), pp. 69–92; Bescós Torres, La Sanidad Militar, 2ª Parte, p. 447.
105 Burón, Hospital de sangre, pp. 247–248.
106 Picardo Castellón, M., "Experiencia personal en un hospital quirúrgico de primera línea durante nuestra Guerra Civil", in *Los médicos y la medicina en la Guerra Civil Española: Monografías Beecham* (Madrid, 1986), pp. 177–202.
107 Herraiz Muñoz, M., "Aplicación y avances en el tratamiento de los heridos en la Guerra civil Española", in *Los médicos y la medicina en la Guerra Civil Española: Monografías Beecham* (Madrid, 1986), pp. 279–290, p. 281.
108 Ibid., p. xiii; Welch, C. E., "War Wounds of the Abdomen", *New England Journal of Medicine*, Vol. 237, No. 5 (1947), pp. 156–162.
109 Beneito Lloris, *El hospital Sueco-Noruego*, p. 119; Bastos Ansart, M., "Conferencias y resumen de revistas", *Revista de Sanidad de Guerra*, Vol. 1, No. 1 (1937), pp. 27–33.
110 Barbiela, F. F., Bastos Ansart, M., & Ramon Otaola, J., *Manual de Sanidad Militar* (Valencia, 1938); Bastos Ansart, Dos problemas de asistencia a los heridos, pp. 9–14; Bastos Ansart, M., "Varios 'standards' de cirugía de guerra", *Revista de Sanidad de Guerra*, Vol. 1, No. 5 (1937), pp. 173–181; Bastos Ansart, M., "Varios 'standards' de cirugía de guerra: 2. – Tratamiento de las heridas vasculares de los miembros", *Revista de Sanidad de Guerra*, Vol. 1, No. 7 (1937), pp. 257–266; Bastos Ansart, M., "Sobre el pronóstico en las heridas de guerra del vientre", *Revista de Sanidad de Guerra*, Vol. 2, No. 9 (1938), pp. 1–17.
111 Bastos Ansart, Conferencias, pp. 27–33.
112 Gómez Durán, Principios fundamentales, pp. 2–35; Gómez Durán, Principios fundamentales, Parte 2ª, pp. 81–101; López Cotarelo, Organización de los servicios sanitarios, pp. 527–553; Oleo Herraiz, Apostillas a los servicios, pp. 254–261; Cuadrado, F., "Resultados inmediatos en heridas cráneo-cerebrales de guerra", *Revista Española de Medicina y Cirugía de Guerra*, Vol. 3, No. 3 (1940), pp. 203–220; Jolly, *Field Surgery*.
113 Massons, *Historia de la Sanidad Militar Española: Tomo II*, p. 440.

114 Gómez Durán, M., "Impresiones sobre cirugía en los hospitales de sangre en el frente", *Galicia Clínica*, Vol. 9, No. 5–6 (1937), pp. 89–140; Gómez Durán, M., "Puestos quirúrgicos avanzados", *Galicia Clínica*, Vol. 10, No. 3–4 (1938), pp. 37–48; Gómez Durán, M., "Táctica terapéutica de urgencia en fracturas de guerra en el frente", *Galicia Clínica*, Vol. 11, No. 7 (1939), pp. 161–172; Gómez Durán, Principios fundamentales, pp. 2–35; Gómez Durán, Principios fundamentales, Parte 2ª, p. 81; Cotarelo, Organización de los servicios sanitarios, pp. 527–553.
115 Cotarelo, Organización de los servicios sanitarios, pp. 527–553.
116 Massons, *Historia de la Sanidad Militar Española: Tomo II*, p. 434; Santos, Nuestro criterio, p. 653; Gómez Durán, Impresiones, p. 126; Gómez Durán, Principios fundamentales, 2ª parte, pp. 81–101.
117 http://hemerotecadigital.bne.es/details.vm?lang=es&q=id:0004154305, description of the newspaper from the National Spanish library website (last accessed 03. 12. 2014.). Rico Belestá, F., "La Sanidad en Campaña", *Libertad*, Vol. 1, No. 5 (1937), p. 5. *Libertad* was the periodical of 'Division 42' Cuenca, part of the 59th Brigade, an autonomous unit affiliated to the CNT–FAI.
118 Rico Belestá, Sanidad, p. 5.
119 *Libertad*, Vol. 1, No. 5 (1937), pp. 5–6; Nombela Gallardo, D., "El porqué de los hipertrofias cardiacas en la Guerra: Dirigidos a los Jefes de Cuerpo, Division y Brigadas", *Libertad*, Vol. 1, No. 4 (1937), pp. 13–14; Nombela Gallardo, Nuestro Servicio Sanitario, pp. 4–6; Rico Belestá, F., "Servicio Sanitario en Campaña", *Libertad*, Vol. 1, No. 7 (1937), pp. 6–7.
120 Rico Belestá, Sanidad, p. 5.
121 Rico Belestá, Servicio Sanitario, pp. 6–7.
122 Ibid.: Jolly, *Field Surgery*, p. 8.
123 Belestá, Servicio Sanitario, pp. 6–7.
124 Oleo Herraiz, Apostillas a lost servicios, p. 256.
125 Ibid.; Jolly, *Field Surgery*, p. 8; Belestá, Servicio Sanitario, pp. 6–7; Gómez Durán, Principios fundamentales, pp. 81–82.
126 Estellés Salarich, La sanidad del ejército, p. 41; Massons, *Historia de la Sanidad Militar Española: Tomo II*, pp. 312–524.
127 García Ferrandis, La Asistencia sanitaria, p. 21; "El palacio de March, convertida en hospital de sangre", *Mundo Gráfico*, 19.08.1936, pp. 6–7; *La Vanguardia*, 24.07.1936, p. 2.
128 Rico Belestá, Sanidad, p. 5.
129 Ibid.; Boscá, Montseny and Vallina, pp. 95–102; & Jolly, *Field Surgery*, pp. 21–8.
130 Gallardo, Nuestro Servicio, pp. 4–6.
131 Ibid.; & Montserrat, Gómez Ulla, pp. 600–604.
132 Ibid.
133 Martí Boscà, Montseny y Pedro Vallina, p. 9; Martínez Vallina, P., *Mis Memorias* (Córdoba, 2000), pp. 328–330.
134 Álvarez, El Cuerpo de Sanidad Militar, pp. 4–5; *Libertad*, Vol. 1, No. 4–6.
135 *Diario Oficial del Ministerio de Defensa Nacional*, No. 296, Tomo 10 (Barcelona), 10.12.1937, p. 482.
136 Jolly, *Field Surgery*, p. 6; Rico Belestá, Sanidad, p. 5.
137 Bescós Torres, La Sanidad Militar en la Guerra de España (1936–1939), 2ª Parte, p. 448.
138 Graham, *Spanish Civil War*, p. 109.
139 Jolly, *Field Surgery*, p. 230–231.

140 Bescós Torres, La Sanidad Militar en la Guerra de España (1936–1939), 2ª Parte, p. 447.
141 Shumacker, H. B., *Leo Eloesser, MD: Eulogy for a Free Spirit* (New York, 1982), p. 164.
142 Anderson, *Friend or Foe*, pp. 169–171.
143 McNeill-Ross, G., *The Epic of the Alcázar* (London, 1937), pp. 93–94; Pita, R., *Armas Químicas: La Ciencia en Manos de Mal* (Madrid, 2008), p. 105.
144 McNeill-Ross, *Alcázar*, pp. 94.
145 Madariaga Fernández, F. J., "Las Industrias de Guerra de Cataluña durante la Guerra Civil" (Universitat Rovira i Virgili, Tarragona, 2003), p. 348.
146 *ABC* (Sevilla), 5.12.1936, pp. 5–6; *ABC* (Sevilla), 18.12.1936, p. 5; "Fight For San Sebastian", *Times* (London, England), 19.08.1936, p. 10; Our Special Correspondent, "San Sebastian Waiting", *Times* (London, England), 08.09.1936, p. 12; Our Special Correspondent, "The Spanish Struggle", *Times* (London, England), 10.09.1936, p. 12; "Commons and Constitutional Issue", *Times* (London, England), 4.12.1936, p. 7; Our Own Correspondent, "Use Of Poison Gas", *Times* (London, England), 07.07.1937, p. 15.
147 Commons and Constitutional Issue, p. 7.
148 Guindal y Calderero, Problemas de salubridad, pp. 503, 536.
149 Ibid.
150 Ibid., pp. 535–536; Bescós Torres, La Sanidad Militar, 1ª parte, p. 92; Consell de Sanitat de Guerra, Instruccions sobre defensa passiva, pp. 375–383.
151 Balfour, *Deadly Embrace*, pp. 133, 145, 309–310.
152 Ibid., p. 133; Fernández, Industrias de Guerra, p. 349.
153 Balfour, *Deadly Embrace*, p. 133; Fernández, Industrias de Guerra, pp. 349, 358, 415.
154 Schmidt, U., *Secret Science: A Century of Poison Warfare and Human Experiments* (Oxford, 2015), p. 10.
155 *ABC* (Sevilla), 18.12.1936, p. 5.
156 Balfour, *Deadly Embrace*, pp. 131, 145.
157 Pita, *Armas Químicas*, p. 107.
158 Fernández, Industrias de Guerra, p. 360.
159 *Gaceta de la República: Diario Oficial*, No. 124, 04.05.1937, p. 542; *Gaceta de la República: Diario Oficial*, No. 133, 13.05.1937, p. 688; *Gaceta de la República: Diario Oficial*, No. 135, 15.05.1937, p. 716; *La Voz*, 05.10.1936, p. 3; *ABC* (Madrid), 12.01.1937, p. 7; *ABC* (Madrid), 07.05.1937, p. 8; *ABC* (Madrid), 08.05.1937, p. 8; *ABC* (Madrid), 12.05.1937, p. 13; "La guerra química III", *Mundo Gráfico*, 02.06.1937, pp. 10–11; *ABC* (Madrid), 30.06.1937, p. 4; *ABC* (Madrid), 10.07.1937, p. 6; "La Cruz Roja y la guerra: La labor de los comités locales, los consultorios gratuitos, los puestos de socorro, las patrullas antigás", *Mundo Gráfico*, 08.09.1937, p. 10; *Mi Revista*, 19.07.1937, p. 72; Sarto, J. D., "Actividades de la Cruz Roja Española: Cómo se prepara a la población civil para su defensa contra la guerra química", *Crónica*, 30.01.1938, p. 5; *Crónica*, 06.03.1938, p. 3.
160 Calderero, Problemas de salubridad, p. 537; Balmori, Servicios sanitarios de antigás, pp. 49–63; *ABC* (Sevilla), 11.06.1938, p. 18.
161 Balfour, *Deadly Embrace*, pp. 128–130, 309–311.
162 Massons, *Historia de la Sanidad Militar Española: Tomo II*, pp. 514–515.
163 Martí Boscà, Algunos Hombres Buenos, p. 153; Vallina, *Mis Memorias*, p. 333.

164 Ibid.; Torres, La Sanidad Militar, 1ª parte, p. 92; Browne, History of Anaesthesia, pp. 65–67.
165 Torres, La Sanidad Militar, 1ª parte; Calderero, Problemas de salubridad, p. 537.
166 Ibid.; Massons, *Historia de la Sanidad Militar Española: Tomo II*, p. 515.
167 Ibid.; "Tecnicas de actualidad: Defensa pasiva organizada", *Crónica Médica*, No. 110 (1937), pp. 47–79.
168 "La guerra química", *Mundo Gráfico*, 19.05.1937, p. 12; "La guerra química II: Las dificultades para llegar a una prohibición de este terrible medio de lucha", *Mundo Gráfico*, 26.05.1937, pp. 15–16; "Guerra química: Cómo deberá ser protegida la población civil contra el terrible peligro", *Caras y Caretas* (Buenos Aires), No. 2, 14.08.1937, pp. 12–13; *ABC* (Madrid), 10.11.1937, p. 1; "La química como arma de guerra: Como era una nueva guerra?", *Mi Revista*, 01.01.1938, pp. 58–60; Esteva Villarasa, J., "La química como arma bélica", *Mi Revista*, 10.02.1938, pp. 39–41; "Guerra química: Las dificultades para llegar a una prohibición de este terrible medio de lucha", *Caras y Caretas* (Buenos Aires), No. 2, 02.07.1938, pp. 12–13; Matthews, J., " 'The Vanguard of Sacrifice'? Political Commissars in the Republican Popular Army during the Spanish Civil War, 1936–1939", *War in History*, Vol. 21, No. 1 (2014), pp. 82–101; "Una exposición de periodicos murales en Madrid", *Mundo Gráfico*, 01.06.1938, pp. 1–2; *Cultura en el frente*, No. 31, 18.10.1937.
169 Ibid.; *La Voz*, 05.10.1936, p. 3; *ABC* (Madrid), 30.06.1937, p. 4; *ABC* (Madrid), 10.07.1937, p. 6; Calderero, Problemas de salubridad, p. 536.
170 *La Vanguardia*, 03.10.1936, p. 4; *ABC* (Madrid), 23.03.1937, p. 8; *ABC* (Madrid), 09.04.1937, p. 8; *ABC* (Madrid), 29.07.1937, p. 3; *ABC* (Madrid), 07.09.1937, p. 5; *La Vanguardia*, 07.01.1938, p. 4.
171 Archivo de la Diputación Provincial de Valencia (ADPV), D 6.1, caja 30, 1937, Consejería de Sanidad y Asistencia Social.
172 http://hemerotecadigital.bne.es/details.vm?lang=es&q=id:0003258528. Description of the newspaper from the National Spanish library website (last accessed 12.12.2015).
173 *Gaceta de la República: Diario Oficial*, No. 213, 31.07.1936, p. 923; Sarto, Actividades de la Cruz Roja, p. 5; www.todoslosnombres.org/content/biografias/juan-morata-canton (last accessed 12. 11. 2014).
174 Morata Cantón, *Defensa de guerra tóxico química*; Morata Cantón, *Guerra química y bacteriológica*; *La Libertad*, 09.05.1937, p. 3; *Gaceta de la República: Diario Oficial*, No. 135, 15.05.1937, p. 716; Viñuales Fariñas, La ciencia al servicio de la barbarie; España, Servicio de Guerra Química, *Información del servicio de guerra química*.
175 *Gaceta de la República: Diario Oficial*, No. 293, 20.10.1937, p. 293; Beevor, *Battle for Spain*, pp. 272, 275.
176 www.todoslosnombres.org/content/biografias/juan-morata-canton (last accessed 12.11.2014).
177 Sarto, Cruz Roja Española, p. 6; Cantón, *Defensa*.
178 Sarto, Cruz Roja Española, p. 6.
179 *Gaceta de la República: Diario Oficial*, 29.12.1936, No. 364, p. 1150; www.todoslosnombres.org/content/biografias/juan-morata-canton.
180 The *BOE* has thirteen entries detailing appointments of 'sargentos practicantes' between 7.12.1937 and 23.12.1938.

181 Ibid. There are multiple entries that refer to the appointment of MOs in the *BOE*, but these refer to either their appointment, assimilation into the military or promotion.
182 Calderero, Problemas de salubridad, p. 537; Balmori, Servicios sanitarios, pp. 49–63.
183 Calderero, Problemas de salubridad, p. 537.
184 Balmori, Servicios sanitarios, pp. 49–63.
185 Ibid.; Jolly, *Field Surgery*, pp. 6–10.
186 Balmori, Servicios sanitarios, pp. 49–50.
187 Parilla Hermida, Los gases de guerra; Calderero, Problemas de salubridad, pp. 503–539. See also Parrilla Hermida, M., *Los gases de combate: Síntomas, tratamiento y protección* (La Coruña, 1936).
188 *ABC* (Sevilla), 10.07.1938, p. 16; *ABC* (Sevilla), 11.07.1938, p. 18; *ABC* (Sevilla), 14.07.1938, p. 19.
189 *ABC* (Sevilla), 09.06.1937, p. 8; *ABC* (Sevilla), 13.08.1937, p. 7; *ABC* (Sevilla), 09.10.1937, p. 7; *ABC* (Sevilla), 16.02.1938, pp. 9–10; *ABC* (Sevilla), 18.06.1938, p. 7.
190 Hermida, Los gases de guerra, pp. 368–391; Calderero, Problemas de salubridad, pp. 503–539; Tecnicas de actualidad, pp. 74–7.
191 Massons, *Historia de la Sanidad Militar Española: Tomo II*, p. 515.
192 *La Voz*, 05.10.1936, p.3; *ABC* (Madrid), 12.01.1937, p. 7; *ABC* (Madrid), 07.05.1937, p. 8; *ABC* (Madrid), 08.05.1937, p. 8; *ABC* (Madrid), 12.05.1937, p. 13; "La guerra química III", *Mundo Gráfico*, 02.06.1937, pp. 10–11; *ABC* (Madrid), 20.06.1937, p. 4; *ABC* (Madrid), 10.07.1937, p. 6; "La Cruz Roja y la guerra", *Mundo Gráfico*, 08.09.1937, p. 10; *Mi Revista*, 19.07.1937, p. 72; Sarto, "Actividades de la Cruz Roja Española", p. 5; *Crónica*, 06.03.1938, p. 3.
193 Jolly, *Field Surgery*, pp. v–vi.
194 Massons, *Historia de la Sanidad Militar Española: Tomo II*, p. 514.
195 Jolly, *Field Surgery*, p.26; Palfreeman, *Aristocrats, Adventurers and Ambulances*, p. 160.
196 Massons, *Historia de la Sanidad Militar Española: Tomo II*, pp. 440–441; Moreno Fernández-Caparrós, L. A., *Historia de la veterinaria militar española: organización de la veterinaria militar durante la Guerra Civil española, 1936–1939* (Madrid, 2013), pp. 39–42.
197 González Canomanuel, M. A., "El comienzo del transporte aéreo sanitario en España. De la campaña del norte de África (1909–1927) al Servicio de búsqueda y salvamento (1955)", *Sanidad Militar*, Vol. 69, No. 4 (2013), pp. 276–282, p. 278; Pérez Ribelles, V., "La sanidad del aire en Zona Nacional durante la Guerra Civil Española", in *Los médicos y la medicina en la Guerra Civil Española: Monografías Beecham* (Madrid, 1986), pp. 203–210; Paulino Pérez, J., "La sanidad del arma de aviación Repúblicana", in *Los médicos y la medicina en la Guerra Civil Española: Monografías Beecham* (Madrid, 1986), pp. 231–236, p. 235.
198 Canomanuel, El comienzo del transporte aéreo, pp. 276–279.
199 Ibid.; Massons, *Historia de la Sanidad Militar Española: Tomo II*, pp. 434–435.
200 Barona & Bernabéu Mestre, *Ciencia y sanidad*, pp. 20–33.
201 Estellés Salarich, La sanidad del ejército, p. 45; Castellón, Hospital quirúrgico, p. 181.
202 Ibid.
203 *ABC* (Madrid), 28.08.1936, p. 6; *ABC* (Madrid), 29.08.1936, p. 9.

204 Bescós Torres, La Sanidad Militar, 2ª Parte, p. 435.
205 *BOE*, 15.10.1936, No. 3, p. 12; Bescós Torres, La Sanidad Militar, 2ª Parte, p. 435.
206 Fyrth, *The Signal was Spain*, pp. 193–194; *Lancet*, Vol. 2, No. 5902 (10.10.1936), p. 861; *Lancet*. Vol. 2, No. 5907, (14.11.1936), pp. 1195–1196.
207 Fyrth, *The Signal was Spain*, p. 194.
208 Ibid., p. 195.
209 Casanova, *Spanish Civil War*, pp. 137, 158, 161, 166, 170.
210 Brasa Arias & Landín Pérez, El trabajo de las mujeres voluntarias, pp. 184–186; *ABC* (Sevilla), 05.11.1937, pp. 1–5.
211 Casanova, *Spanish Civil War*, pp. 83–85
212 Graham, *Spanish Civil War*, pp. 51–52, 81–82, 87–91.
213 MRCUW, 292.946.15b.11, Report on the Health Mission, p. 33; Álvarez, El Cuerpo de Sanidad Militar, pp. 4–5.
214 "Una Ambulancia Inglésa para el Frente", *La Vanguardia* (01.09.1936), p. 36.
215 Fyrth, *The Signal was Spain*, p.43.
216 MRCUW: 292.946.41.128, pp. 1–2.
217 *La Vanguardia*, 29.11.1936, p. 5; MRCUW: 292.946.41.220, pp. 1–2.
218 Palfreeman, *¡Salud!*, p. 166; MRCUW, 292.946.15b.11, Report on the Health Mission, p. 33; MRCUW: 292.946.41.220, pp. 1–2; MRCUW: 292.946.16a.47, "Bulletin No. 5", p. 4.
219 Calvo García, "La ayuda sanitaria internacional a la República española (1936–1939)", *Sanidad Militar*, Vol. 50, No. 3 (1994), pp. 338–347, p. 341; "Entrega de seis tiendas de campaña y veinticinco ambulancias al Ejército", *La Vanguardia* (09.07.1938), p. 4.
220 Bescós Torres, La Sanidad Militar, 2ª Parte, p. 445; Torres, La Sanidad Militar, 1ª Parte, p. 92; Massons, *Historia de la Sanidad Militar Española: Tomo II*, pp. 439–442; Rojo Fernández, V., "Algunos aspectos durante la operaciones de Teruel", in *Los médicos y la medicina en la Guerra Civil Española: Monografías Beecham* (Madrid, 1986), pp. 139–156, p. 146; Gómez Durán, Principios fundamentales: Parte 2ª, p. 89; Molla, V. M., "Algunas consideraciones sobre cirugía en nuestros frentes de Guerra", *Crónica Médica*, Vol. 41 (1937), pp. 91–110, pp. 88–97; García Ferrandis & Munayco Sánchez, La asistencia sanitaria, pp. 245–249; Álvarez, El Cuerpo de Sanidad Militar, pp. 4–5; Donato, M., "Viaje en un tren hospital", *Estampa* (13.11.1937), pp. 4–5.
221 Bescós Torres, La Sanidad Militar, 2ª Parte, p. 434.
222 Beevor, *Battle for Spain*, pp. 315–322; Thomas, *Spanish Civil War*, pp. 767–773; Preston, *Reaction, Revolution and Revenge*, pp. 279–281; Casanova, *Spanish Civil War*, pp. 173–175.
223 García Ferrandis & Munayco Sánchez, La asistencia sanitaria, p. 246.
224 Ibid.
225 García Ferrandis, Anarcosindicalismo y sanidad, p. 71; Cayón García, F., & Muñoz Rubio, M., "Transportes y comunicaciones", in P. Martín Aceña & E. Martínez Ruiz (eds.), *La economía de la guerra civil* (Madrid, 2006), pp. 229–272, p. 247, fn. 25.
226 García Ferrandis, Anarcosindicalismo y sanidad, p. 71; Álvarez, El Cuerpo de Sanidad Militar, pp. 4–5.
227 García Ferrandis, La cobertura sanitaria, p. 191.
228 Álvarez, El Cuerpo de Sanidad Militar, pp. 4–5.

229 Ibid., pp. 4–5; Nombela Gallardo, Nuestro Servicio Sanitario, pp. 4–6: Rico Belestá, Sanidad, p. 5.
230 Ibid.; García Ferrandis, Anarcosindicalismo y sanidad, p. 71; García Ferrandis & Munayco Sánchez, La asistencia sanitaria, p. 246.
231 Álvarez, El Cuerpo de Sanidad Militar, pp. 4–5.
232 Ibid.; Ministerio de la Defensa, *Historia militar de la Guerra Civil en Madrid: Fuentes primarias* (Madrid, 2014), p. 923.
233 Rojo Fernández, Operaciones de Teruel, pp. 144, 155; Bescos Torres, La Sanidad Militar, 1ª Parte, p. 98.
234 Massons, *Historia de la Sanidad Militar Española: Tomo II*, p. 440.
235 Larraz & Barrola, Los pies de Teruel, pp. 198, 200, 205–206, 207–210.
236 Massons, *Historia de la Sanidad Militar Española: Tomo II*, pp. 439–443; Gómez Durán, Principios fundamentales: Parte 2ª, p. 89; Donato, Viaje en un tren hospital, pp. 4–5.
237 Jolly, *Field Surgery*, pp. 27–28.
238 Bescós Torres, La Sanidad Militar, 2ª Parte, p. 445; Barrola, Los pies de Teruel, p. 198.
239 Graham, *Spanish Civil War*, pp. 105–106.
240 Ferrer Córdoba, P., "La sanidad en la marina repúblicana", in *Los médicos y la medicina en la Guerra Civil Española: Monografías Beecham* (Madrid, 1986), pp. 127–138, p. 130.
241 Ibid., pp. 132–133; Massons, *Historia de la Sanidad Militar Española: Tomo II*, p. 450; *Solidaridad Obrera*, 23.09.1936, p. 3; *La Voz*, 10.02.1937, p. 1.
242 *La Voz*, 10.02.1937, p. 1.
243 Ferrer Córdoba, La sanidad en la marina repúblicana, pp. 133–134.
244 Graham, *Spanish Civil War*, pp. 105–106.
245 Gracia Rivas, La sanidad de la armada, pp. 113–114, 120.
246 Moran Cifuentes, Equipo quirúrgico, p. 174.
247 Ibid., pp. 174–175; Gracia Rivas, La sanidad de la armada, pp. 113–114.
248 Moran Cifuentes, Equipo quirúrgico, p. 175.
249 Ibid.; Gracia Rivas, La sanidad de la armada, pp. 113–114.
250 Gracia Rivas, La sanidad de la armada, pp. 115–116.
251 *ABC* (Madrid), 05.07.1938, p. 3; *ABC* (Sevilla), 14.09.1937, p. 13; Scott-Ellis, *The Chances of Death*, pp. 15–16; Cortada, J. W., *Modern Warfare in Spain: American Military Observations on the Spanish Civil War, 1936–1939* (Washington, DC, 2012), p. 97.
252 *ABC* (Madrid), 05.07.1938, p. 3.
253 Campo Rizo, J. M., "El Mediterráneo, campo de batalla de la Guerra Civil Española: la intervención naval italiana. Una primera aproximación documental", *Cuadernos de Historia Contemporánea*, Vol. 19, No. 55 (1997), pp. 55–87, p. 84, fn. 89.
254 *ABC* (Madrid), 15.10.1938, p. 4.
255 Campo Rizo, El Mediterráneo, campo de batalla, p. 84.
256 Álvarez, El Cuerpo de Sanidad Militar, pp. 4–5.

4 Blood propaganda

Introduction

On Friday 7 August 1936, a little over two weeks after the outbreak of the Spanish Civil War, *La Vanguardia* printed the following short article titled 'An Offer by the Blind'. The article stated:

> West Communist Radio has provided us with the following note: the blind comrades of the communist cell of Radio West have not been able to fight at the front, but disposed to give their lives for the cause and because of the ravages caused to the Popular Front they have offered their blood for transfusions for the wounded in the frontline hospitals.[1]

Seven months later, in March 1937, *ABC*, the Catholic daily newspaper published in Sevilla, reported that 'the valorous Falangist Mari-Luz Larios, daughter of the marquises of Marrales [*sic*], after having given her blood for a transfusion twenty-four hours previously for a wounded man, dived into the sea, saving the life of a youth whose boat had capsized'.[2] The previous month in Madrid, an elderly woman in mourning had presented herself at the offices of the Canadian Blood Transfusion Institute housed in Madrid.[3] Damian Esfera, a newspaper correspondent and the unnamed 'medic' he was interviewing 'looked' surprised when she offered to donate some blood for storage. Noting their surprise, she explained that although 'she knew she was old and that her blood might not be of much use', her son had been killed at Talavera, and maybe an injection of her blood might have saved him. It was for this reason, she explained, that she was offering herself, 'so that another mother might save her son, thanks to her donation'.[4]

The above accounts serve as examples of how, from the very start of the conflict, the use of propaganda was central to the dissemination of information in the recruitment of donors (and frequently in promoting an ideological position), relating not just to blood donors, but also in highlighting the importance of different methods of blood transfusion. These methods, whether direct arm-to-arm blood transfusion or the use of stored blood were in fact built on developments that occurred during WWI, and came to fruition early in the Spanish Civil War.[5]

The traditional technique of blood transfusion most common at the start of the conflict was direct arm-to-arm transfusion. The donor's medical history was checked – initially by oral confirmation alone, then later by screening the blood – to exclude those with syphilis and those who had 'suffered from malaria'.[6] A cannula (a hollow needle) was then placed into the vein in the arm of the donor. This was connected by a length of tube, with a valve in the middle to regulate flow and direction, to a cannula placed in the vein of the recipient, who then received a quantity of blood from the donor, which usually totalled about 300–400 millimetres of blood. Techniques and apparatus did vary, but this was the basic principle of the technique, and this remained the most common method of blood transfusion throughout the conflict.[7] Although stored blood was to contribute towards saving lives, the arm-to-arm method was still the main means by which blood was transfused during the conflict. This resulted from the sheer amount of battlefield and civilian casualties, but also because numerous surgeons favoured the traditional method, which they considered a safer technique.[8]

What made Spain different at the time to other nations, was the parallel acceleration in both the Insurgent and Loyalist Zones of methods for storing blood and delivering it to the front in far greater quantities than had been achieved previously. This came as a result of the advancement in recent developments in the preservation of blood. Practices were similar on both sides (with stored blood usually destined for use in the most gravely wounded), regardless of whose service was involved, or perceived differences in the services offered.[9] Nevertheless, the role of the blood donor in the opposing zones reflected different ideological approaches regarding the donation of blood. In the Republican Zone, giving blood was frequently phrased as an anti-fascist activity suitable for both women and men, whereas in the Insurgent Zone the donation of blood was clearly linked to traditional notions of Catholic womanhood, closely tied to a woman's perceived role as a nurturer subordinate to men.[10]

A little over a month after the outbreak of Civil War, the first mobile blood transfusion service of stored blood opened in Barcelona under the direction of Federic Durán-Jordà. The following month in San Sebastian, Carlos Elósegui established a similar service in the Insurgent Zone.[11] The service set up by Dr Durán-Jordà in Barcelona under the auspices of the Partit Socialista Unificat de Catalunya (Unified Socialist Party of Catalunya or PSUC) and the UGT in August 1936, initially delivered stored citrated blood to Republican troops on the Aragón front. The service set up by Dr Carlos Elósegui also provided conserved blood across a wide front and is credited with having provided 25,000 transfusions, by far the largest number recorded for any one service.[12] It was the establishment, however, of the institute in Madrid in late December 1936 by the renowned Canadian thoracic surgeon Norman Bethune that would come to dominate the historiography of blood transfusion during the conflict, with Bethune claiming that it was 'the first unified blood transfusion service in army and medical history'.[13]

This domination of the historiography arose partly from Madrid, and its place at the heart of much of the international propaganda thanks to its iconic resistance to Franco's forces and his fascist allies in the winter of 1936/1937. It was on this front, on the outskirts of the city, that Bethune and the institute first supplied blood.[14] Bethune, nevertheless, after just four months as head of the institute in Madrid, was recalled to Canada due to conflicts within the unit, apparently caused by Bethune's determinedly individualistic approach, which led to the Spanish government bringing it under its own control.[15] He was replaced by Vicente Goyanes, who had worked with Elósegui under Spain's leading expert on haematology and malaria, Gustavo Pittaluga, in the fledgling blood transfusion service at the prestigious National School for Health in Madrid prior to the war. It was Pittaluga who had first organised the blood transfusion service in Madrid after the outbreak of the conflict.[16]

By closely examining the role played by Bethune, this chapter aims to place his contribution within a wider historical context examining the part played by propaganda in this process. It will also highlight the part played by Durán-Jordà (who became the head of the unified blood transfusion services of the Republic in July 1937) and Elósegui in providing blood transfusion of stored blood during the Spanish Civil War.[17] By examining the historiographical threads that have been woven around Bethune, and that place him at the forefront of developments, it is the intention of this chapter to address the imbalance in the historiography that have side-lined some important Spanish contributions, although the historian Linda Palfreeman in the recently published *Spain Bleeds* (2015) does challenge several of these misconceptions.[18] By focusing on the role that propaganda played in the creation of this distorted historiography (not a focus of the recent work by Palfreeman), whether in print media or film, and by examining how it served as an ideological backdrop upon which the blood transfusion services projected their competing claims, this chapter aims to demonstrate how propaganda was an effective tool in targeting audiences not only at an ideological level, but also in the recruiting of blood donors and as a fundraising tool.

Histories of the Spanish Civil War have tended to emphasise the contribution of foreign medical volunteers to the Republican war effort. With many of these histories written outside of Spain, and with gaps in the Spanish archives due to the destruction of important sources, the limited medical focus on the conflict frequently represents international over national perspectives on the conflict. This has often resulted in the marginalisation of the contribution made by Spanish medical personnel, especially those in the Insurgent Zone. To counter this misleading narrative and to better understand how blood transfusion developed during the conflict, and the important role that propaganda played in the process, a historiographical reappraisal is needed. Although Spain was divided, the evolution of the blood transfusion service emerged from developments and shared experiences of doctors who had either trained together in Spain, or were influenced by international developments in blood transfusion, within a specifically Spanish context.

Although propaganda has been defined above in the introduction, and more widely there is a broad understanding of what is meant by 'propaganda', it is worth briefly outlining how the term is further defined for this present study. As used here, it echoes closely Edward Corse's definition of the term in *A Battle for Neutral Europe: British Cultural Propaganda during the Second World War* as being 'used in very broad terms to cover any attempt to influence others and reinforce or change other people'.[19] This interpretation can be delineated further. A leading historian on propaganda, David Welch, offers the following definition:

> An attempt to disseminate propaganda must be both conscious and deliberate. The 'purpose of the propaganda' is therefore the key. Propaganda is an attempt at targeted information with an objective that has been established a priori. Propaganda is best seen as the deliberate attempt to influence public opinion through the transmission of ideas and values for a specific purpose, not through violence or bribery.[20]

Here it has an additional meaning, in that propaganda used in relation to health, specifically blood transfusion, often included educational elements within its framework. This was aimed at both the education and training of other transfusionists and donors, and the promotion of conflicting ideologies in relation to the provision of this life-saving technique. Thus, a further category can be added to Corse's broad definition of propaganda, one that can be defined as 'educational propaganda'.

A clear example that illustrates this definition can be found in the booklet *Cartilla sanitaria del combatiente* (*Health Primer of the Combatant*), published by the Propaganda and Press Section of the Republican Medical Services in August 1937. The advice in this booklet includes information on proper hygiene, teeth cleaning, prevention of sun-stroke, avoiding blood-borne diseases and the importance of only drinking clean water, and is accompanied by text that compares the struggle of the Republic with the French resistance to the Prussian invasion in 1792. It also contains idealised images of the anti-fascist combatant, as well as caricatures of those soldiers who stray from this ideal, such as the whoring soldier or the drunk. Health promotion and education is central to the message contained in this booklet but this message is placed within an ideological context that emphasises that only healthy anti-fascist combatants can hope to vanquish their 'ideologically unsound' opponents.[21]

The historiography of blood transfusion and the Spanish Civil War

The evolution and development of blood transfusion techniques during the Spanish Civil War has given rise to claims of it being the first such service ever established. Chief among these claims is the exaggerated role that Bethune apparently played in the establishment of these facilities.[22] Bethune's own part in the establishment of such claims was by no means a small one; alongside his reputation as a gifted Canadian chest surgeon, he was also known for a somewhat abrasive manner and for being an accomplished self-publicist. His desire to establish a Canadian blood transfusion institute that could compete with the English Hospital at Grañen and the Scottish Ambulance Service as an anti-fascist Canadian national symbol, led to the creation of the service in Madrid.[23] The work of the institute was skilfully promoted by Bethune in letters, radio broadcasts and in the film *Heart of Spain* (1937), and was also heavily promoted in the fundraising tour he undertook when he was recalled from Spain in May 1937.[24] Combined, these had the effect of drawing attention away from developments taking place elsewhere in Spain. It also resulted in the role played by Dr Goyanes Alvarez who succeeded Bethune in Madrid after his departure from Spain, being largely ignored.[25]

The emphasis on Bethune that has come to dominate the history of mobile blood transfusion arose from his understanding of the importance of propaganda. Radio and newspapers were used by both sides in recruiting blood donors, but it was Bethune, through his shortwave radio broadcasts for the Republican Government to North America and participation in the propaganda film *Heart of Spain*, that received much of the publicity outside of Spain.[26] It was his engagement with mass media and his later death as a hero of the left that would ensure that it was his footprint that would remain the most visible after the Spanish Civil War had ended.

The use of print and broadcast media was an important facet of propaganda surrounding blood transfusion. Newspapers, radio broadcasts (which, apart from shortwave transmissions, were aimed at the local population due to their limited range) and films were employed to recruit blood donors and to reinforce competing ideologies in relation to donation. Posters, a powerful propaganda tool used in public health campaigns, seem to have enjoyed a strictly limited use in relation to blood transfusion.[27] The blood transfusion units in Madrid and Barcelona, in recruiting for and in the promotion of their facilities, often linked the giving of blood and the work they were doing as an anti-fascist service by those who donated their blood. By contrast, in the Insurgent Zone, calls for blood were often linked to the reinforcement of traditional Catholic gender roles, with women the focus of much of the publicity.[28]

With the exception of what is a growing corpus of work on Norman Bethune, in part due to his reinvention as a national hero of Canada, but also due to his legendary status in China, where he ironically died of septicaemia (blood poisoning) in 1939, little has been written outside of Spain about the important contribution made by Spanish doctors to the development of a modern blood transfusion service within Spain.[29] Nicolas Coni, in *Medicine and Warfare: Spain, 1936–1939*, refers to the roles played by Durán-Jordà and Elósegui, yet Bethune nonetheless dominates this narrative.[30] Even within Spain, the work done by Durán-Jordà and Elósegui is largely forgotten outside of medical circles. This is perhaps not surprising in a country where open discussion of the Spanish Civil War is still a sensitive subject.[31]

Historians interested in reconstructing the relationship between propaganda and the blood transfusion services are faced with a difficult task. Bethune, due to the status he enjoyed and continues to enjoy in Canada and China, has been the focus of much of the literature relating to blood transfusion.[32] Bethune himself was acutely aware of the role that propaganda could play in advancing his own communist perspective in relation to the Canadian medical effort, but particularly his dominant role in the development of the mobile blood transfusion unit based in Madrid. His engagement beyond the narrow readership offered by medical journals meant that his extensive promotion of the Madrid service over that of Barcelona received much of the attention.[33]

A clue to his ability to manipulate and utilise different forms of media is to be found in his personal background. Bethune was born in Ontario in 1890, and served two tours of duty during WWI, the first as a stretcher-bearer, the second as an MO. A talented writer and artist, he began to develop these skills while confined to two sanatoriums after contracting tuberculosis in 1926. It was during his confinement at the Trudeau Sanatorium near New York in 1927, that he drew a coloured mural on brown paper called *The TBs Progress*, which covered twenty metres of the walls of his cottage.[34]

His interest in art continued throughout his life. He once boasted that he could paint a picture that was good enough to be accepted for the spring 1935 exhibition of the Montreal Museum of Fine Arts. Although untrained, he produced a painting that was accepted, *Night Operating Theatre*, completing it – according to his wife – in two afternoons. It was this combination of artistic ability and 'egotism' that meant that he preferred to be at the centre influencing events, rather than on the periphery.[35]

It was while confined to the sanatorium that he became increasingly dissatisfied with the treatment of a disease that often resulted in death. He pushed for and received radical treatment that involved collapsing the diseased lung. This resulted in the disease being halted within six weeks and affected his own approach to treating the disease in others. This led him to develop an interest in social medicine, as he observed that it was the poor who most frequently died from TB.[36]

During his period as chief thoracic surgeon at the Sacré Coeur Hospital in Montreal, Canada, in 1933, and as part of a campaign to promote the setting up of a social medicine programme, he wrote a radio play about tuberculosis, *The Patients Dilemma; or, Modern Methods of Treating Tuberculosis*, subsequently broadcast on Canadian radio. In the letter he sent to Dr John Wherrett, Executive Secretary of the Canadian Tuberculosis Association, which accompanied the first draft of the play, he wrote: 'I think you will agree with me that the radio has never been exploited to its fullest extent in the education of the public – & the general practitioner'. It was this understanding of the value of education and propaganda that would result in the radio broadcasts he later made in Spain, and in his role in the making of the film *Heart of Spain.*[37] It would also lead to one of the most striking propaganda booklets of the conflict (Image 4), *The Crime on the Road Malaga – Almeria* (1937).

Part of its importance lies in the fact that there were few external witnesses to the flight of the refugees from Malaga after the city's fall in February 1937. Arthur Koestler, the journalist and writer, was a witness to the start of the exodus, as was the British zoologist Sir Peter Chalmers Mitchell.[38] Franco, however, concerned to avoid the kind of international outcry that had resulted from international press reports on the massacres in the bullring in Badajoz after its capture the previous August, took the step of banning all war correspondents from Malaga.[39] Effectively, apart from the refugees themselves and their pursuers, there were few independent witnesses from either side to this tragic flight, which makes the testimony of Bethune and the accompanying photos one of the few contemporary documents that survives.

Written by Bethune, with photographs by his assistant the Canadian architect Hazen Sise, it originated from their experiences, in the company of Thomas Worsley (a driver of the vehicle alongside Sise), en route to the Malaga battlefront with the intent to deliver blood in the specially adapted ambulance. Instead of completing this task, however, the three used the ambulance to help scores of refugees in their 175-kilometre flight.[40] Bethune left a typescript in which he recorded having covered 2,488 kilometres over 85.8 hours between his drive south from Barcelona on 5 February 1937 and his return to Madrid on 16 February. This document provides further evidence for the validity of *The Crime on the Road Malaga – Almeria* as a historical source and also stands testimony to the ground he and his team covered in aiding the refugees.[41]

Heart of Spain, *The Crime on the Road Malaga – Almeria*, newspaper articles, medical journals, photographs and the letters sent to the Canadian Committee to Aid Spanish Democracy (CASD) are all used here to help reconstruct the propagandistic role that blood transfusion played in the broader context of promoting certain ideologies.[42] However, it is when this material is placed alongside the sources specific to the Spanish personalities involved that a clearer and more comprehensive picture emerges about developments relating to the transfusion of blood and the role that propaganda played in this process within Spain. Through an engagement with the Spanish sources in conjunction with those on Norman Bethune, and information gleaned from other literature, such as the *BMJ* and the SMAC archive held at the Modern Record Centre at Warwick University, it becomes possible to build a fuller and more rounded picture of just how important blood transfusion was, not just to the wounded, but also as a fundraising tool on both sides of the conflict.[43]

The political discourses arising out of conflicting nationalist and left-wing ideologies expressed through propaganda, propaganda which, at times, was sophisticated and subtle, was often aimed at the education of different sections

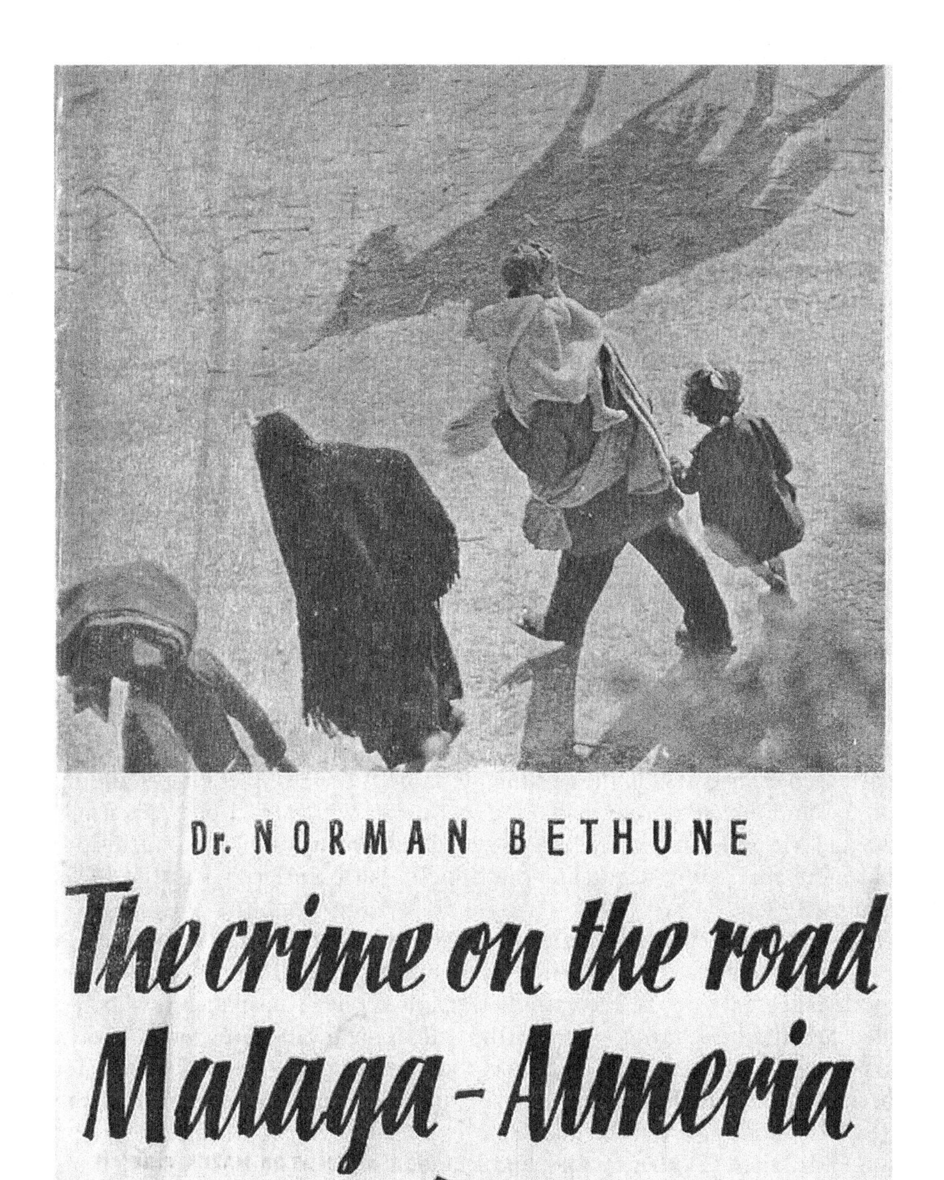

Image 4 Bethune, *The Crime on the Road Malaga – Almeria* (Spain, 1937), frontispiece. Source: Bethune, N., *The Crime on the Road Malaga – Almeria: Narrative with Graphic Documents Revealing Fascist Cruelty* (Spain, 1937).

within society. An exploration of the importance of 'Blood Propaganda', not only highlights the important Spanish contributions made in furthering developments in the field of mobile blood transfusion, but also highlights its role as an ideological tool.

With regards to the Spanish sources, it is primarily the medical journals, the monograph from 1937 by Durán-Jordà titled *The Service of Blood Transfusion at the Front: Organisation-Apparatus*, newspapers and the films *Transfusió de Sang* (English title: *Blood Transfusion at the Front*), *Blood Bank Service in Spain* and *Defenders of the Faith*, which contains a short section on the Insurgent blood service, that form the core of materials necessary for the reconstruction of the Spanish contribution to blood transfusion.[44] Contemporary newspapers from within Spain, which almost invariably seek to promote the vested interests and the political agendas of their proprietors (this being especially true during warfare), also offer invaluable insights into the competing discourses surrounding the propaganda of blood.

The origins of modern blood transfusion

Before examining the role that propaganda played in relation to blood transfusion during the Spanish Civil War, it is worth taking a brief look at how modern blood transfusion evolved. Although innovation was an important aspect of developments within Spain during this period, many of these claims have been exaggerated in the existing literature.[45] For a proper understanding of the undoubtedly groundbreaking work that was carried out, this needs placing within a context relating to new developments in blood transfusion, but more specifically research and advances that occurred during the 1920s and the 1930s.

James Blundell, an obstetrician at Guy's and St Thomas' Hospitals in London, is credited with having given the first blood transfusion of the modern age. In 1818, he successfully transfused one of his patients, who had bled heavily after having given birth, with human blood (previous known experiments had been with animal blood). Although blood groups had not been identified at this stage, his technique was successful enough that the death of those who did die due to having been given the wrong blood type were attributed to other factors, and Blundell went on later to report on his findings in *The Lancet* in 1828.[46]

Techniques in blood transfusion continued to develop with the invention of the hypodermic syringe in 1853, which would facilitate later transfusion techniques. A development that was to prove of importance was the discovery by the Belgian, Adolph Hustin, in 1914, shortly before the outbreak of WWI, that sodium citrate worked as an anticoagulant.[47] It was not until the war itself, however, that blood transfusion became more widely practised, with the direct arm-to-arm method by far the most common method applied. With the development of anticoagulant-preservative solutions, blood depots were established in a few British Casualty Clearing Stations. The presence of these early blood banks contributed towards saving lives, although this is not well documented. The main impetus for this change in practice was prompted by Canadian MOs' addition of citrate to blood to facilitate arm-to-arm transfusion, and by the publication in British medical journals of their findings that demonstrated the greater efficacy of blood over saline for the treatment of haemorrhagic shock.[48] Unfortunately, this practice was not widely established. Many men ended their lives in the 'moribund wards', where those believed to be unfit to survive surgery were sent, and where 'nursing sisters attempted to keep them comfortable until they died'.[49]

The first blood donor service was established by the civil servant Percy Oliver in London. Oliver, secretary of the Camberwell Division of the British Red Cross, organised a system for recruiting donors who could be called upon to give fresh blood at local hospitals. A scheme was devised whereby each donor was tested to establish their blood group and to screen for syphilis. This work was expanded when Sir Geoffrey Keynes, an eminent surgeon from St Bartholomew's Hospital, was appointed as a medical advisor.[50] There were soon blood donor centres in New York and Paris, and in 1936 these were recorded as having carried out 6,686 and 6,298 transfusions respectively.[51] Centres of this type did not become common in Spain until after the outbreak of the Civil War. In Barcelona in 1935 there were only 128 transfusions recorded, which took place in hospitals and clinics, all by the direct arm-to-arm technique, with 83 of the donors being family members.[52]

As blood transfusion became more commonplace, many people lost their fear of what had been an unfamiliar practice and by the outbreak of the Spanish Civil War, Madrid had two departments of haematology, one in the hospital of the Red Cross, where Dr Elósegui was based, and the other in the School of Health under the auspices of Professor Pittaluga. Both of these organisations were able to successfully recruit donors locally for direct arm-to-arm transfusions through appeals over the radio and in the press, and with the onset of the conflict, were able to rapidly organise their own blood transfusion centres, and then blood banks due to the presence of the rudimentary infrastructure required.[53] The institute set up by Bethune by the end of 1936 had 1,000 donors on its books, mainly recruited through 'propaganda de radio y prensa' (radio and press advertising – in Spanish 'propaganda' translates literally as advertising), and these were the main means of recruiting donors (albeit locally) throughout Spain during the conflict.[54] During the two and a half years that the service in Barcelona was in operation, there were up to 28,900 donors registered.[55]

A development that was to prove of interest to Durán-Jordà was the use of stored citrated blood from cadavers, pioneered in the Soviet Union by Sergei Yudin in 1930 as result of a shortage of donors.[56] This use of blood from cadavers had grown out of earlier experiments on preserving body tissue through refrigeration. Between 1930 and 1940, there were more than 2,500 reported cases of transfusion using this method in the Soviet

Union. It was then dropped in part due to technical reasons, but mainly due to objections on moral grounds, although this technique was widely reported upon, with Yudin visiting Britain, Germany and France in 1933. It was in France in 1933 that his monograph *La Transfusion du sang de cadavre à l'homme* was published.[57] Although cadaveric blood transfusion was seen by most doctors as an ethically unsound practice, Yudin's monograph had an influence on the renewal of interest in finding ways to store blood in the mid-1930s. This was particularly true among doctors in an unsettled Europe concerned with the wider use of civilian transfusions should another major European conflict break out.[58]

Advances within Spain not only built on developments in techniques that preceded the conflict but, in the context of the above, did bring about innovations that would save the lives of many wounded civilians and combatants. It would also have an influence, through Durán-Jordà's relationship with Janet Vaughan, a haematologist and radiobiologist at the Hammersmith Hospital, involved in providing medical aid to the Spanish Republic through her involvement with SMAC, on the establishment of a national blood transfusion service in Britain. It was due to her invitation that Durán-Jordà was able to flee Barcelona shortly before it was taken by Franco's troops on 26 January 1939, and come and stay with her in London as an invitee of the British Red Cross. Vaughan, convinced that war was imminent after the Munich agreement of 1938, and concerned that London and other British cities might experience the same mass bombing of civilians experienced in Madrid and Barcelona, drew up plans with the aid of Durán-Jordà and other colleagues for a service similar to that of Barcelona.[59] This plan was accepted by the British government, with Vaughan made head of the North-West London depot for the duration of WWII.[60] A further three blood depots were established in the outer suburbs of London after the outbreak of the war, as well as the Army Transfusion Service in the South-West of England, for the storage and transportation of the blood.

If the Spanish experience with the transfusion of conserved blood had an influence on the development of a similar service in Britain, it also seems likely that it influenced French efforts in this area. However, both countries also built upon their own experience, and the developments of the inter-war years in the building of these services meant that at the start of WWII they were fairly well placed to supply growing quantities of blood to the civilian population and the military.[61]

Russia was also well placed to build upon their own inter-war experience in relation to stored blood and by 1943 in Moscow, 2,000 pints of blood a day were being drawn, citrated and then despatched to frontline hospitals where it could be stored in ice houses for up to eighteen days.[62] Unfortunately, this was not to be the case in Germany, where resistance by doctors to the transfusion of conserved blood meant that in September 1939 there were no blood banks in Germany.[63] It was not until March 1940 that guidelines for transfusions were first circulated.[64] Nevertheless, the German military made efforts to identify the blood types of all its active combatants, with this information printed on their health cards and identity tags, and recruited donors for arm-to-arm blood transfusions from reserve troops stationed near frontline hospitals.[65]

Advances in the provision of conserved blood during the Spanish Civil War resulted from the needs of civilians and combatants involved in 'total war'. The conflict accelerated these developments and influenced advances beyond its own borders. However, it is almost certainly the case that without Spain's conflict or the ensuing World War, these developments would have occurred regardless, as they came out of practices largely developed during the inter-war peace, and not out of the war itself. The interest alone from medical practitioners such as Yudin during this period into the life-saving properties of blood, would have provided sufficient impetus to spur further developments, but blood as a symbol has a much broader cultural significance, and this in turn drives further enquiry. This broader significance was not lost on the propagandists of the day, and it is the symbolism, both religious and cultural, and its relationship with propaganda, that is explored in the following section.

The symbolic power of blood

There were deep-seated cultural and iconographical based notions tied to the giving and receiving of blood in Spain, with the blood-letting sacrificial spectacle of the bullfight a popular event linked to festivals and religious holidays. The bleeding heart of Jesus, with the bloodied nails through the torn flesh of his hand and feet, and the Eucharist, were visible manifestations in churches throughout Spain of the sanctity of blood.[66] An unusual expression of this can be found in a newspaper article from the *ABC* of Sevilla by M. Siurot, published 27 August, 1938, titled 'Los Moritos' (Little Moors).[67] The article begins by describing the anti-atheist credentials of the 'moors' (i.e., their own religiosity) and their 'hatred of the communists'. Siurot then goes on to state how the 'Moritos' were in Spain:

> because they feel themselves fellow companions in their zeal for our struggle, because they have been infiltrated by our blood and our civilisation, and we have been infiltrated by theirs as well. In the eight centuries of the Reconquest, blood and Arabic civilisation … has co-penetrated the races, a transfusion of blood and ideas, a grand civilisation realised by the phenomenon of a moral osmosis.[68]

Similar sentiments are expressed by the right-wing American film director Russell Palmer in the film *Defenders of the Faith*, made in 1938, during a scene where representatives from all sections of the armed forces are gathered to celebrate the second anniversary of the Insurgency on 18 July 1938. In reference to the presence of the Regulares and a common religiosity, Palmer describes them as, 'Moors from Spanish Morocco. Mohammedans, devout, they are renowned for their hatred of communism. The Spanish Moors consider the reds anti-religious because they have defiled and burnt the churches of Spain'.[69]

Alongside this discourse on the sanctity of blood and religiosity existed more romantic notions to do with the sharing of blood. Patience Darton, who worked at the cave hospital in Bisbal de Falset during the Ebro Campaign, volunteered her services to SMAC at the outbreak of the Civil War, and went to nurse in Spain in February 1937. She talked about her experiences during the conflict in an interview about her life in 1993.[70] Patience Darton, whose memory is a little hazy on some points, recalled that

> the Spanish were very romantic about blood transfusion ... blood transfusion of bottled blood started in Spain ... they were very romantic about it, they thought that if they shared our blood, you were half-brothers and so on. We used to do a lot of arm-to-arm stuff, after having tested to see what type you were, what kind of A, B, C, or D.[71]

Hers were the memories of a person in their eighties, and have to be treated with caution, but her reference to the prevalence of arm-to-arm transfusion as the preferred method of transfusion do have some basis in fact. Goyanes, in the *Revista de Sanidad de Guerra* from 1938, reported that out of the 3,000 blood transfusions gathered in his statistical database, seventy per cent had been given by this method.[72]

Hazen Sise, interviewed by Rod Langley for a radio programme about Bethune for Canada Radio International on 26 January 1967, commented that 'the Spanish had an almost mystical feeling about blood ... to do with the corrida (the bullfight)', also noting with reference to Bethune that 'he realised the value of the service being Canadian from a propaganda viewpoint back in Canada'.[73]

Blood as a symbolic motif was a central component of Spanish Catholicism. Catholicism, in turn, was an integral part of Spanish culture in its broadest context. Also culturally entrenched in sections of Spanish society, was an anti-clericalism that had its roots in the early nineteenth century and which had at its core a symbology of blood. By the turn of the twentieth century, this symbology was based in the millenarian hopes and expectations of the anarchist movement (although by no means restricted to it), sections of which saw the bloodletting of the clergy as an important step towards their utopian revolutionary goals.[74] Nearly 7,000 of the clergy were to be killed, mainly at the start of the Spanish Civil War, after the breakdown in law that accompanied the start of the conflict in the Republican zone. An explanation offered by some of those involved in the killing was the need to purify Spanish society so that the revolution could be achieved.[75]

Thus, the bleeding heart of Jesus, the crown of thorns, the Eucharist, Marian devotion and iconography, with the powerful motif of the sacrificial and sanctified blood of Christ at its core, with the crucifixion itself tied to notions that the sacramental blood of Christ when taken as part of the ritual of transubstantiation is a spiritual blood transfusion that can lead to absolution, were not only potent symbols of devotion, but embodied a symbolism of the oppression of the church which from the start of the conflict had identified itself with the Insurgency. Anti-clericalism could take many forms, but in Spain it reflected a perception by sectors of society that the church had betrayed Christ who had shed his blood for the poor. This led to veneration turning to destruction, which in turn led to scenes such as the mock execution by firing squad outside Madrid of a monolithic statue of Christ by Republican militiamen.[76]

Notions to do with the sanctity of blood being tied to religion and the idea of sharing blood establishing a link with the donor were also important factors in the recruitment of blood donors and contributed to the efficacy of propaganda in disseminating different ideologies in relation to blood and its donation. This was no more evident than early in the conflict when a Falangist battalion of blood donors was created with the sole purpose of providing transfusions at the front, and for whom the blood, as embodied in their conservative Catholicism, was a potent symbol of their faith.[77] On the same fronts where Durán-Jordà and Pittaluga's institute were delivering blood, Lorenzo Gironés, a professor in internal medicine from the University of Santiago de Compostela, joined Franco's forces and recruited a battalion of male Falangist volunteers with the purpose of giving their blood in direct arm-to-arm transfusions at the front.[78] He was assigned the rank of MO, and put in charge of the Blood Transfusion Team of the Seventh Army Corps, which was soon to become the Army Corps of Galicia.[79] He recruited only men, as women in the Insurgent zone were not allowed near the frontline unless they were nurses.[80] Gironés, with the help of his aides, Doctors Pintos Pérez, Monterroso, Leiro and Monteis, and the battalion of Falangist blood donors, facilitated hundreds of arm-to-arm transfusions on the Aragón Front and at the hospital in Getafe. Gironés was a strong advocate of the direct method of transfusion, preferring this technique over that of using conserved blood, and argued that the latter should only be used in frontline hospitals where there was no civilian population or reserve troops from which to recruit donors.[81]

The 'soldiers of blood', whose sole purpose in going to the front was as blood donors, were not to last long.[82] The group created by Gironés were disbanded, partly because transfusion services were placed under the control of Elósegui, but also because Franco, keen to create a single party state, was intent on limiting the power of the Falange. Franco set about this in October 1936 when he was declared Generalissimo and Head of State, and achieved his aim in April 1937, when the Falange, the Carlists, Renovación Española and other right-wing groups were fused into the Falange Española Tradicionalista y de las Juntas de Ofensiva Nacional Sindicalista (FET y las JONS) with Franco as leader.[83]

The role of film

The direct recruitment methods favoured by Gironés were never going to be successful enough to recruit the necessary number of volunteers at the front in what was becoming an increasingly bloody conflict. Radio appeals, effective in large urban centres such as Barcelona and Madrid, and to a lesser degree regionally, were nevertheless of limited use due to their restricted range but also because the mass ownership of radio was uncommon in Spain, although people would congregate in bars and other locations to listen to broadcasts. The radio sets of suspected dissidents were confiscated by both sides, and the powerful shortwave broadcasts were predominantly aimed at the outside world with only the more expensive sets within Spain able to receive these transmissions.[84] Newspapers, alongside radio, were a useful medium for recruiting donors locally, but with Spain divided, a national press did not exist. As such, film, easy to distribute, was the ideal vehicle for reaching both national and international audiences. It is the role of film that forms a central focus of this chapter, as it was this powerful medium with its extensive reach that would internationalise the propaganda surrounding blood transfusion. These campaigns also helped raise considerable sums in medical aid, with those in defence of the Republic providing a vital lifeline in the face of an imbalanced non-intervention policy that favoured the Insurgents.[85]

In a SMAC report on the International Conference for Medical Aid to Spain, held in Paris in July 1938, the French delegate reported on 2,640,000 Francs that had been raised in France since the start of the conflict. The majority of this money, he reported, had been spent 'on actual material ambulances or personnel sent to Spain' (89.6 per cent), with a further 3.6 per cent spent on propaganda. He also stated: 'Two films – "Heart of Spain" and "Victory of Life", have been bought, which are successfully being shown at meetings etc. They estimate to receive back about half of the cost of the films and count the balance against propaganda.'[86]

Victoire de la Vie was a forty-nine-minute 'documentary' film about the Republican medical services directed by Henri Cartier Bresson, the internationally renowned photographer, in conjunction with Herbert Kline, and was produced by the CSI, the organisation in Paris through which most medical aid to Spain was channelled.[87] A sophisticated propaganda film, *Victoire de la Vie* also includes schematic drawing animation to demonstrate varying levels of provision and distribution of care.[88] A well-produced film with a high standard of cinematography, it is a less strident piece than *Heart of Spain*. This is underscored by its use of a predominantly mournful orchestral score, *Victoire de la Vie* op. 167, by the French composer Charles Koechlin. Its subject matter ranges the spectrum from childcare in hospitals to military medicine. It has a more straightforward style than contemporary films, with much of its footage seemingly reflecting a more realistic version of care of the wounded, and it is a film that rewards close study. It was first screened in Paris in June 1938 at the Salle Pleyel *Soirée de Gala*, where it was to be shown a further two times. Interestingly, Durán-Jordà does appear briefly in the film outside a military hospital in Barcelona, but only as an unnamed figure standing next to Julio Lozano Bejerano, Chief of the Republican Military Medical Services.[89]

Heart of Spain, produced by Frontier Films in collaboration with the Canadian Committee to Aid Spain, and the North American Committee to Aid Spanish Democracy, with narration by John O'Shaughnessy (of whom little is known), focuses its attention on the defence of Madrid, American medical aid and the work of the institute for blood in the capital.[90] It received its first of many screenings in North America in Vancouver in Canada on 1 August 1937.[91]

In January 1938, in the supplement to the *BMJ*, Dr Ellis of the Royal Society of Medicine, was reported as having shown the film '*Blood Transfusion at the Front*, by Dr Frederic Durán-Jordà' in London.[92] Ellis was to show this film on at least one other occasion three months later, when it was also coincidentally being screened at the Publi Cinema in Barcelona.[93] The original title of the film, *Transfusió de Sang*, was in Catalan, as was its narration, indicating that it was made with a Catalan audience in mind.[94] The British Film Institute (BFI) holds the only known surviving copy of the film *Blood Bank Service in Spain*, which was also made by Laya Films in 1937, and which, until recently, was thought to be the same film under a different name. It in fact turns out to be an entirely different film, and is a 16-millimetre short of ten minutes duration, and although it is about the same service, its footage is almost entirely different and focused on the technical aspects of blood transfusion.[95] However, very little is known about this film.[96] Due to the lack of supporting evidence for the screening of *Blood Bank Service in Spain*, it is *Transfusió de Sang* that is the main focus of the enquiry here, as at this stage it is not known whether *Blood Bank Service in Spain* was shown to an audience, although its existence and its almost exclusive focus on technique would suggest that it was likely seen by a medical audience, albeit a limited one.

During the autumn of 1938, the only known full-length documentary colour film to have been shot in Spain during the Civil War, Russell Palmer's *Defenders of the Faith*, had its first limited screenings in cinemas in the US. A film made in support of Franco, the 'Bishops Committee' is listed as the production company, with the film sponsored by the organisation the 'Relief of Spanish Distress'.[97]

What follows here is an examination of each of the three films that deal, in whole or in part, with blood transfusion. There is a synopsis for each of the films discussed, with these synopses written in a manner designed to reflect their respective visual and narrative messages. The propagandistic elements of the films are analysed, as well as the medical and educational messages embedded within the propaganda, with the aim of constructing a narrative that demonstrates how propaganda and health could be intricately intertwined and used to promote differing ideological viewpoints.

Heart of Spain

The first half of the film *Heart of Spain* is primarily concerned with the defence of Madrid, and depicts both civilian and military life. The film opens with the titles scrolling over the photographic still of a traumatised mother holding a child beneath a sky filled with enemy planes. The scene then shifts to stock film shot by Roman Karmén and Boris Makaseiev, two Soviet cinematographers despatched to Spain at the start of the conflict to record footage. The intention was for this footage to be shown in the Soviet Union and Spain as part of the Comintern's backing of a Popular Front perspective of resistance to fascism, a theme that the film reflected.[98]

References to blood, whether shed by civilians or soldiers, forms a central motif throughout much of the film. This is evident in a scene where Commandant Lister, a Galician communist, addresses the troops. As part of his address he stridently announces that 'this is the season when olives turn blood red in the sun, it seems that even the olives are bleeding now, but some day after our victory, there will be no more violence, no more bloodshed in Spain'.[99] He goes on to stress in his address that

> some of us may die before that time, but others must live for greater work than this ... remember this officers, when you take these men into action, remember they are your brothers. If their blood is spilled, it is the blood of your brothers.

Following these various sacrificial allusions to blood and further footage of fighting, the film turns its attention to care of the wounded. 'An American ambulance unit, two hundred yards behind the trenches, on roads crossed by shellfire', is seen driving across the plain to attend to the wounded injured in the fighting near Madrid. The ambulance is then shown 'speeding the wounded to operating tables where surgeons work in difficulties unknown in times of peace'. After a brief scene that shows surgery in progress in a mobile operating theatre, the scene shifts to the interior patio of an 'American hospital', where 'side by side – the mother bombed in her home – the son shot at the front' recline on stretchers in the hospital courtyard.

The scene then cuts to footage of Salaria Kea, an African American nurse who served with the Abraham Lincoln Brigade, and who is shown changing the dressing of a wounded soldier who is missing part of his arm.[100] Unlike the largely bloodless casualties shown earlier in the film, his amputated stump is revealed, with its poorly approximated skin edges, with the narrator stating, 'this man was struck by an Italian explosive bullet – don't turn away – this is neutrality – this is non-intervention'.

Following further scenes of the wounded at the hospital, the final third of the film turns its attention to blood transfusion, which opens with footage of large queues outside the Madrid Blood Institute. Scenes follow of enthusiastic volunteers willingly climbing onto beds so that their blood can be taken, stored and then refrigerated. The camera lingers in close-up on the blood labels then zooms out to focus on outstretched arms, tourniquets applied, needles piercing the inside of the elbow flexion as blood is collected from donors whose fists clench and unclench to facilitate the flow of blood.[101]

The narrative structure of this section of the film takes as its focus an upright but elderly woman, Hero Escobedo, who appears to be in mourning (she is dressed in black), and Norman Bethune. Bethune is shown having just taken her blood, although interestingly there is no visible puncture mark. The commentary that follows this scene states: 'each new donor asks the same question, will my blood spoil, will it surely be used – can I meet the one to whom it will be given?', a discourse remarkably similar to that found in the *ABC* of 9 February 1937, and indicative of Bethune's influence on the propaganda originating from the institute.[102] Scenes follow of Bethune showing Hero Escobedo around the institute, and as he labels her blood he explains that the label records her name, 'the date July 14, and your blood grouping – group IV'.[103] The date of 14 July given in the commentary is in fact a fabrication, as Bethune by this stage had already left Spain. A possible reason for this is that, with the first public screening of *Heart of Spain* taking place in Canada at the beginning of August 1937, the film's producers could give the impression that the films content reflected up-to-date events.[104]

Footage then follows of the register being brought out by Celia Greenspan, Bethune's laboratory technician, and together they show Escobedo where the blood has been recorded.[105] The footage that follows is of the storage of the blood, more shots of donors from whose arms blood 'is tapped pint by pint, a great human reservoir that flows towards exhausted veins', before cutting to a blood fridge being loaded into the 'ambulance' and heading off to the front.[106] This vehicle is then shown arriving at its 'destination, one of the six frontline hospitals established under Dr Barsky of the American Medical Bureau'. The closing scenes portray a young patient, Enrique Galan, being given a transfusion with the blood 'from the heart of Spain', donated by Hero Escobedo, who bends over him, smiles and kisses him on the forehead. The film closes with forearm after forearm being placed on arm boards, fists clenched ready to pump blood into the waiting bottle that fills before the viewer's eyes.[107]

The reason for such a description of the film, is to demonstrate that, although the film's avowed aim was to show the defence of Madrid, the symbolic heart of Spain alluded to in the title, and to promote the North American organisations supplying medical aid to the Republic, it was a film that sought to influence its audience through the use of selective images. At its core is a message of Canadian and international solidarity with the Spanish Republic; a Popular Front solidarity which through combined action can make 'Madrid the tomb of fascism', a phrase frequently used by Bethune in letters and broadcasts.[108]

The film's main aim, apart from that of raising funds for medical aid, was as a vehicle to 'oppose international fascism', and to promote Frontier Films' ethos of a 'committed social-economic-political stance, and a wise, mature, integrated worldview'.[109] This ethos was reflected in the production company's initial brochure, which accused Hollywood of misusing film's 'great power' and stated that Frontier Films had entered 'the field to produce films that will yield this power consistently on the side of progress'.[110] With the film still awaiting completion upon Bethune's return to Canada, he was initially unable to screen it during his fundraising tour of North America (the tour included addressing crowds in both the US and Canada), with the consequence that much of the accompanying media attention centred around him. Some 8,500 people alone turned out for his opening address at the Mount Arena in Montreal on 18 June 1937.[111]

Heart of Spain showed to a full house of 3,000 people when it was first screened by Bethune at the Orpheum Theatre in Vancouver, Canada, on 1 August 1937.[112] Although there are no exact figures for money raised from the screenings in North America, at one meeting that Bethune addressed, where he described his experiences on the road between Malaga and Almeria, nearly $2,000 was raised.[113] Despite the attendance of large crowds at many of the gatherings, North America was still in the grip of a depression, and in Sudbury on 11 July 1937 only $22.40 was raised from a crowd of 700 people.[114]

The film was also screened outside of North America. The organising secretary of SMAC 'whilst in Paris had seen the film' and 'advised its purchase for propaganda work ... but the cost would be about £150' so 'it was decided to get detailed costs, and if possible get a copy here for viewing'.[115] This would suggest that it had been successful in raising funds in France, but again there seem to be no figures relating to sums raised. This may be as the result of the destruction of French archives in bombing raids during WWII, but this is merely a tentative hypothesis and future research may possibly reveal some data relating to how many people saw this film in France and how much money was raised.[116] A French version of the film titled *Spaniens Hjärta* with Swedish subtitles was also shown in Sweden as part of fundraising efforts and was distributed by the Swedish Aid Spain Committee.[117] The Madrid Film Institute has also recovered another French version of the film with its original title of *Coeur d'Espagne*, which consists of the last roll of footage looking at blood transfusion.[118] Together, these two copies provide additional information, albeit scanty, as to the wider dissemination of this film.

Heart of Spain was never intended as a medical film; nevertheless, if this was the only surviving testimony to such techniques then this would undoubtedly contribute to its historical value. Its strength, however, lies in the successful portrayal of the events it sets out to describe and its sophisticated use of propaganda to propagate its anti-fascist Popular Front message. This led to the film's other purpose as propaganda being met, that of being seen by many thousands throughout North America, but also in France (and possibly in other countries involved in raising money for medical aid, such as Sweden), and as a consequence not only promoting the core ideology of the film but fulfilling one of its key goals of raising money to facilitate further international medical participation and aid to the beleaguered Spanish Republic.[119] Although there is no evidence at present for *Heart of Spain* being shown in Britain during the conflict, propaganda efforts in the form of leaflets, booklets, posters and film were an important aspect of fundraising in Britain, and by the end of the conflict more than £2,000,000 had been raised in Britain, with the majority of this money going towards medical and food aid for Spain.[120]

Transfusió de Sang

The film *Transfusió de Sang* by Frederic Durán-Jordà, made at some point during 1937, was a nine-minute short, shown in cinemas in Barcelona. It was also screened at least twice to medical audiences in Britain, once at the end of 1937 and again in the spring of 1938.[121] The British medic Dr Ellis left a contemporary description of the film, after a screening for a medical audience in April 1938. He described the film as demonstrating 'the organisation of a blood transfusion service under conditions of modern warfare, and illustrates the Durán-Jordà method of storage and distribution of blood'.[122] He describes the interior of a blood transfusion lorry shown in the film as 'containing a generator, two refrigerators, and room for two stretchers'.

Ellis, as can be reasonably expected given he was writing a description for a medical journal, focuses on the film's medical aspects. This, however, is not strictly speaking a 'medical film', as the production company, Laya Films, principally produced propaganda films for cinema consumption with the aim of promoting a left-wing Catalan perspective, neither explicitly anarchist or communist, in defence of the Republic.[123]

It is arguably the accompaniment of the image and the word that makes cinematic propaganda more effective than the moving image alone, as a specific message can be more directly delivered. This becomes evident when comparing this film with *Blood Bank Service in Spain*, a silent 16-millimetre short. This was a popular format for 'medical' films as it was relatively inexpensive, and could be accompanied by a lecture to better explain its contents.[124] Apart from the opening scenes of *Blood Bank Service in Spain*, which contains its only overt political message – the camera focuses in on the letters CNT-FAI on the side of a crate of potatoes being loaded onto a truck – it is a film about 'advanced' blood collection and transfusion techniques. The film is shot almost entirely in close-up, a visual device similar to that used in 'research' films made in Nazi Germany at the time. The technique was intended to 'stress particular details under investigation', and in this case gives added emphasis to the scientific nature of the film's content.[125]

In contrast, the political message of *Transfusió de Sang* is clearly 'spelt out', with the narration tied closely to the imagery seen on screen.[126] The film's opening shot focuses its lens on the visually striking side of the converted fish-truck, with its graphic of three donors, each representing the main Catalan political factions, having their blood collected by a white-coated medic. There then follows images of technical staff in a lab with a variety of apparatus consisting of a wide assortment of glass utensils and tubes, before shifting to footage of the preparation of a blood donor and the extraction of her blood (almost all the donors shown are female), which is then shown having sodium citrate added. Following on from this is footage of the blood being mixed with other donated blood in the lab, a technique favoured by Durán-Jordà, so as to minimise adverse reactions during transfusion caused 'by hematic groups insufficiently determinate, the number of which varies according to different authorities'.[127] After further technical scenes, followed by stock footage of warfare, a female receptionist is shown receiving a phone call with a request for blood to be delivered to the front. The footage that follows shows medics or technicians jumping into the converted fish truck, which then sets off for the frontline.[128]

The van is shown arriving 'at the front' where a man lies on a stretcher awaiting a transfusion. The blood, in its vacuum sealed elongated glass ampoule is shown being placed in a flask to warm to '36–40° centigrade', so as not to exacerbate any shock symptoms present in the wounded patient by transfusing refrigerated blood.[129] The blood is then transfused and the film closes with footage of a hospital train and of a military hospital with the commentary emphasising that the blood is available for transfusion in all of these locations.

The commentary, that runs almost continuously throughout the film, after a brief opening anti-fascist preamble, states that it is 'to the directors of the Servei de Transfusió de Sang and its collaborators, such as its anonymous donors of blood, that this film is dedicated, as an homage to their civic heroism in contributing to its great results'. It then goes on to stress the egalitarian nature of the service by stating that 'the blood is extracted from voluntary donors without distinction of sex, age, political or syndicalist ideology'. The commentary then goes on to describe the transfusion techniques shown in the film, how the blood is collected, citrated, bottled, mixed and stored, and also emphasises the cleanliness and sterility of these procedures. The service is then described as ready to respond to 'all the petitions from the front for the injection of fresh blood into the veins of the wounded soldiers'. In its closing narration, it describes how the 'Servei de Transfusió de Sang', created by Durán-Jordà, had been set up by a 'political syndicalist party', the PSUC (controlled by the Partido Comunista de España, the Spanish Communist Party or PCE) 'who then later passed it onto the Generalitat'. It also states that the Catalan Parliament had then passed this on to the Republican Army Health Corps so that its 'benefits can be extended to all soldiers'.[130]

This commentary, with the exception of its educational element, the description of the technical aspects of blood donation and transfusion, has a clear propagandistic message. This message, however, does distort certain information. Thus, having been created by the PSUC (with the aid of the UGT), until its assimilation into the Republican Army Health Corps, it is unlikely that the blood transfusion service willingly supplied blood to 'all soldiers', as the POUM militias were hated by the Stalinist-controlled PCE, with only slightly less ire reserved for the anarcho-syndicalist militias of the CNT.[131]

There is evidence that supports this argument, as the booklet by Durán-Jordà, *The Service of Blood Transfusion at the Front: Organisation-Apparatus*, states on its opening page that the PSUC and the UGT 'thought it advisable that its own columns ... and the Field Hospitals controlled by these two organisations, should have a Service for the transfusion of preserved blood'.[132] Even after its assimilation, its benefits could not be extended to all soldiers, as for reasons mentioned previously, such as the sheer number of casualties, resistance to the use of conserved blood and an inability to supply on such a large scale, it was just not possible to offer this service universally within the Republican Zone.

This documentary short, which combines propaganda and education, is illustrative of how propaganda could be used to target more than one audience. Whether this is the result of Durán-Jordà targeting the general public within Spain so as to keep up the supply of donors – arguably the main purpose of the film – while at the same time trying to attract the attention of the medical community outside of Spain is difficult to establish. What does appear to be certain is that it did catch the eye of both these audiences. Part of this success can be attributed to Durán-Jordà's wider engagement with print media including journals and newspapers, which ensured that there was contemporary interest in his work.[133]

Bearing in mind the interest from figures in the medical community in Britain, what is perhaps harder to explain is how his contribution seems to have been so quickly forgotten. Janet Vaughan does not reference his work directly after May 1939, when she expressed her gratitude to 'Dr. Duran-Jorda [*sic*] for the information he has given me about his experience with stored blood in the Spanish War', except for one citation of his work in a journal article she wrote in October 1940. A possible explanation for this may lie in the fact that Durán-Jordà frequently referred to the work of Yudin in his writing.[134] With the Nazi-Soviet Pact of August 1939, any connection of the new national blood transfusion service, however nebulous, that attributed any of the work it carried out as having anything to do with research originating in the Soviet Union may well have been reason enough for him to be sidelined.[135] Another reason may be found in the complicated processes involved in his system of blood collection and conservation with its delicate vacuum-sealed large glass ampoules.[136] The system used by Bethune with its simpler and more robust 'milk bottle' type containers, was also the method used in

Britain, when during the panic in September 1938 caused by the Munich Crisis, refrigeration units and a large supply of obsolete milk bottles were located in preparedness for war, and it was this type of container that was used by the British during WWII.[137]

Nevertheless, the contribution made by Durán-Jordà to the transfusion of conserved blood was an important one. This is evident in the articles he wrote and the two films made about the service. Further evidence for this is to be found in the inclusion of footage from *Transfusió de Sang* in the film *Blood Transfusion*, made by the Ministry of Information in Britain in 1941. In the commentary that accompanies this brief section, it is stated that 'stored blood was given its first test under practical conditions in the Spanish Civil War of 1936', with Durán-Jordà also mentioned in this commentary.[138] His obituary in the *BMJ* of 20 April 1957, reported that 'with the outbreak of the Spanish Civil War he organised the Blood Transfusion of the Republican Army, using for the first time on a large scale, the civilian population as donors'. It also acknowledges that it was in 1937 that he

> officially took up the post as chief of the service. In this capacity he obtained the highest medical award of the Catalan Government, and was invited to various European countries to lecture and advise on the organisation of national blood transfusion services.[139]

Defenders of the Faith

There is little written in the historiography of cinematography during the Spanish Civil War that includes reference to Russell Palmer and his film *Defenders of the Faith*. What is known is that he was titular head of the Peninsular News Service in New York, an organisation created to promote the Francoist viewpoint in the US. Palmer strongly believed in disseminating a positive propaganda message on Spain that contrasted what was coming out of Great Britain and France, and he spent considerable sums propagating a simple, uncomplicated message to an American middle-class seemingly disinterested in polemical discussion.[140] These positive propaganda elements are clearly visible in the film he shot in Spain, with respect for religion, an organised society, the supposed agricultural abundance of the Insurgent Zone and the care of the wounded by 'saintly' nuns, carefully chosen images that purport to portray everyday normality of life in insurgent occupied territory.

The main focus of this enquiry into the film is the four minutes and forty-one seconds that deal with the blood transfusion service set up by Elósegui. Palmer states in the commentary that this 'system had been in operation since the very start of the conflict'. Officially recognised under the title, 'servicios de transfusión de sangre conservado en el suero IHT' (Blood Transfusion Services of Conserved Blood in IHT Serum) on 22 January 1937, it had in fact been in existence since September of the previous year.[141]

IHT was an effective anticoagulant combining sodium citrate and other constituents, first devised by the Institute of Haematology and Blood Transfusion in Moscow in the early 1930s. At first glance, these initials would seem to be a reference to constituents of the serum, however, this was not the case, as they referred instead to the institute in Moscow itself.[142] Not surprisingly, this detail is missing from *Defenders of the Faith*, which highlighted the WWI origins of blood conservation. However, the initials did appear, first in the *Boletín Oficial del Estado* of 22 January 1937 that first reported on the services official recognition, and then in the *ABC* of Sevilla of 23 January 1937, although there was no explanation of its origins.[143] Its absence thereafter, except for an occasional reference in the medical journals, is not surprising as, from the start of the conflict, the Insurgents were portrayed as being engaged in a Catholic Crusade of national liberation against the forces of communism. Its Moscow origins were largely glossed over in the medical journals, which is indicative of how far-reaching Francoist censorship, self-imposed or otherwise, was in the post-war period.[144]

Defenders of the Faith lays claim to be the 'first picture of actual warfare ever to be made in natural colour'.[145] This is difficult to verify, nevertheless, it is a rare and early example of a full-length war documentary in colour.[146] In light of this, its almost total absence from the historiography on propaganda and cinema during the Spanish Civil War is difficult to understand. A possible explanation may lay in the fact that the US President Roosevelt did not officially recognise Franco's government until its official victory on 1 April 1939.[147] Additionally, the US press frequently condemned the Francoist regime as little more than a satellite of Germany. Falangist groups were banned in the US and it wasn't until friction increased between the US and the USSR after the end of WWII that Francoist propaganda could fully show its face across the Atlantic. This may well have led to this film, which was not finished until some point late in 1938, only having restricted and limited screenings.[148]

An important film, it also contains footage of a Muslim hospital where wounded Maghrebi troops can be seen being entertained by Moroccan musicians as they relax in the grounds.[149] Also of interest is footage of a patient with facial injuries with an unusual plaster cast over his head and part of his face, which helps in dating the film, as the cast is shown having written on it, '13.7.1938. Viva España'![150]

The film's approach to blood transfusion is very different to what is encountered in *Heart of Spain* or *Transfusió de Sang*, in that any similarities in the techniques shown are offset by *Defenders of the Faith*'s simpler and more straightforward style. The cinematography frequently involves the use of a static camera with events happening in front of it, or moving across the screen. At other times the camera pans across images seen at a distance. Its simple style is nevertheless effective.

Rarely does it set out to shock. There is footage of an exploratory laparotomy being performed. There is also the aforementioned footage of the wounded soldier with facial injuries, which also shows him after corrective plastic surgery performed under local anaesthetic with his nose completely missing. Although these images are undoubtedly shocking, this does not appear to have been Palmer's intent, as his concern was more with showing the care being received by the wounded, rather than verbally equating it with a communist atrocity, perhaps allowing the viewers to draw this conclusion for themselves.

The section on blood transfusion differs from *Heart of Spain*, in that the footage of soldiers receiving transfusions of stored blood is free of images of mutilation and bloodshed. The commentary that accompanies the opening image of the 'Servicio Oficial de Transfusión de Sangre Conservada (The Official Service for the Transfusion of Conserved Blood)' logo states that 'war is not all destruction, the blood transfusion service of the army exemplifies the conservation of life'. The scene that follows, portrays conservatively dressed smiling young women seated at the doors to a hospital preparing to give 'blood donations for their cause … and although not everyone can give their blood … for these young ladies it is the fifth contribution of this kind'.[151] The claim is made that the initiative for this service comes from the Spanish people itself, whereas in fact it was formally established by military decree.

Women were especially the target of recruitment campaigns for blood donation. They were seen as the ideal candidates as this fitted Insurgent notions of a woman's role being subordinate to that of men, and offering succour to the wounded soldier embodied beliefs central to Insurgent interpretation of Catholic doctrine.[152] This discourse on the female role within traditional Spanish society was an important part of the religious and political ideology of the right in Spain. It was Pilar Primo de Rivera (younger sister of José Antonio), head of the Female Section of the Falange, who was a key figure for promoting this 'traditionalist' view of women. In an address to Falangist women during the conflict, she praised the 'silent labour of those who constantly give their blood for transfusions, in that as women they have been unable to give it at the front'.[153]

Palmer proceeds to make the point that the Blood Transfusion Service had been 'created with very little help from the outside'. This point may well have been made in light of the screenings of *Heart of Spain* in North America in summer 1937, a film that highlighted Canadian and US medical aid; and to give emphasis to the resourcefulness of the Spanish people in creating 'their own' transfusion services without the benefit of external aid.[154]

Palmer states in relation to the facilities established by Elósegui that, 'today it gives a more prompt and efficient service than has been available to the injured in any previous war'. Although at first glance this seems a contentious claim to make, the Spanish medical literature does support this claim. The 'Servicio Oficial de Transfusión de Sangre Conservada' was recorded as having had 30,000 donors and having carried out 25,000 transfusions throughout the conflict, whereas the service of Durán-Jordà had 14,000 active donors and carried out approximately 20,000 transfusions. However, the latter was based in one location, Barcelona, whereas Elósegui had twenty-six teams to extract and conserve the blood, as well as three mobile campaign vehicles with sophisticated equipment, which indicated a well organised service, something the film is keen to stress.[155]

Palmer was also keen to stress the different approach taken by 'Dr Elósegui of the Nationalist Medical Corps', stating that he used 'a unique and different method' of blood extraction. This consisted of a needle attached to the vein filling the bottle directly, as opposed to via a tube, as can be seen in *Heart of Spain* and *Transfusió de Sang*, with the donor gently flexing and clenching her fingers into her palm as per 'the doctor's orders'. These images are in stark contrast to the vigorous clenching of the fist to facilitate blood flow that is seen in *Heart of Spain.* The donated blood is described by Palmer as the 'fountain of life', blood that may take up to two weeks to reach its destination, and once there 'restore strength and vitality to some shell-torn soldier at the front'.[156]

It is at this point that the film claims that:

> previously, blood transfusion had been impossible to realise without there being direct contact between the blood donor and the receiver of the blood, but in 1914 it was discovered that thanks to the use of an anticoagulant it was possible to conserve blood in its natural fluid form for an indefinite period of time.

There is no mention here of the important work carried out by Yudin, but it does pay homage to the work carried out in WWI, and does not set out to claim that Elósegui invented this method. The footage continues with a scene of the bottled blood being placed into a fridge in a mobile blood transfusion vehicle before being driven off.

In what appears to be a carefully staged scene, the camera then cuts to the female volunteers encountered earlier being awarded medals and certificates for their contributions.[157] This section of *Defenders of the Faith* closes with a white-coated medic preparing blood transfusion equipment, with Palmer stating that 'in cases of extreme loss of blood or terrific shock a prompt transfusion may be the only means of saving lives' and that this should be given 'as close as possible to the actual line of battle'.[158] An apparently wounded young soldier on a stretcher is shown being given a blood transfusion.

If the three films are examined together, they all differ slightly in their portrayals of blood transfusions. *Transfusió de Sang* is specifically about blood transfusion and the delivery of this service to the front. *Heart of Spain* dedicates the initial part of its story to the emblematic struggle for the defence of Madrid, before turning its attention to the work carried out by Bethune in the capital. Palmer's film dedicates only a short section to the Official Blood Transfusion Service of Conserved Blood created by Elósegui. One thing that unites all three films, however, is their attempt, through the medium of the moving image accompanied by dialogue, to highlight the efficiency and organisation of their own services. All three demonstrate an awareness of the importance of film as a medium for promoting ideologies and raising funds within the area of their immediate relevance, but also as a means for the wider dissemination of ideological viewpoints outside the area of conflict, whether it be in wider Europe or across North America.

These films also stand testimony to the important work carried out by the respective transfusion services and are important visual records. What sets *Heart of Spain* apart is the positioning of Bethune as the main focus of the camera in its section on blood transfusion, whereas neither Elósegui nor Durán-Jordà appear in their respective films. Bethune's presence in *Heart of Spain* demonstrated his understanding of the importance that the visible presence of a figurehead could play in maximising the propagandistic value of the issues he was keen to promote. Bethune, in defence of his beliefs was keen to place himself centre-stage, and evidence of this can be found in the extensive collection of photographs that contain Bethune, held at both the Imperial War Museum and the Marx Memorial Library in London.[159]

The image and the word

Blood as a symbol of both death and regeneration was part of the cultural fabric of Spain, but also of those societies where Catholicism had been a shaping force in national identity, such as in France and the French-speaking parts of Canada.[160] Bethune, although from a Presbyterian family in Canada, where iconography and the bleeding heart of Jesus would have had little place, nevertheless understood how to use blood's symbolism for propaganda purposes, not only from the point of view of his role as a transfusionist but also its graphic impact both pictorially and in print. Although this is evident in *Heart of Spain*, which engages directly with the symbolic meaning of blood, equally important from a propaganda viewpoint was Bethune's willingness to engage closely with themes of suffering in printed form, in the booklet, *The Crime on the Road Malaga – Almeria* (see Image 4 above).

Despite being about the desperate plight of an estimated 100,000 refugees who fled Malaga after its fall in February 1937, this booklet also focused on the role that Bethune played alongside Hazen Sise and Thomas Worsley in helping refugees, with the blood delivery ambulance an important element in the narrative. Here the printed word is accompanied by the vivid unspoken power of the understated images of refugees fleeing Malaga rather than await an uncertain fate, and where 1,574 people alone were executed in the seven weeks after its fall, that serves as vehicle for this powerful message.[161]

The predominant strength of *The Crime on the Road Malaga – Almeria* lies mainly in its use of twenty-one black and white images in the main text to portray the suffering of the refugees, with the lens of Hazen Sise concentrating on children, women and the elderly, eschewing the showing of blood. To accompany these words and the text of the introduction there are four

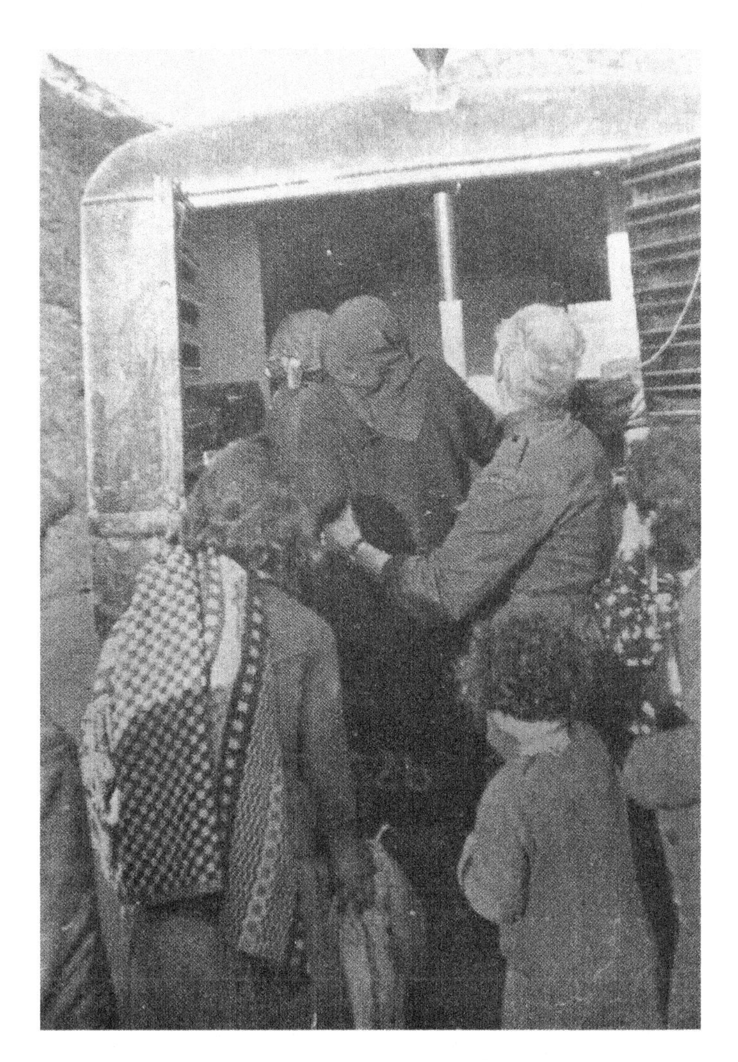

Image 5 Bethune assisting refugees into ambulance, February 1937.
Source: Bethune, N., *The Crime on the Road Malaga – Almeria: Narrative with Graphic Documents Revealing Fascist Cruelty* (Spain, 1937).

small photographs showing Bethune. One of these images (Image 5) shows Bethune helping refugees into the ambulance, and alongside the other images of Bethune, are seemingly placed there to reinforce his humanitarian and anti-fascist credentials. It is the simplicity of the images of the refugees that highlight the desolate condition of what Alardo Prats, the anarchist journalist who wrote the introduction, described as 'the frightened exodus of a whole town, who preferred death a thousand times rather than submit to the criminal tyranny of fascism'.

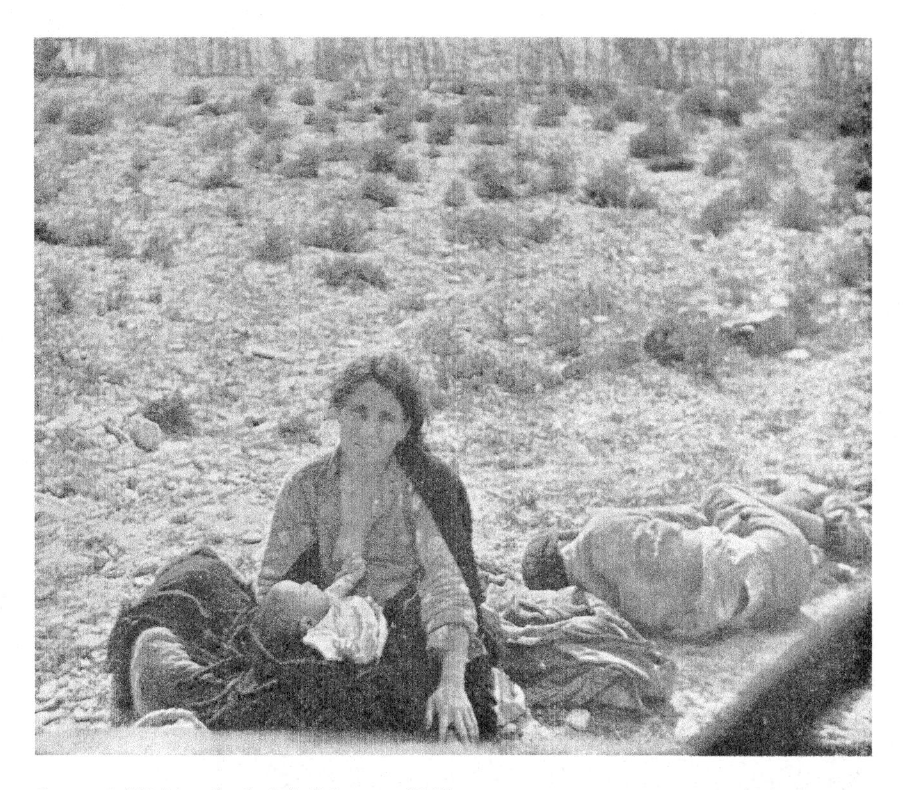

Image 6 'Waiting for help', February 1937.
Source: Bethune, N., *The Crime on the Road Malaga – Almeria: Narrative with Graphic Documents Revealing Fascist Cruelty* (Spain, 1937).

One of its most compelling images is that of a forlorn woman by the roadside 'waiting for help', a baby asleep in her lap, her chest half uncovered, giving the impression that she has just recently succoured her child (Image 6). Also to be seen is a young man asleep on his side on the ground at the roadside, while on the other side of her is her meagre bundle of visible possessions. Although none of the photos, at least in their surviving form, are of a particularly high quality, the bony outline of her sternum and chest are clearly visible, and her small breast seems hardly capable of having produced much milk.[162]

A photograph of the same woman, not included in the booklet was exhibited at the Sala de Exposiciones Alameda, in Málaga in 2004 (Image 7).[163] In this image, which, like the previous photograph, appears to have been taken from the ambulance, the woman's arm still cradles the baby, but now instead of looking directly towards the camera her other hand covers her face.

A striking feature of the booklet is the similarity between some of its images and the series of black and white etchings by Goya, *Los Desastres*

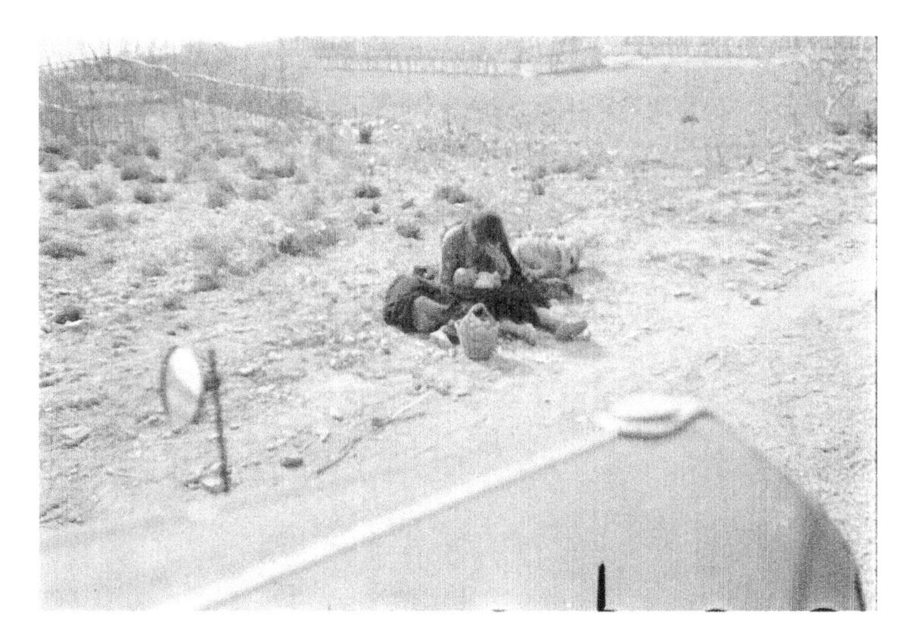

Image 7 Hazen Sise, Woman 'waiting for help' (Spain, 1937). Centro Andaluz de Fotografía in Almería, 2004.

Source: Images supplied courtesy of Jesús Majada Neila.

de la Guerra (*The Disasters of War*). These were a series of eighty-two etchings created between 1810 and 1815 that dealt primarily with the War of Independence of 1808–1814, and included several works depicting refugees. One such similarity can be seen between the photograph by Hazen Sise of the woman 'waiting for help', and print number sixty by Goya, 'There are none who will succour them' (Image 8). This print depicts a woman, her hand covering her face, three figures prostrate on the ground surrounding her.[164] Although one woman is seated and the other standing, both images share a similar sense of desolation and there are similarities in the text describing their plight.

Peter Chalmers Mitchell, a witness to the flight of refugees fleeing Malaga from advancing Italian troops, drew comparisons in *My House in Malaga* with what he witnessed to what he had seen in pictures by Goya. He observed of their initial flight that they were

> hurrying, pushing, groaning, screaming, faces mottled with grey and green and dull red, fear and misery turning them into one of Goya's most dreadful pictures. Goya, who saw these things more than a century ago, the dispossessed of the earth driven only by dull, almost animal, instincts of flight![165]

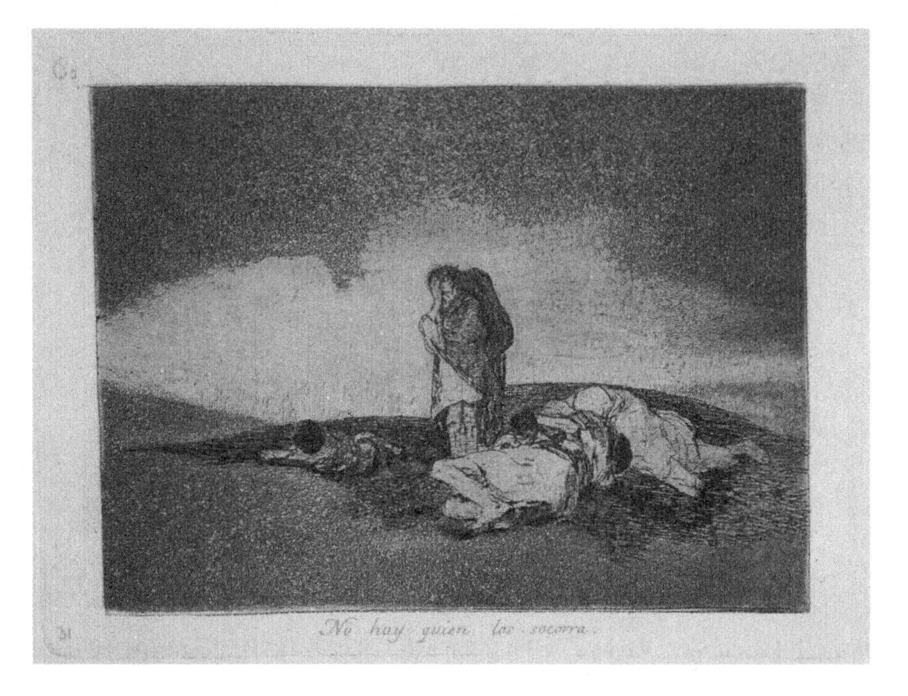

Image 8 Goya y Lucientes, *Los Desastres de la Guerra*, plate no. 60. 'There are none who will succour them.'

Source: *Los desastres de la guerra*, plate No. 60, (1st edition, Madrid: Real Academia de Bellas Artes de San Fernando, 1863).

The similarity with Goya is also evident in the last image to be found in the booklet (Image 9). This photograph shows a group of three young women seated on bundles with a small girl, having just recently arrived in Almeria, sheltering next to a low wall.

The arrival of the refugees in Almeria was accompanied by a major bombing raid on the centre of the town where many of the refugees were congregated. It is this event, according to the caption, that the group is sheltering from. Plate number fifty-two from the *Desastres de la Guerra* series shows a huddle of three women and a girl next to the lower segment of a ruined wall (Image 10). These two images are remarkably alike in their composition, although the caption that accompanies the image by Goya reads 'they did not arrive in time'. This is essentially what Bethune was stating in the caption in the booklet. Having arrived in a city that was supposed to represent safety, they were nevertheless subject to bombing and machine-gunning and were anything but safe.[166]

The similarities in the images described above, accidental or not, point to a recurring and pervasive imagery of warfare and suffering that comes

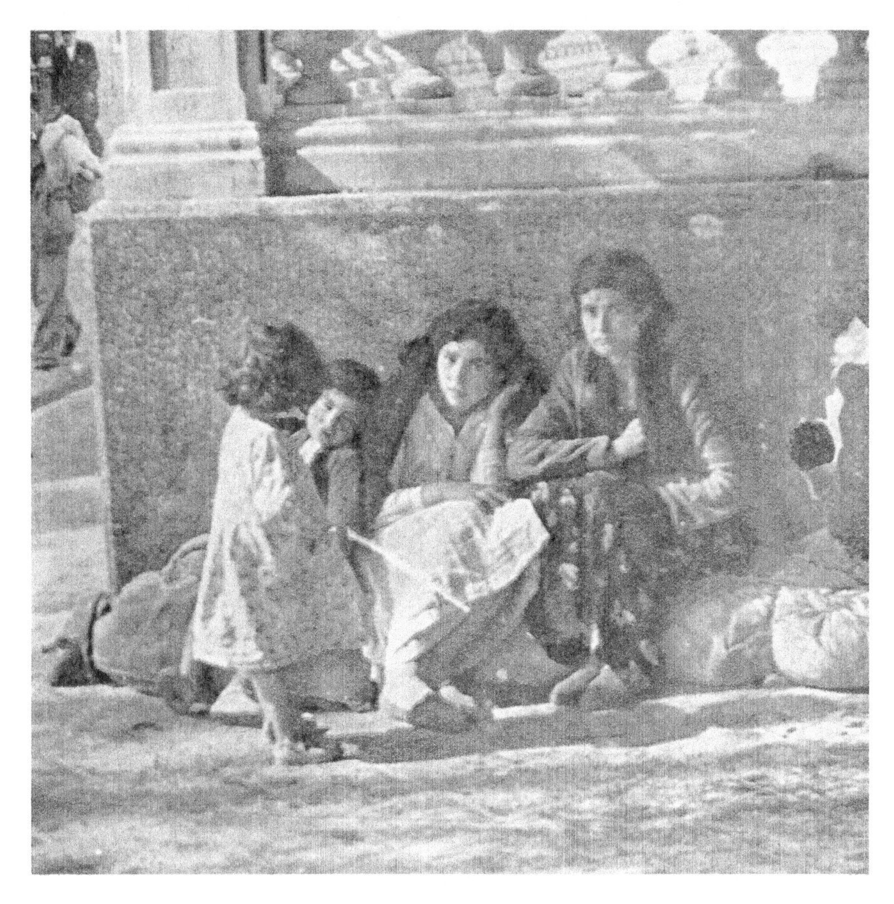

Image 9 'In Almeria international machine gunning also fiercely pursues the defenceless inhabitants of Malaga.'

Source: Bethune, N., *The Crime on the Road Malaga – Almeria: Narrative with Graphic Documents Revealing Fascist Cruelty* (Spain, 1937).

through Goya's and Sise's images. The comparison, therefore, with Goya is valid in that both Bethune and Goya used images of the suffering of refugees to advance their own arguments against the perceived tyranny of totalitarian aggression.[167] The suffering that they seek to portray is further linked by the expression of common themes, with these images additionally serving as visual records of traumatised victims of warfare.

The photographs by Sise also serve as an important visual source for the flight of refugees from Malaga as there is little contemporary graphic evidence relating to this event. The picture of a child (for example), her back to the camera, a discarded doll on the ground besides her, is an emotive and powerful propaganda image (Image 11).

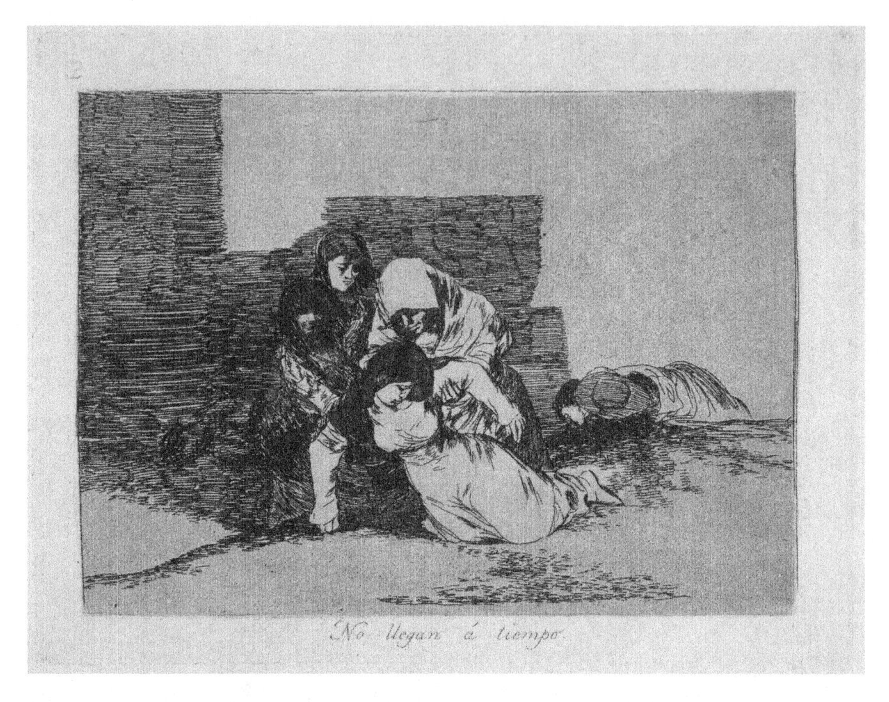

Image 10 Goya y Lucientes, *Los Desastres de la Guerra*, plate no. 52. 'They did not arrive in time.'

Source: *Los desastres de la guerra,* plate No. 52, (1st edition, Madrid: Real Academia de Bellas Artes de San Fernando, 1863).

In the English version the text reads simply, 'Nothing matters now – not even her doll'. The Spanish version on the other hand reads, 'Abandoned? Lost? The girl is suffering to the extreme of forgetting or even scorning yesterday's treasure.'[168] Both of these captions are designed to heighten the perceived despair of this image, the 'discarded' doll an important motif. A closer inspection, however, reveals that by her feet is a piece of sugar cane (an important crop in South-Eastern Spain at the time).[169] The child, whose hands are unseen, has these raised to the lower part of her face, and a photo not included in the booklet shows this indeed to be the case (Image 12).

These two images are of historical interest in that it can be compared to an earlier image in the booklet of refugees outside a house (Image 13), with a caption that reads, 'Sugar cane their only sustenance' with the caption in the Spanish version of the booklet alluding to it being a 'scarce' food source.[170] These photographs thus convey the scant food resources that were available to the refugees.

The image of the refugees outside the house resting while eating provides further evidence on the physical state of the refugees (Image 13). If the feet of

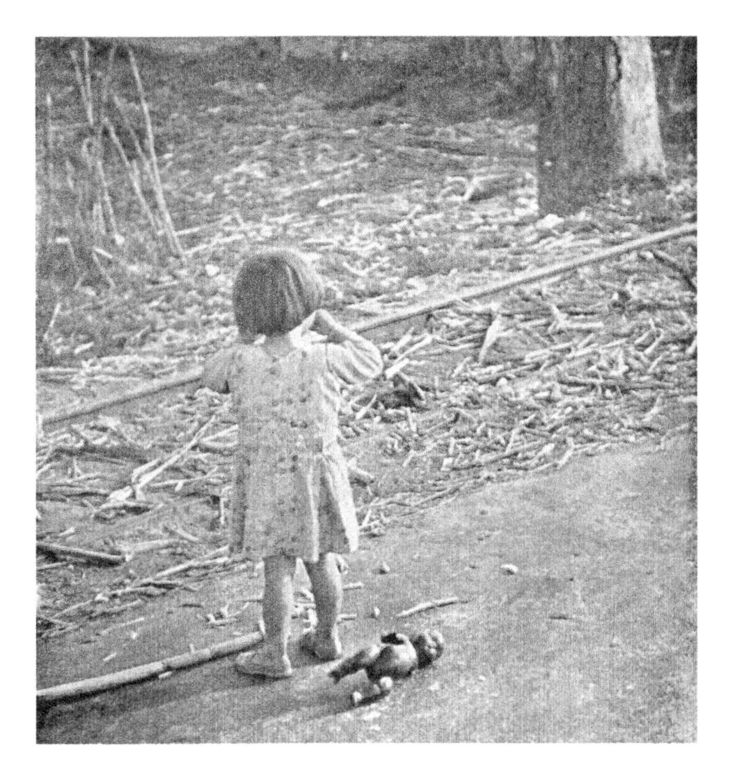

Image 11 'Nothing matters now – not even her doll', February 1937.
Source: Bethune, N., *The Crime on the Road Malaga – Almeria: Narrative with Graphic Documents Revealing Fascist Cruelty* (Spain, 1937).

the woman seated at the front of the picture in the centre are examined closely there is evidence of the damage done to them by the trek. Ángeles Vásquez León's own experience as a refugee, who fled the fall of Malaga, reflects this and many of the experiences to be found in the booklet. At one point, Ángeles was forced to stop walking as her feet were so swollen and cut that walking became impossible. She was only able to reach Almeria through the aid of a retreating militiaman who carried her there on his horse.[171]

It is left to the propagandist pen of Bethune in his four-page narrative to more fully describe the desperate plight of the refugees. He described how, alongside Worsley and Sise, he had arrived in Almeria at five o'clock on 10 February 1937, 'with a refrigeration truckload of preserved blood from Barcelona', with the intention of proceeding to 'Malaga to give blood transfusions to wounded'. They soon abandoned the idea of delivering the blood from Barcelona due to being unable to proceed through the mass of refugees on the narrow coastal road. They decided instead to aid the children among the refugees by assisting as many as they could by ferrying them in the

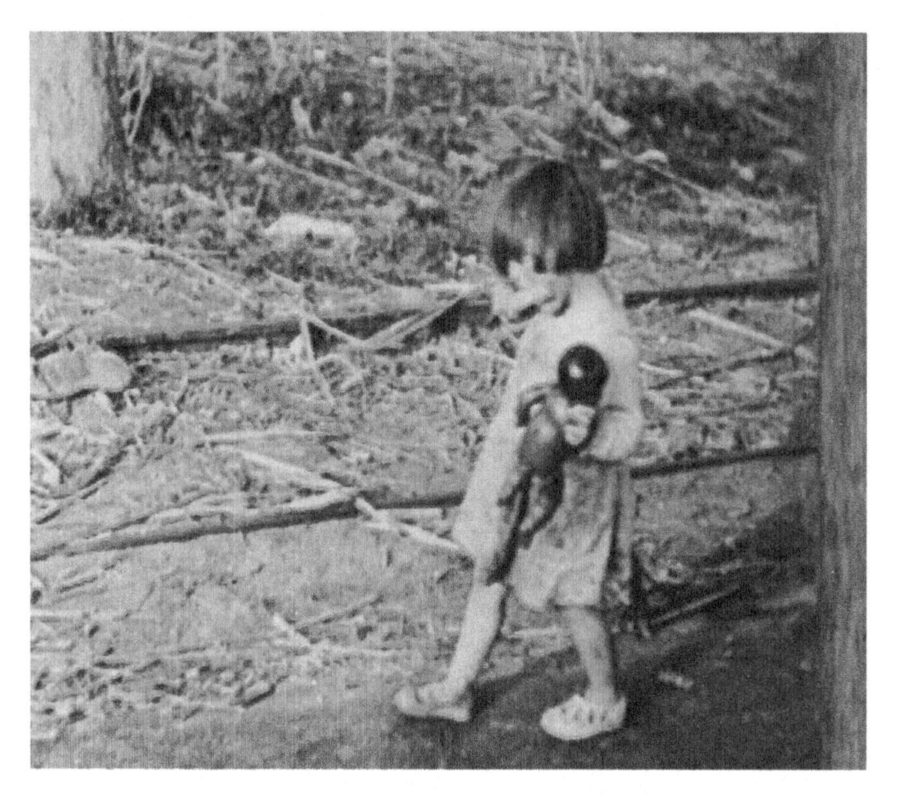

Image 12 Hazen Sise, 'Child eating sugar cane' (Spain, 1937).
Source: Image supplied courtesy of Jesús Majada Neila.

ambulance to Almeria. This proved to be more difficult than they anticipated as they were 'besieged by a mob of frantic mothers and fathers' who all wanted their own children rescued, and this rule was quickly abandoned.[172] Bethune emphasised their plight by stressing the moral dilemma he faced by having to choose between 'a mother silently watching us with great sunken eyes carrying against her open breast her child born on the road two days ago' (a possible reference to the woman in Image 6), and 'a woman of sixty unable to stagger another step, her gigantic swollen legs with their open varicose ulcers bleeding into her linen sandals'.[173]

The stark, vivid descriptions of the refugees, with blood and suffering important motifs in describing their plight, demonstrated Bethune's ability to target his audience through the use of emotive language and images. He presented certain verifiable facts, exaggerated it is true, but cleverly constructed to achieve maximum impact and even to shock. It was this skill at weaving true events into a targeted narrative that makes *The Crime on the Road*

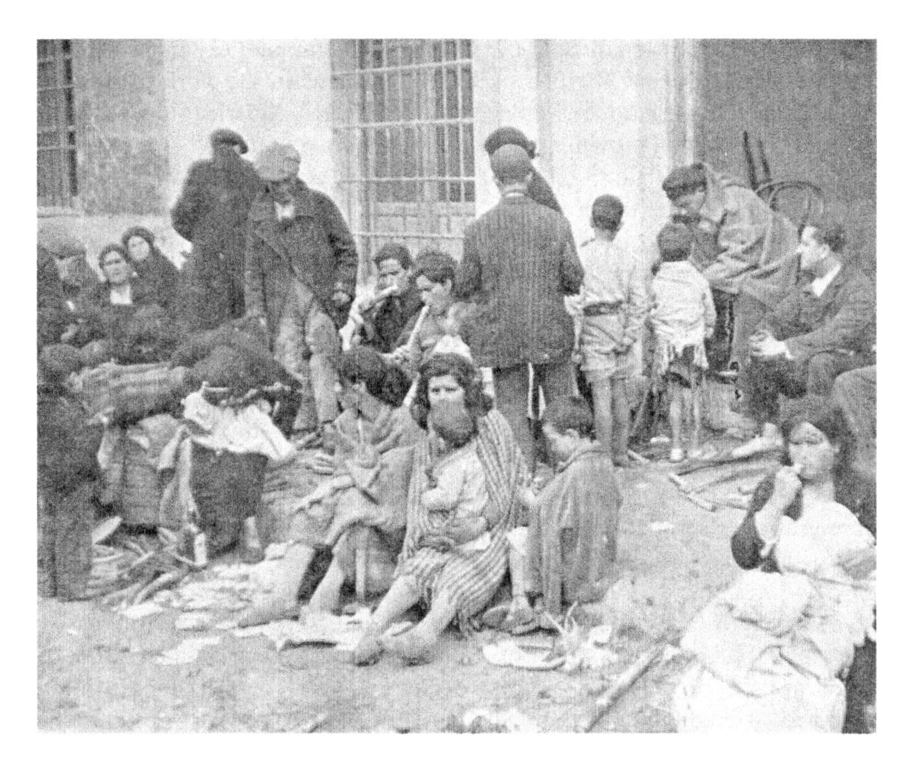

Image 13 'Sugar cane their only sustenance', February 1937.
Source: Bethune, N., *The Crime on the Road Malaga – Almeria: Narrative with Graphic Documents Revealing Fascist Cruelty* (Spain, 1937).

Malaga – Almeria such an effective piece of propaganda.[174] Unfortunately, its wider effectiveness as propaganda can only be partially judged, as there are no figures for how widely it was disseminated. However, there was also a French version of the booklet, and the fact that it was printed in at least three widely spoken languages would indicate that is was meant for wider distribution.[175] Although the booklet provides evidence of Bethune's skill as a propagandist, it is also a testimony to the humanitarian assistance given by Bethune, Sise and Worsley to the refugees during an exodus that is estimated to have cost at least 3,000 lives.[176]

Medical journals and propaganda

Medical journals, more commonly associated with a scientific approach, were also used for propagandist purposes. The booklet *Service of Blood Transfusion at the Front: Organisation-Apparatus*, 'a scientific article intended for general distribution' written in English (there was also a shorter Catalan version), was aimed at the dissemination of Durán-Jordà's technique to the wider medical community outside of Spain.[177] One of the communities targeted would undoubtedly have been the British doctors involved in the work of SMAC, but another possible target would have been North American doctors and associated personnel providing medical care within Spain.[178]

The booklet, with one or two exceptions, is constructed along similar lines to many of the medical journals cited throughout this chapter. These exceptions, however, are very much indicative of its attempt at targeted information that emphasised the organisational qualities of the PSUC in 'organising and developing a service of Blood Transfusion at the Front'. This can be seen in the reference to 'Emergency Hospital No, 18, with all the auxiliary services necessary to a nosocomium, including a research laboratory'. The booklet then goes on to describe the technical aspects of blood collection and conservation, and the fact that 'at the present time we have on file, duly classified, 3014 persons' with 'as many more in the process of classification, this being due to a veritable crusade carried on by our friends and comrades in several large factories'.[179]

A similar approach is taken by Durán-Jordà in an article he wrote for the *Revista de Sanidad de Guerra* of December 1937, which dedicated fifty of its pages to nine articles that he either wrote (seven) or co-wrote (two), all related to citrated blood.[180] Both works described the scientific aspects of blood transfusion, and both works stressed the need for the administration of stored citrated blood to be taken out of the hands of experts. Thus, in the booklet, Durán-Jordà wrote:

> if we have achieved anything practical in our Service, it is the simplification of the technique of the transfusion ... we have now placed this operation within the grasp of any auxiliary worker who is an expert on endovenous [*sic*] injections.[181]

He used the same argument in the journal, where he also stated that 'our experience of a year of fighting with hundreds of transfusions carried out, has led us to believe that we have achieved this objective'.[182]

The works examined above form part of a diverse corpus of materials concerned with not only the recruitment of blood donors but also disseminating ideological viewpoints through an intelligent approach to propaganda. By appropriating a respected format such as that of the journal and by the use of the journal itself, views could be expressed through a sophisticated use of print that had the chance of targeting different communities, and thus reaching a wider audience than that offered by a political pamphlet or booklet.

Conclusion

The blood transfusion services, established shortly after the outbreak of the Spanish Civil War, were to make a valuable contribution to saving lives during a bloody and savage conflict that cost hundreds of thousands of lives. Significant advances were made in the provision of citrated blood and in its delivery to the front. These advances were by no means restricted to one side. A combined estimated total of 45,000 blood transfusions with conserved blood were carried out by the respective services of Durán-Jordà and Elósegui between August 1936 and April 1939, but these figures do not include the transfusions carried out by the centres in Madrid, Valencia, and Linares.[183] These figures, however, should be viewed within the context of the total number of blood transfusions carried out during the conflict, including the arm-to-arm transfusion technique, the use of which was significantly higher than that with conserved blood. Nevertheless, the efforts expanded in trying to save lives through blood donation owed a considerable debt to research and work carried out since the discovery of sodium citrate's properties as an anticoagulant at the start of WWI.[184]

What set Spain apart in the development of improved and innovative blood transfusion techniques was the deployment of this propaganda not only as a tool in promoting recruitment of donors but also as a means of propagating differing ideologies. At the centre of the dissemination of these contesting ideologies were cultural notions embedded deep within Spanish society, which drew upon religion and sacrificial motifs in reaching beyond the moveable borders of a divided Spain.

Norman Bethune, through a combination of his forceful personality and a masterly manipulation of propaganda, placed himself at the centre of these developments. His role, while undoubtedly an important one, was part of the continuity of change that had its roots in the nineteenth century. Nevertheless, through a skilful use of virtually all of the tools of propaganda at his disposal, he not only promoted the work of the Madrid blood transfusion services, but used this promotion to push a Popular Front humanitarian agenda at the centre of international aid.

Bethune's understanding of the role that propaganda could play was part of a much wider movement in the use of mass media in fighting a propaganda war that defined the battlegrounds between the broad and often uneasy coalition of the left against Francoist Catholic nationalism. The fact that it was Bethune who came to represent the important progress that took place within Spain in relation to blood transfusion stands testament to the power that propaganda could wield when used effectively to target national and international audiences.

Due to the predominance of non-Spanish authors in the historiography of the Spanish Civil War, which arguably persisted until after the fall of the Francoist dictatorship and the slow opening of the archives previously only accessible to those interested in the 'official version of the Civil War', international medical efforts have often overshadowed the work of Spanish medical personnel. The Republican propaganda that has left such an indelible imprint on how the historiography was formulated, played an integral part in mythologising the contribution of the International Brigades during the conflict. These myths, with their feet so firmly rooted in the propaganda of the day, make an exploration necessary that restores the balance between national and international efforts and challenges the argument which highlights that medical contributions originated primarily outside of Spain, with the part played by Bethune in the development of a mobile blood transfusion service overshadowing the important part played by Durán-Jordà and Elósegui in the development of these services.

Many of those who did contribute towards advances in medical practice and towards the organisation of medical services in the Republican Zone during the Spanish Civil War, at the end of the conflict were either purged from their posts or fled into exile, rather than await an uncertain fate. Both Durán-Jordà and Josef Trueta were able to find sanctuary in Britain but hundreds of thousands of their fellow countrymen fled the Insurgent advance on Catalunya, and made their way across the Pyrenees to France.

It is the experience of these refugees and the vanquished within Spain that forms the central focus of the next chapter. The trauma that refugees had faced for much of the war was at least mitigated in part by a common struggle and reasonable access to medical care. The experience of defeat, by contrast, for both the refugees in France and the vanquished within Spain was to be one of an imposed trauma, where medical cover was scant, disease rampant and hunger the common lot of the defeated. The situation within Spain itself was exacerbated further still as Franco and the new dictatorship continued its long campaign of punishing the 'reds', well into the post-war period.

Notes

1 *La Vanguardia* (edición general), 07.08.1936, p.11.
2 *ABC* (Sevilla), 27.03.1937, p. 15; Beevor, *Battle for Spain*, pp. 16–18, 40–41.
3 *ABC* (Madrid), 09.02.1937, p. 8; Stewart, R., & Stewart, S., *Phoenix: The Life of Norman Bethune* (Montreal, 2011), p. 161.
4 *ABC* (Madrid), 09.02.1937, p. 8.
5 Schneider, Blood Transfusion, p. 188.
6 Stewart & Stewart, *Phoenix*, p.169; Durán-Jordà, F., *The Service of Blood Transfusion at the Front: Organisation-Apparatus by Frederic Duran-Jorda, Technical Chief of the Service, Director of Emergency Hospital No. 18* (Barcelona, 1937), p. 8.
7 Giangrande, P. L. F., "The History of Blood Transfusion", *British Journal of Haematology*, Vol. 110, No. 4 (2000), pp. 758–767., p. 761; Franco Grande et al., *Historia de la anestesia*, pp. 217–218.
8 Franco Grande et al., *Historia de la anestesia*, pp. 216–218.
9 Ibid., pp. 214–216.
10 *ABC* (Madrid), 23.01.1937, p. 4; *ABC* (Madrid), 24.01.1937, p. 4; *ABC* (Madrid), 25.02.1937, p. 14; *La Vanguardia* (edición general), 04.10.1936; *La Vanguardia* (edición general), 16.10.1936; *La Vanguardia* (edición general), 04.05.1937; *ABC* (Sevilla), 05.12.1937, p. 25; Gollonet Megías, A. & Morales López, J., *Rojo y Azul en Granada (más datos por la historia de la guerra civil española), Ilustraciones fotográficas ... cuarta edición* (Granada, 1937), pp. 169–171; *ABC* (Sevilla), 05.12.1937, p. 25; Primo de Rivera, P., *4 Discursos de Pilar Primo de Rivera* (Madrid, 1939), p. 34.

11 Franco Grande et al., *Historia de la anestesia*, pp. 234–235.
12 Stewart & Stewart, *Phoenix*, p. 169, Durán-Jordà, *The Service of Blood Transfusion at the Front*, p. 5; Hernández Giménez, J., "La transfusión sanguínea en el ejército", *Ejército: Revista Ilustrada de las Armas y Servicios*, No. 67 (1945), pp. 13–20., p. 15.; *ABC* (Madrid), Miércoles 18.03.1981, p. 97; Bernabéu Mestre, El papel de la Escuela Nacional, p. 71; Giangrande, The History of Blood Transfusion, p. 762; *BOE*, No. 94, 22.01.1937, p. 180; *ABC* (Sevilla), 23.01.1937, p. 10.
13 Stewart & Stewart, *Phoenix*, p. 171; Hannant, L., *The Politics of Passion*: Norman Bethune's Writing and Art (Toronto, 1998), p. 150. There was also a centre that transfused conserved blood in Valencia, and one in Linares in Southern Spain, but little is known about this service. See Franco Grande, A., Cortes, J., Alvarez, J., & Diz, J. C., "The Development of Blood Transfusion: The Contributions of Norman Bethune in the Spanish Civil War (1936–1939)", Canadian Journal of Anaesthesia, Vol. 43, No. 10 (1996), pp. 1076–1078.
14 Graham, *Spanish Civil War*, p. 42.
15 Hannant, *The Politics of Passion*, pp. 157–158.
16 *ABC*, Madrid, 18.03.1981, p. 97 (Obituary of Carlos Elósegui); Bernabéu Mestre, El papel de la Escuela Nacional, pp. 65–89.
17 Puyal, C. H., & Mur, M. C., "Notas históricas sobre el hospital de sangre número 18 de Barcelona (1936–1939)", *Gimbernat: Revista Catalana d'història de la medicina i de la ciencia*, Vol. 27 (1997), pp. 173–184, p. 176.
18 Palfreeman, *Spain Bleeds.*
19 Corse, *A Battle for Neutral Europe*, p. 6.
20 Cull et al., *Propaganda*, p. 318.
21 "Jefatura de Sanidad del Ejército de Tierra", *Cartilla sanitaria del combatiente* (Madrid, 1937).
22 Preston, P., "Two Doctors and One Cause: Len Crome and Reginald Saxton in the International Brigades", *International Journal of Iberian Studies*, Vol. 19, No. 1 (2006), pp. 5–24, p. 18; Allen, T., Allen, J., & Gordon, S., *The Scalpel, the Sword: The Story of Doctor Norman Bethune* (Toronto, 2009), p. 9; Shepard, D. A. E., & Levesque, A., (eds.), *Norman Bethune: His Times and His Legacy* (Ottawa, 1982); and www.thecanadianencyclopedia.com/articles/norman-bethune (last accessed 07.11.2013), all emphasise Bethune's contribution over that of Durán-Jordà and Elósegui.
23 Hannant, *The Politics of Passion*, p. 131.
24 Stewart & Stewart, *Phoenix*, p. 208; *Heart of Spain*, Director: Herbert Kline (Frontier Films, 1937).
25 Goyanes Álvarez, V., "La transfusión de sangre en el Sector Centro", *Revista de Sanidad de Guerra*, Vol. 11, No. 12 (1938), pp. 159–176; Hannant, *The Politics of Passion*, p. 157.
26 Hannant, *The Politics of Passion*, pp. 128–129; Stewart & Stewart, *Phoenix*, pp. 223–225; Franco Grande, A., Diz, J. C., Aneiros, F. J., Cortés, J., & Alvarez, J., "The 'Servicio Hispano-Canadiense de Transfusión de Sangre' in the Spanish Civil War (1936–1939)", *Bulletin of Anaesthesia History*, Vol. 17, No. 2 (1998), pp. 14–16; *Heart of Spain.* The film was made in collaboration with Leo Hurwitz, Paul Strand, the Hungarian photographer Geza Karpathi and the American newspaper correspondent Herbert Kline.
27 Díaz-Plaja, F., *La vida cotidiana en la España de la Guerra Civil* (Madrid, 1994), pp. 320–321; Fundación Pablo Iglesias, *Carteles de la Guerra* (Madrid, 2008), an important collection of posters that contains public health posters but none for blood transfusion.

28 *ABC* (Madrid), 23.01.1937, p. 4; *ABC* (Madrid), 24.01.1937, p. 4; *ABC* (Madrid), 25.02.1937, p. 14; *La Vanguardia* (edición general), 04.10. 936; *La Vanguardia* (edición general), 16.10.1936; *La Vanguardia* (edición general), 04.05.1937; *ABC* (Sevilla), 05.12.1937, p. 25; Gollonet Megías & Morales López, *Rojo y Azul en Granada*, pp. 169–171.

29 Tse Tung, M. [Zedong, M.], *Quotations from Chairman Mao Tse Tung*, trans. Barnstone, W. (San Francisco, 1972), pp. 171–172; Lynch, M., *Mao* (London, 2004), pp. 177–178. During the Cultural Revolution in China, *The Little Red Book* by Mao, which contained a brief article titled, 'In Memory of Norman Bethune', became prescribed reading across China, and thus ensured Bethune's status as a figure of national importance. Lethbridge's *Norman Bethune in Spain* and Palfreeman's *Spain Bleeds* are the most recently published books that examine Bethune's role in Spain. He is also remembered in Andalucía in Spain, where his assistance in aiding refugees fleeing the fall of Málaga in February 1937 is commemorated. See Stewart, R., & Majada, J., *Bethune en España* (Madrid, 2009).

30 Coni, *Medicine and Warfare*, pp. 75–78.

31 Renshaw, L., *Exhuming Loss: Memory, Materiality and Mass Graves of the Spanish Civil War* (Walnut Creek, 2011), pp. 20–21.

32 Hannant, *The Politics of Passion*; Allen et al., *The Scalpel, the Sword*; Stewart & Stewart, *Phoenix*; *Bethune*, Director: Donald Brittain (National Film Board of Canada, 1964); Beevor, *Battle for Spain*, pp. 200–202.

33 Stewart & Stewart, *Phoenix*, p. 182.

34 Hannant, *The Politics of Passion*, p. 22.

35 Ibid., p. 75.

36 Ibid., pp. 13–14, 22, 51–52, 75.

37 Ibid., pp. 51–52, 150–151, 135–144 (radio transcripts).

38 Koestler, A., *Spanish Testament* (London, 1937); Chalmers Mitchell, *My House in Málaga*; Preston, *Spanish Holocaust*, p. 177.

39 Preston, *Franco*, p. 218.

40 Bethune, N., *The Crime on the Road Malaga – Almeria: Narrative with Graphic Documents Revealing Fascist Cruelty* (Spain, 1937), published in English, Spanish and French, un-paginated; Preston, *Spanish Holocaust*, p. 177.

41 Typescript of mileage by Norman Bethune, date unknown but written before his departure from Spain in May 1937, from the family archive of the Goyanes family (I am grateful to Avelino Franco Grande for granting me access to these papers).

42 The letters sent to the CASD are reproduced in Hannant, *The Politics of Passion*.

43 MRCUW, SMAC papers, from the archive folder: Spanish Rebellion: Medical Aid 1937–1940.

44 Durán-Jordà, *The Service of Blood Transfusion at the Front*; *ABC* (Madrid); *ABC* (Sevilla); *La Vanguardia*; *Ejercito: Revista Ilustrada de las Armas y Servicios*; *Cientifica Medica*; *La Cronica Medica; Revista Sanidad de Guerra* (May 1937 to May 1938 Republican); *Revista Española de Medicina y Cirugía de Guerra* (post May 1938 an Insurgent publication); *Semana Medica Española; Boletín del Colegio Médico de Pontevedra*, 31.12.1939, pp. 8–11; the films *Transfusio de Sang* (Laya Films, 1937), *Blood Bank Service in Spain* (Laya Films, 1937), Palmer, *Defenders of the Faith* (1938).

45 Hannant, *The Politics of Passion*, p. 10; Preston, Two Doctors and One Cause, p. 18; Lozano, M., & Cid, J., "Pioneers and Pathfinders; Frederic Durán-Jordà: A

Transfusion Medicine Pioneer", *Transfusions Medicine Reviews*, Vol. 21, No. 1 (2007), pp. 75–81, p. 77

46 Giangrande, The History of Blood Transfusion, p. 760.

47 "A Brief History of Blood Transfusion", www.ibms.org/go/nm:history-blood-transfusion (last accessed 03.04.2014), pp. 2–6 (article originally published in the November 2005 issue of *Biomedical Scientist*, the journal of the Institute of Biomedical Science),.

48 Harrison, M., *The Medical War: British Military Medicine in the First World War* (Oxford, 2010), p. 105; Pelis, K., "Taking Credit: The Canadian Army Medical Corps and the British Conversion to Blood Transfusion in WWI", *Journal of the History of Medicine and Allied Sciences*, Vol. 56, No. 3 (2001), pp. 238–277, pp. 253–254.

49 Klein, H. G., Spahn, D. R., & Carson, J. L., "Transfusion Medicine 1: Red Blood Cell Transfusion in Clinical Practice", *The Lancet*, Vol. 370, (04.08.2007), pp. 415–426, p. 415; Pelis, Taking Credit, pp. 249–250.

50 Giangrande, The History of Blood Transfusion, p. 762.

51 Schneider, Blood Transfusion, p. 207.

52 Lozano & Cid, Pioneers and Pathfinders, p. 76.

53 Schneider, Blood Transfusion, pp. 197–207; Franco Grande et al., The 'Servicio Hispano-Canadiense de Transfusión', p. 15.

54 Franco Grande et al., The Development of Blood Transfusion, pp. 1076–1078.

55 Lozano & Cid, Pioneers and Pathfinders, p. 77.

56 Ibid., p. 76; Durán-Jordà, *The Service of Blood Transfusion at the Front*, p. 7; Saxton, R. S., "The Madrid Blood Transfusion Institute", *The Lancet*, Vol. 230, No. 5949 (1937), pp. 606–608.

57 Alexi-Meskishvili, V., & Konstantinov, I. E., "Sergei S. Yudin: An Untold Story", *Surgery*, Vol. 139, No. 1 (2006), pp. 115–122, p. 119.

58 Ibid.; Schneider, Blood Transfusion, p. 210.

59 Schneider, Blood Transfusion, p. 210.

60 MRCUW: 292/946/42/102, p. 1; "Medical Aid for Spain", MRCUW: 292/946/42/104, p. 1; "St. Pancras and Holborn Spain Week, 22–28 January, 1938" (SMAC leaflet that includes, 'Tuesday, 25th January. 8 p.m. Lantern Lecture by Dr. Janet Vaughan on the British Medical Unit in Spain'); Vaughan, J., "War Wounds and Air Raid Casualties: Blood Transfusion", *BMJ*, Vol. 1 (1939), pp. 933–936; Doll, R., "Vaughan, Dame Janet Maria (1899–1993)", in *Oxford Dictionary of National Biography* (Oxford, 2004); online edition., May 2010, www.oxforddnb.com/view/article/42277 (last accessed 09.04.2014); Beevor, *Battle for Spain*, p. 379.

61 Schneider, Blood Transfusion, p. 213.

62 Swan, H., "S. S. Yudin: A Study in Frustration", *Surgery*, Vol. 58, No. 3 (1965), pp. 572–585, p. 578.

63 Ibid., p. 215; Navarro Carballo, *Frederic Duran i Jorda*, pp. 276–278.

64 Schneider, Blood Transfusion, p. 215.

65 Navarro Carballo, *Frederic Duran i Jorda,* pp. 276–7.

66 Mateos Royo, J. A., "All the Town is a Stage: Civic Ceremonies and Religious Festivities in Spain During the Golden Age", *Urban History*, Vol. 26, No. 2 (1998), pp. 165–189.

67 *ABC* (Sevilla), 27.08.1938, p. 4.

68 Ibid.

69 Palmer, *Defenders of the Faith*; *ABC* (Sevilla), 19.07.1938, p. 3.

70 Palfreeman, *¡Salud!*, pp. 141–144; MRCUW: 292/946/42/16, p. 1., "Reports Received from Mrs Leah Manning and Circulated to the Committee in Accordance with Resolution 10th August 1938"; British Library Sound Archive (BLSA), *Andrew Whitehead Interviews with Political Radicals*, C1377/47.
71 BLSA, C1377/47.
72 Goyanes Álvarez, La transfusión de sangre, p. 168.
73 BLSA, *Norman Bethune: Spain and China,* phonographic recording on vinyl, 1976 (missing shelfmark).
74 Brenan, G., *The Spanish Labyrinth: An Account of the Social and Political Background of the Spanish Civil War* (Cambridge, 1943). pp. 43, 152–155.
75 Ledesma, J. L., "Enemigos seculares: La violencia anticlerical (1936–1939)", in J. de la Cueva & F. Montero (eds.), *Izquierda obrera y religión en España, 1900–1939* (Alcalá de Henares, 2012), pp. 219–244, pp. 221, 238.
76 Vincent, M., "The Keys of the Kingdom: Religious Violence in the Spanish Civil War, July–August 1936", in C. Ealham & M. Richards (eds.), *The Splintering of Spain: Cultural History and the Spanish Civil War, 1936–1939* (Cambridge, 2005), pp. 68–92, p. 80.
77 M. Burleigh, *Sacred Causes: The Clash of Religion and Politics, from the Great War to the War on Terror* (London, 2006), pp. 139–140; Franco Grande et al., *Historia de la anestesia,* p. 217.
78 Franco Grande et al., *Historia de la anestesia*, p. 217.
79 Navarro Carballo, *Frederic Duran i Jorda*, p. 242.
80 There were still a few women armed and fighting in support of the Republican Government at this stage. The artist and political activist Felicia Browne was the first recorded female foreign national reported killed in action in Spain and was shot dead by Insurgents on the Aragón Front in late August 1936. See: Buchanan, T., "Browne, Felicia Mary (1904–1936)", *Oxford Dictionary of National Biography* (Oxford, 2005), online edition, January 2008, www.oxforddnb.com/view/article/92459 (last accessed 09.04.2014).
81 Navarro Carballo, *Frederic Duran i Jorda*, p. 243.
82 Franco Grande et al., *Historia de la anestesia*, p. 217.
83 Ibid.; Carr, *Spain, 1808–1975*, pp. 673, 675–676; Beevor, *Battle for Spain*, pp. 7, 20, 255. The Carlists were supporters of the rival Bourbon claimant to the throne. Renovación Española were supporters of Alfonso XIII who had been forced to abdicate in 1931.
84 Davies, A., "The First Radio War: Broadcasting in the Spanish Civil War, 1936–1939", *Historical Journal of Film, Radio and Television*, Vol. 19, No. 4 (1999), pp. 473–513, p. 486.
85 Overy, R., "Saving Civilization: British Public Opinion and the Coming of War in 1939", in D. Welch & J. Fox (eds.), *Justifying War: Propaganda, Politics and the Modern Age* (Basingstoke, 2012), p. 187; Fraser, *Blood of Spain*, pp. 127, 135, & 216.
86 MRCUW: 292/946/42/15, p.3., Report on International Conference for Medical Aid to Spain.
87 Henri Cartier-Bresson/Filmographie, www.henricartierbresson.org (last accessed 17.03.2014).
88 *Victoire de la Vie* (Henri Cartier Bresson and Herbert Kline, 1937), www.parcours.cinearchives.org/les-films-731-94-0-0.html (last accessed 15.01.2014); Schmidt, U., *Medical Films, Ethics, and Euthanasia in Nazi Germany: The History of Medical*

Research and Teaching Films of the Reich Office for Educational Films– Reich Institute for Films in Science and Education, 1933–1945 (Husum, 2002), p. 43.

89 Orledge, R., *Charles Koechlin (1867–1950): His Life and Works* (Luxemburg, 1981), pp. 170–171.

90 Crusells, M., "El Cine durante la Guerra Civil Española 1936–1939", *Comunicación y Sociedad*, Vol. 11, No. 2 (1998), pp. 123–152, p. 151; British Film Institute (BFI) Online Film Catalogue, http://explore.bfi.org.uk (last accessed 17.03.2014); Alexander, W., "Frontier Films, 1936–1941: The Aesthetics of Impact", *Cinema Journal*, Vol. 15, No. 1 (1975), pp. 16–28, p. 16.

91 Stewart & Stewart, *Phoenix*, p. 224.

92 *BMJ*, 1938; 1: S1.

93 Ellis, R. W. B., "Blood Transfusion at the Front", *Proceedings of the Royal Society of Medicine*, Vol. 31, No. 6 (April, 1939), pp. 684–686; *La Vanguardia* (edición general), 01.04.1938, p. 8. It is likely that the film shown was *Transfusio de Sang* rather than *Blood Bank Service in Spain*, as the report by Ellis is closer in its description to *Transfusió de Sang*.

94 *Transfusió de Sang*.

95 *Blood Bank Service in Spain* (BFI Viewing Copy: 8091 780 A).

96 Extensive enquiries by the author, which has included corresponding with archivists at the British Red Cross, British Medical Association and the Wellcome Library and Archive, have been unable to shed further light on the audience for this film or why or for whom it was made.

97 Catalogue entry for *Defenders of the Faith* at http://explore.bfi.org.uk/4ce2b70a16b83 (last accessed 09.04. 2014).

98 Sánchez-Biosca, V., *Cine y Guerra Civil Española: Del mito a la memoria* (Madrid, 2006), pp. 73–74, 85–92.

99 *Heart of Spain*.

100 www.alba-valb.org/volunteers/salaria-kea (last accessed 17.01. 2014). Salaria Kea also briefly appears in *Victoire de la Vie*.

101 *Heart of Spain*.

102 Ibid.; *ABC* (Madrid), 09.02.1937, p. 8

103 *Heart of Spain*.

104 Stewart & Stewart, *Phoenix*, p. 208.

105 Hannant, *The Politics of Passion*, p. 134. Letter to CASD from Bethune. 17.12.1936.

106 *Heart of Spain*.

107 Ibid.; Carrol, P. N., *The Odyssey of the Abraham Lincoln Brigade: Americans in the Spanish Civil War* (Stanford, 1994), p. 103.

108 Hannant, *The Politics of Passion*, pp. 134–194.

109 Alexander, Frontier Films, p. 20.

110 Ibid.

111 Stewart& Stewart, *Phoenix*, pp. 214–215.

112 Ibid., p. 224.

113 Ibid., p. 215.

114 Hannant, *The Politics of Passion*, p. 186.

115 MRCUW: 292/946/43/56 p. 4.

116 "Memory of the World: Lost Memory – Libraries and Archives destroyed in the Twentieth Century", prepared for UNESCO on behalf of IFLA by Hans van der Hoeven and on behalf of ICA by Joan van Albada (Paris, 1996).

117 Amo García, A., & Ibáñez Ferradas, M. L. (eds.), *Catálogo general del cine de la Guerra Civil/edición a cargo de Alfonso del Amo García; con la colaboración de M. Luisa Ibáñez Ferradas* (Madrid, 1996), pp. 544–545; Swedish Film Institute Database: www.filminstitutet.se/en/ (last accessed 04.04.2014).
118 Amo García & Ibáñez Ferradas, *Catálogo general del cine*, pp. 544–545.
119 Crusells, El Cine durante la Guerra Civil, p. 151; MRCUW: 292/946/42/15, p.3., SMAC, Report on International Conference for Medical Aid to Spain; Stewart & Stewart, *Phoenix*, p. 224; Alexander, Frontier Films, p. 20.
120 Overy, Saving Civilization, p. 187.
121 Ellis, Blood Transfusion at the Front, pp. 684–686; *La Vanguardia*, 01.04.1938, p. 8.
122 Ellis, Blood Transfusion at the Front, pp. 684–686.
123 Crusells, El Cine durante la Guerra Civil, pp. 130–131.
124 *Blood Bank Service in Spain*; Schmidt, U., *Medical Films*, pp. 24, 44, 70.
125 Schmidt, *Medical Films*, p. 43.
126 *Transfusió de Sang.*
127 Durán-Jordà, *The Service of Blood Transfusion at the Front*, p. 14. This is a reference to the as yet unknown rhesus factors, proteins on the surface of the blood cell, which were discovered by Landsteiner and Wiener in 1940. See “A Brief History of Blood Transfusion”, www.ibms.org/go/nm:history-blood-transfusion, pp. 2–6 (last accessed 30. 03. 2014).
128 *Transfusió de Sang.*
129 Durán-Jordà, *The Service of Blood Transfusion at the Front*, p. 14.
130 *Transfusió de Sang.*
131 Ibid.; Durán-Jordà, *The Service of Blood Transfusion at the Front*, p. 7; Beevor, *Battle for Spain*, p. 108.
132 Durán-Jordà, *The Service of Blood Transfusion at the Front*, p. 7.
133 Ibid., p. 7; Durán-Jordà, F., “El Servicio de Transfusión de Sangre de Barcelona: Técnicas y utillaje”, *Revista de Sanidad de Guerra*, Vol. 1, No. 8 (1937), pp. 307–321, p. 308; *La Vanguardia* (suplemento), 04.09.1938; Durán-Jordà, *The Service of Blood Transfusion at the Front.*
134 Durán-Jordà, *The Service of Blood Transfusion at the Front*, p. 7.
135 Calvocoressi, P., & Wint, G., *Total War: Causes and Courses of the Second World War* (London, 1972), pp. 86–90; Vaughan, War Wounds, p. 936; Dubash, J., Clegg, O., & Vaughan, J., “Changes Occurring in Blood Stored in Different Preservatives”, *BMJ*, Vol. 2, No. 4162 (1940), pp. 482–484, p. 484.
136 Durán-Jordà, *The Service of Blood Transfusion at the Front*, pp. 1–20.
137 Schneider, Blood Transfusion, pp. 212–213.
138 The Wellcome Library, Moving Image and Sound Library, *Blood Transfusion*, Ministry of Information, Britain, 1941. Shelfmark: 4423D
139 *BMJ*, Vol. 1, No. 5024 (20 April, 1957), pp. 903–962, p. 953.
140 Moreno Cantano, A. C., “Proyección propagandística de la España franquista en Norteamérica (1936–1945)”, *Hispania Nova: Revista de Historia Contemporánea*, No. 9 (2009), pp. 93–118.
141 *BOE*, No. 94, 22.01.1937, p. 180; *ABC* (Sevilla), 23.01.1937, p. 10; Franco Grande et al., *Historia de la anestesia*, p. 214.
142 Vaughan, War Wounds, p. 934.
143 *ABC* (Sevilla), 23.01.1937, p. 10.

144 Blanco Rodríguez, Historiografía, p. 749; Elósegui, C., "Editorial: El Instituto Español de Hematología y Hemoterapia", *Semana Medica Española*, Vol. 1, No. 3 (1942), pp. 231–241; Hernández Giménez, La transfusión sanguínea en el ejercito, p. 15; González Romero, A., "Transfusión de sangre", *Boletín del Colegio Médico de Pontevedra* (1939), pp. 8–11.
145 Bentley, B. P. E., *A Companion to Spanish Cinema* (Woodbridge, 2008), p. 79.
146 *Defenders of the Faith.*
147 Graham, *Spanish Civil War*, p. 166.
148 Moreno Cantano, Proyección propagandista, pp. 93–118.
149 *Defenders of the Faith.*
150 Ibid. 'Viva España', translates as 'Long Live Spain'.
151 *Defenders of the Faith.*
152 Gollonet Megías & Morales López, *Rojo y Azul en Granada*, pp. 169–171; *ABC* (Sevilla), 05.12.1937, p. 25; Primo de Rivera, *4 Discursos de Pilar Primo de Rivera*, p. 34.
153 Payne, S. G., *The Franco Regime, 1936–1975* (London, 1987) p. 187; Primo de Rivera, *4 Discursos de Pilar Primo de Rivera*, p. 34.
154 Goyanes Álvarez, La transfusión de sangre, pp. 159–161; *La Vanguardia*, 22.05.1938, p. 8.
155 Massons, J. M., "L'Obra de Frederic Duran I Jorda Viscuda Per Mi", *Revista de la Real Academia de Medicina de Catalunya*, No. 21 (2008), pp. 52–55, pp. 54–55; Franco Grande et al., The 'Servicio Hispano-Canadiense de Transfusión', pp. 15–16; Franco Grande et al., *Historia de la anestesia*, pp. 234–235.
156 Palmer, *Defenders of the Faith.*
157 Ibid.; *ABC* (Sevilla), 08.04.1937, p.14.
158 Palmer, *Defenders of the Faith.*
159 IWM, Vera Elkan Collection; MML, the International Brigade Memorial Archive (IBMA), Boxes: 29 and 33.
160 Hannant, L., "'My God, Are They Sending Women?': Three Canadian Women in the Spanish Civil War, 1936–1939", *Journal of the Canadian Historical Association/Revue de la Société historique du Canada*, Vol. 15, No. 1 (2004), pp. 153–176, pp. 163, 166, 176.
161 Bethune, *The Crime on the Road Malaga – Almeria*; Preston, *Spanish Holocaust*, pp. 177–178. For an account of this flight by an early figure in challenging the silence within Spain on confronting the past, see Vásquez León, *Un boomerang en Jimena de la Frontera*, pp. 73–101.
162 Bethune, *The Crime on the Road Malaga – Almeria*. As the Málaga-based historian Jesús Majada Neila has observed, this figure bears more than a passing resemblance to the woman cradling a dead baby in Picasso's *Guernica* from 1937. This figure may well have served as inspiration for Picasso, as Málaga was his birthplace.
163 Images 6 and 11 by Hazen Sise, and the photos from *The Crime on the Road Malaga – Almeria*, provided courtesy of Jesús Majada Neila, curator of the exhibition: Norman Bethune: El crimen de la carretera de Málaga-Almería (febrero 1937), Centro Andaluz de la Fotografía, Junta de Andalucía, 2004.
164 Goya y Lucientes, F. de, *Estampas, Desastres de la Guerra*, plate no. 60 (1810–1815). Available to view at https://commons.wikimedia.org/wiki/Los_desastres_de_la_guerra (last accessed 03.04.2014).

165 Chalmers Mitchell, *My House in Málaga*, p. 266.
166 Preston, *Spanish Holocaust*, p. 178; Vásquez León, *Un boomerang en Jimena de la Frontera*, p. 97; Bethune, *The Crime on the Road Malaga-Almeria.*
167 Goya y Lucientes, F. de, *Estampas, Desastres de la Guerra*, plate no. 52 (1810–1815).
168 Bethune, N., *El crimen del camino Málaga-Almería: Relato con documentos gráficos reveladores de la crueldad fascista* (Spain, 1937).
169 Martín Rodríguez, M., "La industria azucarera española 1914–1936", *Revista de Historia Económica*, Vol. 5, No. 2 (1987), pp. 301–324.
170 Bethune, *El crimen del camino Málaga-Almería.*
171 Vásquez León, *Un boomerang en Jimena de la Frontera*, pp. 73–101.
172 Bethune, *The Crime on the Road Malaga – Almeria.*
173 Ibid.; Vásquez León, *Un boomerang en Jimena de la Frontera*, pp. 73–101.
174 Bethune, *The Crime on the Road Malaga-Almeria*; Beevor, *Battle for Spain*, pp. 200–202; Fraser, *Blood of Spain*, p. 313; Vásquez León, *Un boomerang en Jimena de la Frontera*, pp. 73–101; Preston, *Spanish Holocaust*, pp. 177–178.
175 Bethune, N., *Le crime sur la route Malaga-Almeria: Narrative avec documents graphiques révélant la cruauté fasciste* (Spain, 1937).
176 Bethune, *The Crime on the Road Malaga-Almeria*; Vásquez León, *Un boomerang en Jimena de la Frontera*, pp. 73–101; Preston, *Spanish Holocaust*, pp. 177–178.
177 Durán-Jordà, *The Service of Blood Transfusion at the Front*; Durán-Jordà, F., *El servei de transfusió de sang al front: Organització-utillatge* (Barcelona, 1937).
178 Ibid., p. 7; Franco Grande et al., The 'Servicio Hispano-Canadiense de Transfusión', p. 16.
179 Durán-Jordà, *The Service of Blood Transfusion at the Front*, pp. 7, 13–14, 17–20.
180 Durán-Jordà, El Servicio de Transfusión de Sangre de Barcelona, pp. 307–308; Lozano & Cid, Pioneers and Pathfinders, p. 80.
181 Durán-Jordà, *The Service of Blood Transfusion at the Front*, p. 17
182 Ibid.; Durán-Jordà, El Servicio de Transfusión de Sangre de Barcelona, p. 308.
183 Massons, L'Obra de Frederic Duran I Jorda Viscuda Per Mi, pp. 52–55; Franco Grande et al., The 'Servicio Hispano-Canadiense de Transfusión', pp. 15–16; Franco Grande et al., *Historia de la anestesia*, pp. 214–218; Franco Grande et al., The Development of Blood Transfusion, pp. 1076–1078.
184 Schneider, Blood Transfusion, pp. 188, 192–193, 211, 213.

5 The end of the Spanish Civil War and the trauma of post-war Francoism

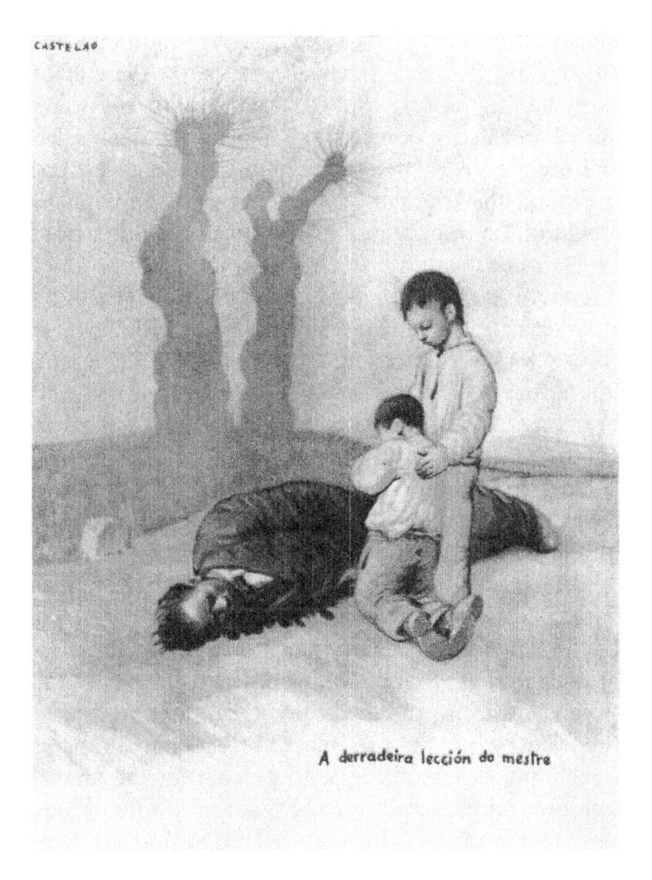

Image 14 Alfonso Daniel Rodríguez Castelao, 'A derradeira lección do Mestre' (The Teacher's Last Lesson), 1938.

Source: Alfonso Daniel Rodríguez Castelao *Galicia Mártir: Estampas* (Oficinas de Propaganda CNT-FAI (Valencia, 1937).

Introduction

On 1 April 1939, the Spanish Civil War 'officially' ended following the unconditional surrender of the Republican forces.[1] With the fall of Madrid as a result of surrender rather than conquest, the Second Republic, born with so much hope out of the elections that followed the abdication of Alfonso XIII in 1931, was at an end.[2] The repression that was to follow was harsh, and it was made even harsher for many of the victims who endured further suffering during the terrible 'hunger years' that followed the war when food was scarce, disease widespread and access to medical care similar to, or worse, than it had been since before the birth of the Republic.[3]

With the defeat at the Ebro in November 1938 and the devastating blow this dealt to the Republican Armies of Spain's North-East, Catalunya fell within two months, with the Insurgents capturing Barcelona at the end of January 1939, forcing nearly half a million people to flee into exile in France. The conditions encountered in hastily constructed internment camps led to widespread disease and high levels of mortality among the refugees. For those who stayed on in France, the traumatic experience of the Civil War soon segued into a continuation of war's traumatising effects resulting from French participation in WWII. For the majority of Spaniards, exile in France was temporary. Many of the refugees were fleeing the immediate danger of an advancing army rather than seeking permanent residence beyond the Spanish borders. However, for those who were seeking asylum outside of Spain, French policy towards the refugees on the whole was dictated by cost, and was therefore principally concerned with their return to Spain, regardless of the fate that awaited them there.[4]

It is the impact on medical provision occasioned by the fall of Catalunya and the end of the Spanish Civil War, the flight of refugees into exile and the impact that the defeat and loss of between fifteen to twenty per cent of the medical profession to exile or 'depurificación' had on healthcare in the immediate aftermath of the war that form the focus of this chapter.

Despite the warning signs evident in December 1938 that a large number of refugees would make their way to France following the collapse of the Catalan Front, French policy, unwisely, was predicated on a more prolonged Republican resistance followed by an eventual mass surrender to Franco's forces. Therefore, the French authorities did little to prepare for the arrival of nearly half a million refugees on French soil in the space of less than three weeks.[5] Republican forces in fact fought a well-organised retreat and as a consequence much of the army of the Levant passed over into France. Here, it was disarmed and its soldiers incarcerated in concentration camps, with initially little or no shelter or sanitary facilities, and treated as prisoners of war.[6] Nevertheless, not all of the army in the north was able to flee, and concentration camps at Reus and Tarragona were hastily constructed to accommodate the 116,000 Republican soldiers and prisoners captured by Francoist forces. By March 1939, seventy new camps had been built to accommodate the ever-increasing number of captured Republican soldiers in Spain, bringing to a total of 190 the number of Insurgent prison camps at the end of the Spanish Civil War.[7]

The experience of the interned soldiers and that of the many thousands of civilians, including women and children, subjected to the repressive measures of the Francoist penal system, echoed that of their compatriots in France. They too were subjected to life in unhygienic and insanitary environments, exposed to extremes of weather, hunger and work in labour battalions, although for the hundreds of thousands interned in Spain, the Franco Regime actively pursued a widespread policy of reprisal and punishment.[8] This involved being subjected to political purges and processes of 're-education' and re-Catholicisation, which were imposed upon the defeated, facilitated, as it were, by a number of repressive and retroactive laws that allowed for prosecution of Republicans for 'offences' dating back to October 1934.[9]

Among the refugees who crossed over into France and those who fled to North Africa at the end of March 1939, following the collapse of the Central Sector, on the few ships in port in Almeria willing to take them were a number of doctors and other medical staff. A census of the refugees carried out in France in the summer of 1939 included 1,500 medical professionals, from doctors to nurses and pharmacists.[10] Many of those who fled beyond French shores never returned. Britain only allowed in 329 Republican exiles, eleven of whom were medical practitioners, but many more made their way to Mexico and the Americas, although there were also a number of Republican exiles who ended up in Nazi concentration camps, with the majority of these sent to the Mauthausen concentration camp in Austria.[11]

Although the Spanish Civil war was to continue for another two months after the fall of Catalunya, the hard-fought battles that had been so costly in terms of human lives throughout the course of the war, were over. Only 300 of the 5,146 who fled the central zone and who arrived in Oran in the early spring of 1939 required immediate hospitalisation. These caused little strain on the Algerian capital's hospitals, although typhus did break out aboard the overcrowded *Stanbrook* as a result of the refusal by the French authorities to allow disembarkation for three weeks of its 2,638 passengers.[12] This chapter therefore focuses primarily upon the impact that the Francoist victory had on healthcare at the end of the war and in the immediate post-war period through an analysis of events in the Catalan Provinces, across the border in France, and through an examination of the terrible effects that the purges and loss of medical personnel to exile had more widely across Spain.[13]

The Spanish Civil War 1936–: An ongoing conflict?

Victory for Franco in the spring of 1939 heralded the start of a dictatorship that was to last for nearly forty years. Helen Graham, however, has argued that the Civil War did not end with Franco's pronouncement that, 'on this day, with the capture and disarming of the Red Army, the National troops have achieved their final military objectives ... The war is over.' For Helen Graham, 'the war still rumbles on'.[14]

In at least one sense this is an accurate statement as, to this day, there are still definable battle lines. The heirs and apologists of Franco seem intent on denying a voice to the victims of the Insurgency and post-war Francoism with a distorted discourse of the collective culpability and inevitable tragedy of civil war.[15] The Association for the Recovery of Historical Memory, and the State Federation of Forums for the Recovery of Memory, the main Spanish groups bent on challenging the 'inevitability' discourse, desire to allow the victims in unmarked graves across Spain first and foremost an identity in its most literal sense, and, more widely, for this identity to be tied to the defence of the Second Republic against an illegitimate coup that led to the long-lived dictatorship.[16] It is also part of an ongoing battle that took its current shape at the turn of the twenty-first century and which is, in part, aimed at addressing the trauma inflicted upon the defeated as a result of Franco's victory in the Spanish Civil War, and the legacy of this trauma for their descendants. This battle is centred upon gaining recognition for the past victims of the conflict and the post-war repression to be recognised as victims of the Francoist regime. Franco's war of attrition against his enemies did not stop with victory on the field of battle in the spring of 1939, despite the sounding of the death knell of the Republic in the pronouncement of 1 April 1939, as the remnants of the Republic – as embodied by its supporters within Spain – were made to taste the full bitterness of their defeat.[17]

The capacity for reconciliation and 'rehabilitation' of the traumatised, whether living or dead, has been hindered by the amnesty law passed by the Spanish parliament in 1977, which in part was the result of fear of a new civil war, and which made it impossible for perpetrators of human rights violations to be prosecuted.[18] Included in the law, which applied to political acts and crimes committed prior to 15 December 1976, was a clause that provided a complete amnesty 'for crimes and misconducts that may have been committed by the authorities, officials and public security forces on the occasion of the investigation and prosecution of acts covered by this law'.[19] Although the wording of the law effectively exonerated both sides from crimes committed during the Civil War, including those who were part of the Francoist apparatus of repression during and after the Civil War, the law failed to take into account the widespread prosecution of Republicans following the decree *La Causa General: Informativa de los delictivos y otros aspectivos de la vida en la zona roja desde el 18 de Julio hasta la liberación* (*General Proceedings: Report on Criminal Events*), which was promulgated in April 1940.[20] This decree, alongside the *Law of Political Responsibilities* of 9 February 1939 (which allowed for 'crimes' to be prosecuted dating back to 1934), meant that countless Republicans paid the price of the Francoist victory by being imprisoned, deprived of their possessions or sentenced to death, despite the majority being innocent of any crime, whereas the perpetrators of

Francoist crimes were later protected from prosecution by the new amnesty law of 1977 in the post-Franco era.[21]

Additionally, hundreds of thousands of Republicans were forced to bear the physical legacy of defeat after the war, through incarceration in internment camps and in forced labour battalions where malnutrition and disease was rife.[22] Rape, which had been used systematically as a tool of war by the Insurgents, became a widely used weapon of repression during the interrogation of female prisoners in the post-war period. Widely attributed to the 'savage Moor' during the conflict, the use of rape was in fact widespread among other frontline units such as the Legionnaires, and with Falangists and other rightist elements in the rear-guard, and its continued use in the post-war period resulted in physical injuries and lasting mental trauma for its victims.[23]

Republican women in particular, bore the brunt of the 'positive eugenics' programme of the new regime, under the leadership of the military psychiatrist Juan Antonio Vallejo Nájera, Director of the Psychiatric Services of the Insurgents during the conflict.[24]

The programme was based on environmental rather than biological ideas of eugenics. Although influenced by the racial ideas on eugenics coming out of Nazi Germany, Nájera's focus was on finding the 'red gene' with the aim of pathologising 'left-wing ideas'.[25] Intent on 'cleansing the race', his 'Catholic' approach ruled out the use of sterilisation to achieve his aims, and this in turn led him to developing the idea of separation as a means of eradicating the 'red gene'. He had particularly harsh views on what he termed 'female revolutionary criminality', and his close links to both Franco and his wife Carmen Polo, and his ideas on punishments and 'treatments' for the defeated, meant that his views were popular among the military hierarchy in the post-war period.[26]

Women seen as of a 'degenerative propensity' were separated from their children, with lasting traumatic implications for mothers and infants alike, with wider effects felt within family networks with fathers and relatives also traumatised by the actions of the new regime.[27] Children of 'red' parents deemed unfit to raise their offspring were sent to state institutions where they were often brutally treated, and their collective experience was all too frequently informed by physical and mental mistreatment, with medical provision often withheld or entirely absent.[28]

Thirty years after the passing of the amnesty law, the statute 52/2007 was enacted during the premiership of the socialist leader José Luis Rodríguez Zapatero. Commonly known as the Law of Historic Memory, it was aimed at providing 'definitive reparation and recognition for those who suffered in the civil war' and the subsequent Francoist dictatorship, such as the mothers and infants who had been separated as a result of the eugenics policy.[29] It was also the aim of the legislation to facilitate the process of addressing the legacy of this trauma by pledging state aid to identify mass graves of the Spanish Civil War, establishing norms whereby these could be investigated as part of a process of reconciliation.[30]

This, unfortunately, has since come to nothing, as the current government (at the time of writing) has not allocated any funds towards this end since 2012, despite calls from the United Nations for the government of Spain to adapt these investigations as official state policy.[31] To this day, there are still the remains of at least 30,000 bodies of an estimated 150,000 victims of the Francoist Civil War and post-war repression buried in unmarked pits across Spain, with Spain second only to Cambodia in the numbers of victims who lie in unmarked graves. Spain is also the only democratic country in the world where 'governmental bodies have failed to investigate their own extrajudicial killings'.[32] Less than 400 of the 2,382 recognised burial sites so far have been investigated, and with open and frank discussion of the Spanish Civil War still taboo for many in Spain, the echoes of the conflict are still felt in Spain today.[33]

Trauma and its legacy

Trauma, whether physical trauma occasioned by injury or psychological trauma induced by participation in conflict as a combatant or civilian, can have lasting and damaging effects.[34] Additionally, the use of terror as a systematic weapon of war by Franco and many of his generals, and the accompanying use of rape as an instrument of social control not only inflicted physical injuries on victims but lasting psychological injuries too.[35] The level of trauma varied according to an individual's experience of it, and this was also true for many of the refugees who, as participants in the conflict, whether passively or actively, bore the added burden of a disconnect from familiar surroundings, people, and home.[36] Additionally those refugees affected were the direct sufferers of traumatic memory as a lived experience, whether the trauma was induced by psychological injury, physical injury, or by both.[37]

A lasting impact of war is also how it affects the memory of those traumatised by the conflict. The psychological scarring left by war can manifest itself in many ways, but it is the painful and at times vivid recall people have of these events (filtered through their own experience and perspectives) that is one of war's lasting legacies.[38] This is important, as the effect of such conflicts are not confined by the timeframe within which they took place but have long-term effects, particularly for those denied the chance to articulate their suffering, an important part of healing. This is also important as the fixing of an autobiographical memory in the minds of those exposed to such trauma can serve as additional evidence that allows for further exploration of the widespread impact that war can have on the collective psyche of a nation, especially the defeated part denied expression of their suffering.[39] This type of evidence may have a limited applicability in wider historical contexts, but with psychological trauma also under the microscope here, its validity is significantly enhanced as it becomes an important measure through which to analyse reactions to war and defeat.[40]

Treatments dictated by physical trauma have to a large degree been the central subject that has informed the discussion at the heart of this book, as the aim has been to explore medical responses to injury at an organisational, personal and cultural level. Whether a wounded Moroccan amputee, a combatant who survived due to a blood transfusion or a disabled veteran with a partially paralysed arm saved from amputation by the closed plaster method, physical trauma often has a lasting effect on the life affected by such an event. Even a wound resulting in a mild disability, such as the loss of part of a hand or a foot, a common injury during the conflict, can have lasting effects on how a person is able to live their later life. However, the psychological trauma occasioned by defeat, exile, incarceration and repression, although less visible and therefore less easy to quantify, also has a real and lasting effect that can span decades.[41]

An important issue that should be addressed when tackling the relevance of the long slow burn of the aftermath of the Spanish Civil War, and of its dying bloodless battles (depending upon whether the war is accepted as over or not), is the issue of trauma, specifically in relation to the losers who bore the brunt of the harsh encompassing repression of Francoism. To try and separate physical from psychological trauma – to try, in other words, to only look at the visible wounds and scars of warfare – is to deny the injuries inflicted upon the body politic of the defeated part of the nation. It is for this reason that in this concluding chapter an examination of the closing months of the war and immediate post-war period is also required as the delivery of healthcare to the traumatised defeated was a contested battleground. This was true whether applied to those in the internment camps of France and North Africa, the villages of Andalucía, or the concentration camps and prisons of the new regime, through which 400,000 people had passed by 1947.[42]

The unequal trauma of defeat

The unequal nature of the conflict during the final months of the war, the inequities imposed upon the defeated as a result of the post-war purges, and the continuation of the campaign by Franco to 'eliminate' communism and freemasonry within Spain after the war, means that the discussion within this chapter is focused upon those who found themselves on the losing side. However, it is important in any such discussion to consider that, despite there being clear victors and vanquished that emerged from the conflict, the war in Spain was first and foremost a civil war. Therefore, although it was the defeated Republicans who bore the brunt of an imposed trauma, the suffering experienced by both vanquished and victors during violent conflicts, or their immediate aftermath, are often complicated and exacerbated even further when the conflict in question is a civil war.

In nations where reconciliation is missing from a post-civil war dialogue, it is not only the defeated whose trauma is denied a voice. The denial to those on the winning side of the right to care or mourn for family, friends or members of the community perceived as being on the 'wrong side' of such conflicts, ensures that the trauma of the 'winning side' of a nation that has been at war with itself is suppressed and therefore this trauma has a wider impact and spread across that society.[43] This impact was less on the Francoist side when it came to mourning the dead, as it was possible to recover many of the bodies of the Insurgent fallen. The public reburial and the active commemoration of the fallen through the construction of memorials and processions to honour the 'martyrs' who had given their lives to save Catholic Spain ensured the victors had a public outlet for their mourning.[44] As Peter Anderson has noted, 'the form in which the Francoist dead were remembered as heroes or martyrs who had sacrificed their lives to purify "Spain" of its Republican enemies struck a deep chord with the regime's support base and offered much solace'.[45] The following case study examines how participation in public rituals associated with Holy Week served not only to celebrate victory configured within an expressly Catholic discourse, but also served as a ritualised expression of grief and suffering for the 'victors' tied closely to the sanctified image of the crucified Christ.

Gloriously mutilated: Christ the amputee

Grieving for the victors, as previously mentioned, had a number of public outlets. Perhaps the most unusual manifestation of this was a religious procession first held in Málaga on Maundy Thursday 1939, five days after the official end of the Spanish Civil War, which continued to be performed annually until 1976, a year after Franco's death.[46] The procession involved the National Confraternity of the Mutilated of the Christ of the Miracles carrying a 'desecrated' early eighteenth-century wood sculpture of the crucified Christ through the streets of Málaga on a plinth, to the apparent rapture and devotion of the gathered citizens (Image 15).[47] The life-size crucifix, which had sat high on the wall in the Church of the Tabernacle in the centre of Málaga, was the subject of an iconoclastic attack after the outbreak of the Civil War. A militiaman had climbed a ladder intending to hack down the statue, but, given the height of the crucifix, only managed to sever the right leg above the knee and the foot of the left leg.[48]

These processions are of particular interest as those who processed the Christ were Insurgent veterans disabled during the conflict – 'soldiers of the crusade', members of the Honourable Corps of Gentlemen Mutilated in War for the Fatherland a body founded by the 'gloriously mutilated' veteran and Africanist Millán Astray.[49] Membership was restricted to those 'who had lost parts of their bodies on the field of battle in defence of God and the fatherland'.[50] Through their participation in a sanctified Catholic ritual the veterans were able to parade their disability as the ultimate sacrifice in the defence of religion and country, while at the same time having their own disabilities publicly identified with those of the 'mutilated Christ'. For those who had lost all or part of a lower limb the connection was most obvious. Nevertheless, the crucified Christ in Catholic iconography was and is a potent image of

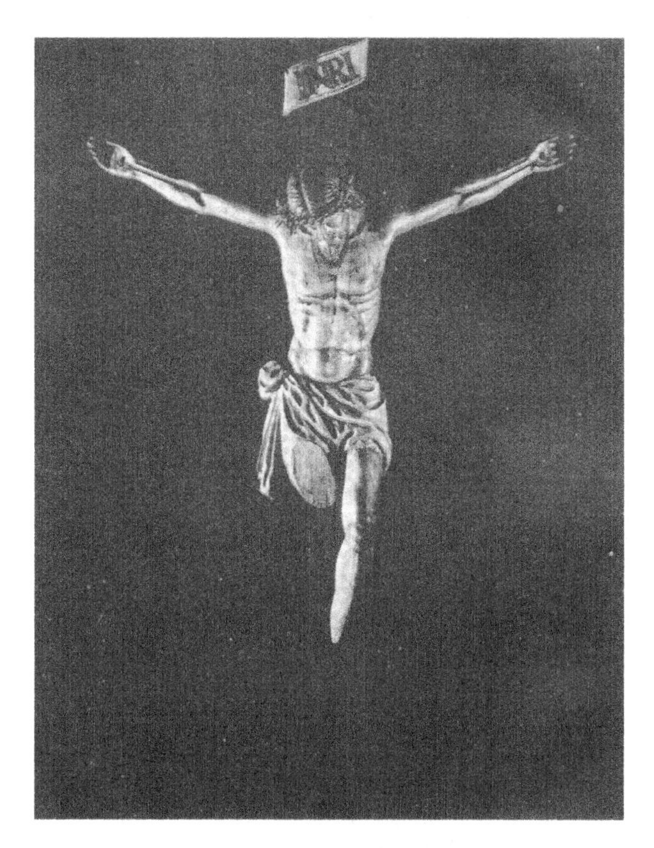

Image 15 'The Mutilated Christ' by Jerónimo Gómez, Málaga 1939.
Source: Image courtesy of Marion Reder Gadow, University of Málaga.

suffering. In a country where re-Christianisation, punishment and reform were central to the new Francoist narrative, reflecting the trauma suffered by Christ through the public display of covered wounds, served both as a validation of the trauma experienced by Francoist veterans and as badges of honour in the service to the fatherland.

Millán Astray, infamous for his cry of 'Death to intelligence! Long live death!', who lost his left arm and right eye in combat in Morocco, made an address during the first Station of the Cross on Maundy Thursday 1939 that encapsulated the above ideas:

> This Christ which the reds have mutilated, the same as they have done to Spain, but who were unable to tear free his heart, soul, or his head, have only been able to mutilate it the same as they have done to us [...] We have been fortunate to shed our blood and give part of our bodies for the Fatherland. You are the most glorious after the dead. We have

> brought out in procession this Christ acclaimed by the multitude through the same streets and plazas that mutilated him.[51]

Ordinarily, desecrated religious statues that could be salvaged were restored so as to reflect the intact corporality of the crucified Christ, however, in this instance Pope Pius XII gave permission for the figure to be left untouched rather than be returned to its 'pristine integrity'.[52] In a similar manner the confraternity of the 'Mutilated Christ' eschewed the traditional robes and capuchóns (pointed hoods) worn by penitents during Holy Week, instead wearing capes over their army and Falangist uniforms and thereby maintaining a clear martial identity that emphasised the origins of their injuries.[53]

The ability of the victors to portray themselves simultaneously as victims of the 'red terror' that threatened to engulf Spain, and as the saviours who, through their own sacrifice, had rescued the nation from the 'Marxist hordes', allowed for ritualised public expressions of grief and suffering denied to those on the losing side.[54] Among the defeated there were some who could also find solace in the victors' identification with sacrifice and loss, as 'public devotions had contestable meanings, even those whose origins can be clearly located in the war itself'.[55] Nevertheless, the prohibition of public mourning for the Republican deceased was an added trauma borne most heavily by the defeated, although with civil war the cause of a national trauma, those among the victors who had lost family and friends on the opposing side were too denied a public outlet for their grief.

The decree establishing the Honourable Corps of Gentlemen Mutilated in War for the Fatherland in 1938 also established full pension rights for those Insurgent veterans classed as totally incapacitated and was enacted in the Insurgent Zone where it overturned the previous national decree established in 1932.[56] With its subsequent ratification in October 1939 aimed at providing employment for disabled members, soldiers who had fought in defence of the Republic were barred from belonging to the new national body that represented disabled veterans and thus from claiming pensions under the dictatorship. It was not until 1976 that the first legislation for establishing pension rights for Republican combatants and their families was enacted.[57]

The Holy Week processions held in Málaga 1976 were the last time that the 'Mutilated Christ' was processed through the streets. The Prelate of Malaga Ramón Buxarrais decided in 1977 that the procession would not take place, apparently due to the unstable political situation. However, by this stage there were also calls by Republican disabled veterans to be admitted to the parade, and it was for this reason, rather than to allow their admission, that the procession with its clear Francoist connections was cancelled.[58]

The 'Mutilated Christ' is still a contested symbol in Málaga today. Despite calls for the procession to be reinstituted as a public parade, the consensus among the religious confraternities and political parties in Málaga is that this should not take place. In a nation where street names and memorials to Francoism are still in evidence, and where the Popular Party regularly obstructs efforts to remove these, the figure of the damaged Christ and the martial origins of the confraternity have proved to be too strongly associated with Francoism for the procession to be reinstated.[59]

This ability of the victors to participate in public rituals that validated their real and perceived sacrifice provided an important outlet for a large number on the winning side who themselves had been traumatised by the war. Nevertheless, this can only be applied to the public expression of grief and suffering, which inevitably has to conform to institutional constructs, whereas private grief is a far more complex experience when arising from the suffering of a civil war and thus not so easily assuaged as this can involve being denied the right to grieve for a relative or friend. It is now widely accepted by psychologists that the subduing of stressful memories related to the experience of suffering mental trauma related to warfare effectively prolongs that trauma.[60] With the suppression of any open discussion of the Civil War that did not reflect accepted Francoist discourses for decades following the conflict, the trauma of both the vanquished and to a lesser degree the victors was suppressed, effectively prolonging the mental suffering of millions of Spaniards.[61]

The beginning of exile: Conflicts in motion

On 16 November 1938, the Battle of the Ebro, the largest offensive of the Civil War, ended in defeat for the Republicans.[62] Casualties on both sides were extensive. Historians differ on the numbers of wounded and killed during the battle; however, total casualties for the offensive were in the region of 100,000, with fatalities for both sides numbering somewhere between 13,000 and 19,000 dead.[63]

The defeat at the Ebro, which came so shortly after British and French capitulation to Hitler over the annexation of the Sudetenland at Munich in September 1938, meant that not only was the retreating Republican Army in the north no longer in a position to effectively resist the advancing Francoist forces due to the superior firepower of the Insurgents, but for a majority of those in Republican Spain, there was no longer any doubt that appeasement signalled the death of the Republic itself.[64]

As a result of the Republican defeat at the Ebro, nearly 40,000 refugees from Aragón and more than 130,000 refugees from those areas of Catalunya that Franco had conquered took refuge in the remaining Republican-controlled area of the Catalan region. For many, however, their stay was to be short-lived. A little over a month after the Republican army had withdrawn across the Ebro, the final Insurgent offensive against Catalunya began.[65] By the time Barcelona fell on 26 January, many of the inhabitants of the swollen Catalan capital had already fled towards the French Pyrenean border.

In a period of less than three weeks 470,000 refugees from Catalunya, over thirty-five per cent of whom were Catalan, crossed over into France.[66] Among the refugees were more than 12,000 wounded soldiers 'under treatment' who formed part of the difficult exodus that made its way along mountain paths and roads before crossing to relative safety in France. The French authorities were reluctant to open their border and initially only allowed civilians to cross, with 150,000 alone making the difficult crossing between 28 January and 5 February 1939. The majority of this first wave consisting of women, children and the elderly were dispersed to requisitioned centres and hastily constructed camps throughout France where they were generally better treated than the refugees who were to follow.[67]

By the middle of February, however, 180,000 of the near half-million refugees who had fled were interned in just two internment camps: the overcrowded beach camps of Argeles sur Mer and St Cypriens in the French Département des Pyrénées-Orientales. The appalling conditions on the exposed beaches where many refugees, predominantly soldiers and men of military age, had little or no protection against the cold winter conditions, except for the clothes and bedding they had brought with them, were greatly exacerbated by poor sanitation and the fact that many of the refugees were suffering from varying degrees of malnutrition.[68] Contaminated water led to dysentery being rife in the camps with scabies also a common scourge, problems not made any easier by the availability of only the most rudimentary of medical cover.[69] There are no reliable figures for the numbers of deaths that occurred in Argeles sur de Mer and St Cypriens during the first few months of their existence, but somewhere between 15,000 and 50,000 people were to die and be buried in the sand at these two camps alone.[70]

For the numerous combatants and civilians in the Central-Southern Zone in March 1939, the only escape was via Republican-held ports on Spain's Levantine coast. The merchant ship *The African Trader* evacuated the first civilians on 19 March 1939, including a number of doctors and nurses.[71] Thousands of refugees also fled Madrid just prior to its capture by Franco's troops. Only 5,146, however, were able to flee the Levantine port of Alicante at the end of March for Algeria on the few remaining ships in harbour, and there were numerous suicides among those trapped in the port who feared the uncertain fate that awaited them. Additionally, with those trapped on the quayside without access to food and water for three and a half days, a number of children died as a result of inanition.[72]

A British hospital ship, *The Maine*, was able to leave Valencia on 28 March 1939 for Marseilles with 200 wounded and a number of medical personnel on board, but this was the only known medical evacuation to have occurred in this sector.[73] Overall 15,000 people were able to flee the Central-Southern Zone for French-held territories in North Africa; however, many thousands more were left to await an uncertain fate in a post-Civil War Spain where thousands were to die, victims of an ongoing repression that was to last for many years.[74]

Among the many thousands of refugees who did not return after the Spanish Civil War had ended were hundreds of doctors whose services were forever lost to Spain, including eminent doctors such as Durán-Jordà, Josep Trueta and Juan Morata Cantón.[75] According to the somewhat imprecise and at times incomplete survey carried out in the summer of 1939 by the Servicio de Evacuación de Refugiados Españoles (Service of Evacuation of Spanish Refugees, or SERE), there were 553 doctors, 503 nurses, 268 pharmacists and 135 dentists interned in French camps in June 1939. However, this figure was in fact considerably higher, as subsequent research has revealed that the number of healthcare professionals who fled Spain by the end of the Civil War was at least twice this number, as the figure of 3,750, doctors, dentists, nurses, medical practitioners, veterinarians and pharmacists provided by Javier Rubio in *Emigración* in 1977 does not includes those names of those missing from censuses and statistics.[76] The SERE report also states that at this stage there were still more than 300,000 refugees in France, although the number could well have been higher as this is based on a figure of 400,000 refugees after the fall of Catalunya, rather than the 470,000 who were known to have crossed into France.[77] By the end of 1939, according to the inaccurate census carried out in the camps, there were 26,000 refugees living beyond European shores, with Mexico, due to its support of the defeated Republic, attracting the largest number of medical exiles, but the majority of Spanish refugees who had made their way across the Pyrenees were either repatriated to Spain or ended up in labour battalions in France.[78] Others were left with little option but to join the French Army or the Foreign Legion, and thousands of Republicans went on to fight with the resistance.[79] Spanish anarchists and socialists of the Leclerc Division were among the first troops to liberate Paris in August 1944, and apart from the few who made their way clandestinely to Spain in the hope of aiding the Spanish resistance to overthrow Franco, the majority went on to live out their lives in exile in France.[80]

By December 1939, an estimated 360,000 refugees had returned to Spain where many healthcare professionals were forced into internal exile as a result of Franco's purges of the professional classes. Nevertheless, there were still at least 140,000 Spanish refugees living in France at the end of 1939 who found themselves unwittingly caught up in a new war against fascism (the figures above include a number of refugees who had sought refuge in France prior to the fall of Catalunya). It should be noted, however, that the accuracy of Rubio's figures are disputed as they were taken from the 1943 publication of the National Service of French Statistics, whose own figures were based on those provided by the Interior Minister in December 1939. It would appear that these figures were distorted for political reasons, and therefore the number of Republican exiles who were faced by nearly six more years of war was likely to have been much higher.[81]

With the mobilisation of large sectors of the French workforce after the outbreak of WWII, the majority of Republicans in France faced the additional trauma of being coerced into French labour battalions or of remaining confined in the camps. Many of those who had made it to North Africa were forced to do hard labour on the Trans-Saharan Railway in Algeria and French

Morocco, and subjected to a strict discipline in punishment camps by the French military authorities for the slightest infraction of draconian rules.[82] However, despite this reversal of French policy towards Spanish refugees that accompanied the start of WWII, Spanish Republicans were viewed with increasing suspicion by the new Vichy authorities after the occupation of France by German forces in 1940. An estimated 9,000 were sent to German and Austrian concentration camps during the occupation of France. The majority, some 7,189, were incarcerated in Mauthausen-Gusen concentration camp in Austria, with the first arriving in August 1940. In all 4,815 were worked and starved to death before the camp was liberated in May 1945.[83]

A result of the flight into exile of important figures from the world of medicine and science was the effect on public health in post-war Spain, where food shortages and widespread hunger were negatively affecting the nation's health.[84] This problem was made worse by the loss on both sides during the conflict of a number of healthcare professionals due to summary executions, although in the Republican Zone this was mainly during the opening months due to the breakdown in order, and those who died in frontline hospitals or in the frequent bombing raids on Republican-held cities.[85]

The impact that the loss of medical personnel to exile, both internal and external, was to have on post-war medicine and science within Spain is shown in the following example. In July 1936, the University of Barcelona had 319 lecturers and documentation survives for 135 of the 141, about forty-five percent, who had sanctions imposed on them after the fall of Catalunya. There were three lecturers from pharmacy, nine from the sciences, eleven from law, forty-one from philosophy and letters, and seventy-one lecturers of medicine, 22.26 per cent of the overall total. Of the scientific and medical elite from universities across Spain as a whole, 22.8 per cent were victims of the purges that restricted their practice or expelled them from their posts entirely, with a further 1.25 per cent jailed.[86]

The Catalan Campaign

The Republican defeat at the Ebro signalled the beginning of the end for the Spanish Republic. The Republican army of the Ebro had lost large amounts of military hardware and with Russian war material held up in France, and the Republican industrial heartland hemmed in and under siege, rearming the defeated army in the north was impossible.[87] After joining up with the Army of the East in Catalunya, the Republican forces were greater in number to the troops arraigned against them, but they lacked sufficient ammunition and were heavily demoralised, with the majority believing that victory was no longer possible. The Insurgent forces not only enjoyed a more than three to one advantage in artillery terms, but also total superiority in the air.

The Insurgent advance on 23 December 1938 was rapid, with Catalunya overrun in little more than a month. Town after town fell in rapid succession, and with the imminent fall of Barcelona forcing a mass flight of refugees towards France, a humanitarian crisis unfolded that the Republican Government was powerless to prevent.[88]

Despite the resistance offered by soldiers who fought in retreating units as they fled towards France, the refugees were victims of continued bombardment from the air and from the sea, and there was little will or strength left to fight among the refugees and wider population where malnutrition was rife.[89]

The bombing of Catalunya: Lessons learned?

The conflict in Spain was notable as being the first full-scale European war of the twentieth century where deliberate aerial bombing by aviation behind the lines was extensively deployed as a weapon of war.[90] Barcelona and other Levantine towns and cities had been the victims of numerous bombing raids since the start of the conflict, carried out predominantly by Italian airplanes based in nearby Majorca. These raids habitually targeted both civilian and military targets, with Barcelona alone the victim of 350 raids during the conflict, leading to significant civilian casualties.[91] These raids varied in intensity, but between the 16 and 18 March 1938, intensive aerial bombing of Barcelona resulted in 1,000 dead and 2,000 wounded. Similarly, the bombing of civilians fleeing territories that had fallen to the Insurgents throughout the conflict, such as occurred during the flight from Malaga to Almeria in February 1937, also resulted in numerous casualties.[92]

It was certain casualties from the bombing raid on Barcelona, among others, that were to serve as case studies for the influential work by the Catalan surgeon Josep Trueta *Treatment of War Wounds and Fractures* first published in 1939, although a Catalan version of the book had first appeared in 1938.[93] The book, with its use of medical photography, stands testimony to the traumatic physical injuries sustained by both civilians and combatants, with forty-one of the forty-eight images used to illustrate serious limb injuries in various stages of healing.[94] The publication of this book, which was concerned primarily with the closed plaster method of treatment, was to prove influential during WWII, where its methods were widely employed, albeit with varying results, on a number of fronts from North Africa to the Pacific.[95]

Between the start of 1938 and the beginning of 1939, a number of hospitals in the region were also the victims of air raids, particularly those in areas lacking aerial defences.[96] The Institute of Childcare of Reus in Catalunya was partially destroyed in the bombing raids of January 1938, and a number of hospitals in Barcelona were regularly evacuated to special hospitals outside the city that had been provided with underground operating theatres.[97] Durán-Jordà, during the heavy bombardments experienced by Barcelona on numerous occasions, was forced to work in a basement room fifteen foot by eight foot, which had been reinforced with concrete one metre thick throughout.[98]

Shortly after fleeing into exile in Britain early in 1939, both Trueta and Durán-Jordà provided oral testimony on the type of protection needed against aerial bombardment to the Intelligence Branch of the Air Raid Precaution Department of the British Home Office.[99] However, with fear of an impending war in Europe of widespread concern among the British populace, close attention had already been paid to civilian bombing in Spain. British doctors who had served in Republican Spain also shared their experiences of bombing and civil defence, and therefore the contribution made by Trueta and Durán-Jordà in sharing their knowledge of air raid precautions should be considered within this wider context.[100]

During the Ebro Offensive and the Catalan Campaign Insurgent aerial bombardment was intensified even further. It was during this period that Republican hospital services near the approaching Insurgent frontline were forced to relocate, partly as a result of bombardment and partly as a result of rapidly shifting battlefronts.[101] For those who fled the Insurgent advance following the fall of Barcelona, their experience echoed that of the refugees who had fled Málaga two years previously; they were bombed and strafed from the air, with those on the coastal road towards Le Perthus also the subject of bombardment from the sea.[102]

Hospitals in retreat: A case study

The Hospital Savinosa in Tarragona, about sixty miles south-west of Barcelona, was an important medical establishment which existed under a variety of names and whose facilities were forced to relocate on a number of occasions.[103] The hospital, which enjoyed extensive orthopaedic facilities, was originally set up at the end of July 1936 by the Spanish orthopaedic surgeon Jimeno Vidal, a skilled practitioner of the closed plaster method who first established orthopaedic facilities in Reus at the Hospital Pere Mata only a few miles from Tarragona.[104] The hospital, a former psychiatric institute, was requisitioned for the Aragón Offensive during the summer of 1937 and its facilities transferred to Tarragona, where a branch line was built from the main railway to facilitate the entrance of hospital trains.[105] Jimeno Vidal was appointed Director of Surgery at the hospital under the command of the Fifth Army Corps, which was led by the hard-line, Moscow-trained communist Enrique Lister.[106]

As a result of preparations for the Ebro Offensive, the facilities and the patients, including those confined to beds in continuous traction devices, were then transferred by a special train to the monastery at Banyoles, 120 kilometres north-east of the Catalan capital and 73 kilometres from the French border.[107] After the initial stages of their treatment, and once they had been stabilised, patients from Banyoles were then transferred to Military Clinic No. 7, a hospital closer to the French border in nearby Olot, a centre also supervised by Jimeno Vidal.[108] By the time of the Catalan Offensive, there were more than 1,000 wounded at the hospital and a number of the patients and staff able to flee made their way to France to escape the advancing Insurgent army.[109] However, the wounded from Olot who made their way into France were initially incarcerated in Vallespir in the French Pyrenees, where the harsh winter conditions at 1,000 metres exacted a heavy toll on the wounded.[110]

Rudolph Matas, a pioneer of vascular surgery of Catalan origin, visited a number of hospitals in Catalunya including the hospital at Banyoles in the late autumn of 1938. During this time he witnessed the closed plaster method being used in a number of well-run hospitals. He was in Catalunya to secure passports for relatives whom he wanted safely transferred to France, a process that was to take him two months.

Although Matas was a vascular surgeon, he was nevertheless cognizant of different approaches within orthopaedic practice and outlined the differences in the application of the closed plaster method as used by Jimeno Vidal and Josef Trueta, namely Trueta's avoidance of the use of skeletal traction (a mechanical traction device) to reduce fractures, an important development as patients could be more easily moved to rehabilitation centres to free-up much needed beds. It was at Banyoles that Vidal shared his latest statistics with Matas on the 6,000 fractures he had treated during the course of the war, including the 500 fractures of the femur. Among this last group there had been only sixteen deaths and five amputations, a marked improvement on previous conflicts.

The importance of the account by Matas, which reflects observations made in the closing months of 1938, is that they indicate that at this stage, in Catalunya at least, Republican medical facilities for the treatment of fracture patients, both civilian and military, seem to have been relatively well organised. Matas also acknowledged in his address that 'statistical compilations of the experience of the military surgeons attached to General Franco's armies have not been collected in sufficient number for general comparison with the Catalonian statistics'.[111]

He argued, however, that since the majority of Spanish surgeons had been influenced by Böhler, an influential Austrian traumatologist, and citing the figures for the Victoria Base Hospital as reported by Captain Arguelles Lopez, which compared with those of Vidal, that it was likely that once the statistics were collated they would be found to be similar.[112]

This advanced orthopaedic care was still available in the increasingly threatened areas of Catalunya right up until the collapse of the Catalan Front. This was, in part, due to the work of surgeons such as Trueta and Vidal, but also due to the efficient hospital reallocation procedures carried out in the face of Insurgent advances.[113] Also of importance was the contribution made by other Catalan surgeons familiar with the closed plaster method in maintaining orthopaedic services in Catalunya at the time. Joaquím Trias i Pujol, a distinguished veteran of the Protectorate, was head of the Military Hospital of Vallcarca in Barcelona throughout the war (appointed by Federica Montseny in January 1937), previously Director of the Health Council of War, and had been responsible for appointing

Jimeno Vidal head of the hospital in Reus.[114] After sending his family to safety in France, Trias i Pujol appointed a fellow Catalan, Moisés Broggi, who had worked previously in Barcelona treating orthopaedic casualties, as his successor to oversee the handing over of the hospital to the Insurgents before fleeing into exile himself.

Trias i Pujol did not return to Spain until 1947, when he was briefly imprisoned for having treated an anarchist guerrilla involved in the post-war struggle against Francoism, with Broggi, who had served with the International Brigades, barred from holding public posts for ten years after the conflict.[115]

Evacuating the wounded

Despite the high level of care for those under orthopaedic treatment, the Catalan Offensive was to have severe consequences for the medical infrastructure of Republican Catalunya. Well-organised services were increasingly tested, although every effort was made to care for the wounded and to evacuate those in need. Nevertheless, the fear of reprisals, born out of the knowledge of what had befallen those who had resisted Franco's forces elsewhere, led to many hospitalised patients with serious wounds also trying to flee, despite the inherent difficulties involved.[116]

A young communist, Teresa Pàmies i Bertran, who later endured the hardships of prison life under Francoism due to her participation in the underground resistance movement, witnessed the fear provoked by the Insurgents' entry into Barcelona in January 1939.[117] Her account, written thirty-five years after the events it described, nevertheless is an example of how a traumatic memory can become fixed in the mind of a person witnessing a traumatising event:

> There is one thing I will never forget: the wounded who crawled out of Vallcarca hospital, mutilated and bandaged, almost naked, despite the cold, they went down the street, shrieking and pleading with us not to leave them behind to the mercy of the victors. All other details of that unforgettable day were wiped out by the sight of those defenceless soldiers … the certainty that we left them to their fate will shame us for ever. Those with no legs dragged themselves along the ground, those who had lost an arm raised the other with a clenched fist, the youngest cried in their fear, the older ones went mad with rage. They grabbed the side of lorries loaded with furniture, with bird cages, with silent women, with indifferent old people, with terrified children. They screamed, they ululated, they blasphemed and cursed those who were fleeing and abandoning them.[118]

The wounded soldiers, of which there were approximately 20,000 in Barcelona, had good reason for wanting to flee, as their injuries marked them out as soldiers who had resisted the Francoist advance and made them prime targets for the repression that was to follow.[119]

Despite the fact that many of the wounded were trapped in Barcelona and unable to flee, there were efforts made right up to the last moment to ensure that those who feared reprisals and wanted to flee were able to be evacuated. Shortly before the fall of Barcelona, a train left the beleaguered Catalan capital for Girona 100 kilometres to the north-west, carrying a number of wounded from the city's military hospitals.[120] On board the train, alongside several surgeons of note, including Josef Trueta, was Ignacio Ponseti Vives.[121] Upon arrival in Girona he was charged with the transfer of the wounded by ambulance from the 'Hospital of Olot' to Prats de Mollo across the French border.[122] The patients, who were transferred with the help of local smugglers who supplied cars and mules after the chauffeur of the ambulance absconded with his vehicle, made their way over the Pyrenees into France, taking three days to reach safety.[123]

Transport was available to a number of those in the military, including soldiers, as the Republican Army in retreat took with it all mobile vehicles (including ambulances and mobile surgical units) and armoury, but this war and medical material was confiscated upon passing into France.[124] Nevertheless, tens of thousands of the wounded who fled to France did so on foot and included a number of upper-limb-fracture patients with their arms in slings or immobilised in plaster.[125] An unfortunate few who were being treated by the closed plaster method and managed to cross over into France ended up losing limbs due to inexperienced French surgeons mistaking the bad smell from the casts for the putrefaction of gangrene. Fortunately, this number was small and the mistake soon rectified, although the literature does not state whether the 'Spanish Method' continued to be used for these types of cases.[126] Nevertheless, the confiscation of medical equipment, both large and small, meant that, with only limited French medical aid available, the chance to alleviate the suffering of the wounded and infirm by utilising experienced Spanish medical personnel and their equipment was lost, and unnecessary deaths were the result.

Shortly before the evacuation of the Military Clinic at Olot early in February 1939, Jimeno Vidal, in his supervisory capacity, paid a visit to the hospital there. Chief among his concerns for both the centres under his supervision was ensuring that medical care continued for those patients who could not be evacuated. It was during his brief absence from the hospital at Banyoles that a contingent of troops from the Lister Brigade who were fighting a retreating action, arrived at the hospital to evacuate the staff there to France.[127]

It was hoped that units fighting defensive actions and the medical staff in Catalunya would be able to rejoin the army of the centre in the central zone after the fall of Catalunya. This was something the advancing Insurgent army was hoping to avoid and this, coupled with the disintegration of Republican resistance in Catalunya, was one of the main reasons for the rapid Insurgent advance.[128]

The soldiers who arrived at Banyoles under the command of Captain Trigo evacuated a total of twenty-three staff from the hospital. Among those evacuated was Gerta Kromarch, the Austrian wife of Jimeno Vidal.[129] Unfortunately, those who were to be evacuated never reached France. On 6 February 1939, the truck carrying the hospital staff set off north-west towards the frontier at Port Bou, but stopped in Vila Sacra, about halfway to their destination, where all twenty-three members of staff from the hospital were executed. It has been suggested that Kromarch was accused of being a traitor, but this does not explain why staff including radiologists and pharmacists were also summarily executed, with the reason for their execution an unsolved mystery.[130]

Jimeno Vidal was subjected to the 'purification' purges at the end of the conflict and was not only stripped of his medical rank but also his university positions. Ironically, for someone who it appears served the Republic willingly in his capacity as surgeon, he then fled to Nazi-occupied Vienna where he went to work with his previous mentor Böhler, and is credited with introducing the 'Spanish Method' into the German Military Health Services in 1940. He was forced to return to Spain after the defeat of Germany in 1945, where he saw out his days working as a traumatologist in a private clinic as he had been barred from public office.[131] His experiences were not atypical of the many Spanish surgeons who suffered the trauma of what often amounted to internal exile within Spain, in that many had to resort to private practice to make a living as within Spain they were barred from public practice.

Repression and incarceration: The persecution of nurses in occupied Catalunya

With the occupation of Catalunya, and because of the flight of a large number of the medical profession, the Insurgents were faced with having to care for large numbers of wounded either unable to flee or unwilling to seek refuge outside of Spain. Priscilla Scott-Ellis and the medical team to which she belonged were able to enter Barcelona a day after its capture, on 27 January 1939, making her ideally placed to record her observations on the delivery of the medical care in or near the city.[132] After serving during a number of campaigns since arriving in Spain in October 1937, which included nursing the wounded from both Teruel and the Ebro Fronts, she decided in January 1939 to join a surgical team of the Moroccan Army Corps in order to nurse closer to the frontline.[133]

Her team, which had been based in Reus after its fall to the Insurgents on 15 January 1939, moved to Sitges, 40 kilometres down the coast from Barcelona, on 24 January 1939. It was there that Scott-Ellis joined them in the early hours of 25 January 1939. Initially she had been unable to locate the new hospital as she first had to find the Medical Service Headquarters, which had moved to Vilanova i la Geltrú due to the rapid Insurgent advance.[134] By the time that Scott-Ellis joined the team there was little work to do in the hospital apart from surgery on two gravely wounded soldiers (a third case was described as inoperable), and the plan was for the team to move to Barcelona the following day.[135]

A concern expressed by Scott-Ellis was that her team would be inundated with work once they arrived in Barcelona where 'the Reds have probably left all their hospitals full of wounded'.[136] This fear, for Scott-Ellis at least, was not realised upon her arrival as she was given leave, but her diary entry for 3 February 1939 when her team were back in Sitges, describes how she acted as a surgical assistant during operations. She also described how the Insurgent medical services were inundated with patients due to 'there being 6,000 wounded Reds in Barcelona' (a conservative figure), and because 'the Red nurses need to be removed', which meant that with many Republican nurses barred from practising, there were not nearly enough Insurgent nurses to replace them.[137]

Nurses removed from their posts were often harshly treated. In Barcelona, fifty nurses were jailed in the women's prison in the Les Corts district between 29 January 1939 and 6 October 1939. One of these women, Eugenia González Ramos, a 20-year-old from Madrid, was executed in the notorious Camp de la Bóta in May 1939.[138] The camp, an old military fort, was the scene of forty-four executions carried out by the Republican authorities in September and October 1936.[139] However, it was after the war, between 1939 and 1952, that 1,717 executions were to take place there, with the killing of González Ramos taking place on 11 May 1939.[140] González Ramos, who was judged by court martial (she had worked in a military hospital) for the crimes of having been a member of the Spanish Communist Party, was denounced by a nun who had concealed her religious identity and with whom she had worked at the clinic. The nun had been promoted to head of nursing after the Francoist occupation and had seen this as an opportune moment to rid herself of one of her former colleagues. Her death was recorded as being due to an internal haemorrhage. However, in this instance this was not as a result of trying to cover up the cause of death, rather it was as a result of a law of 1870 that stated that in cases of violent death, carrying out the death penalty or a death in a penal institution, it was forbidden to enter these details in the civil register.[141] As a result of this law, the true figure of those who were executed while in captivity is difficult to quantify with any exactitude, nevertheless it is now widely accepted that at least 50,000 people were executed between 1939 and 1945.[142]

Denunciation was an important Francoist weapon in the post-war period where it quickly became admissible evidence in court hearings and tribunals, and as such an important means of securing convictions. The huge strain placed upon an unprepared state apparatus unable to cope with the sheer number of the defeated that were required to be 're-educated' and purged led to denouncement becoming the main means by which convictions were secured. The policy of returning people to their homes for investigation and incarceration, a practice that had originated during the occupation of territory during the conflict, also facilitated the widespread use of denunciation as a tool of repression, as localised contexts allowed for allegations to be more specific, although the scope for what constituted a valid denunciation could be very broad.[143] It was enough on occasion to merely have complained about Insurgent air raids and for someone to state before a tribunal that this had been the case, for this to result in imprisonment.[144]

Therefore, from the start the new Francoist State depended on its own supporters (and to a lesser degree those who gave their support to the regime in order to survive) throughout Spain to help carry out its systematic repression of the defeated. The *ABC* of 1 April 1939 stated that 'our triumph allows us to measure precisely the guilt of our enemies ... to achieve this aim Generalísimo Franco requires your unreserved and enthusiastic collaboration', and with so many people imprisoned, and with the judicial system under severe strain, denunciations were the primary means by which convictions were secured.[145]

As a result of the culture of denunciation encouraged by the Francoist authorities, the field for petty actions of vengeance was wide open, contributing significantly towards the trauma of the defeated. Although González Ramos was condemned more than anything for her communist affiliations, she was also condemned for having served in the kitchens of a militia based in Carabanchel early in the war. The denunciation against her helped to secure a conviction. Women who had worked as cleaners or washerwomen for Republican institutions were also denounced and found themselves victims of the purges after the war had finished.

Guilt through association was often also a *de facto* crime. Trinidad Gallego Prieto, a nurse and a midwife who had joined the Spanish Communist Party in 1935, was detained in Madrid in April 1939 and jailed in the Las Ventas Women's Prison. As a well-known communist who had worked as a surgical nurse during the Spanish Civil War, and as someone who had helped set up the Lay Committee for Nurses (Comité de Enfermeras Laicas) in February 1935 to protest against the monopoly of public nursing places by the female religious orders, her family also became suspect. Gallego Prieto was detained on 12 April 1939 while at home, and both her mother and her eighty-seven-year-old grandmother, neither of whom had known political connections, were imprisoned together. The three family members were not released until August 1941, although Gallego Prieto was reimprisoned in 1942. It was during her second period of incarceration in the densely overcrowded prison of Las Ventas that Gallego Prieto was forced to work as a midwife.[146] Many mothers and young infants died in the prison due to the appalling conditions they were kept in. Additionally, there were only two doctors at the prison, with no gynaecologist appointed until 1943. It was also while working at the prison that Gallego Prieto was witness to the disappearance of young infants as a result of the Francoist 'positive eugenics' programme, which under the Franco's dictatorship saw at least 30,000 children taken from their mothers and given (or sold) to 'good catholic parents'.[147] It is likely that many nurses who had qualified during the war (or the much smaller number who had qualified prior to the conflict), rather than face a tribunal in the hope of reintegration into the nascent nursing profession, opted to forgo this uncertain option and returned to civilian life. A number of midwives in Madrid who had held title prior to the conflict, chose not to subject themselves to the arbitrary approval process procedures of the tribunal system after the war. Apart from those who had died during the conflict or who were incarcerated once Madrid fell to the Insurgents, there were those who simply chose not to return to their profession for fear of being purged and a number of midwives went into exile abroad.[148] Forty-six midwifes were purged from their posts in Madrid alone following the war, and this was a pattern repeated among nurses and midwives throughout Spain. This was mirrored in small villages across Spain where a large number of women, from teachers to nurses, were removed from their posts, a process of repression that had existed since the start of the Insurgency in the areas under their control.[149]

It was a combination of the above factors that complicated medical care once Catalunya fell to the Insurgents. As a result of the removal of much of the Republican medical personnel from their posts and the flight of medical staff to France, the Insurgents were faced with the issue of having to treat Republican wounded as well.[150] There were contingents of nurses on standby in the Insurgent rear-guard ready to move into hospitals where there were shortfalls, but it is unlikely that these were sufficient in number to replace those who had fled or were removed from their posts.[151] However, this was, to a certain degree, mitigated by the Insurgents at this stage having far fewer of their own wounded to treat and by the return of the female religious orders to hospitals in Republican-held areas, with nuns being the traditional mainstay of Spanish nursing.[152]

Hospital penitentiaries

It would appear that the wounded left behind in Catalan hospitals in the first instance were reasonably well treated, but the evidence for this continuing beyond the period of immediate occupation either in Barcelona or further afield is sparse and contradictory due to the inflated claims made during the early triumphalist phase of Francoism.[153] What is known, however, is that a number of 'frontline' hospitals were turned into hospital prisons and the prisons of the new Francoist regime had a poor record for the treatment of prisoners and this also seems to have been true of prison hospitals.[154]

Collective punishment of the defeated Republicans was high on the agenda of the new regime. A misplaced belief in Spain's ability to stand alone following the hardships imposed by the Civil War, saw the state pursue autarkical policies, leading to 200,000 people dying of starvation during the early 1940s. If the majority of these deaths were attributable to famine, the endemic diseases that swept across Spain found fertile breeding grounds in the internment camps, prisons, hospitals and prison hospitals of the Francoist regime, with even minor infections capable of killing those whose diets were devoid of proteins and fats.[155] However, despite the state's intention to punish the defeated, nearly three years of Civil War had left much of the Spanish population in dire economic straits, and while those on the losing side were the most severely impacted by disease and famine, the poor throughout Spain as a whole suffered the hardship of what later became known as the 'hunger years'.[156]

During this time, epidemic diseases that had become more manageable through public health schemes prior to the conflict resurfaced throughout Spain.[157] There were epidemics of typhus, a disease that had largely been controlled on both sides during the Spanish Civil War, with 4,000 people affected in Málaga alone in 1941.[158] TB, malaria and diarrhoea also contributed to the large rise in mortality, with diarrhoea the cause of 60,000 deaths, many of them children, during 1941.[159]

Confinement in institutions meant that people whose health had been compromised by war and the often inadequate diet available in besieged Republican areas, were exposed to contagious illnesses that could often be fatal.[160] The women's prison in Segovia, founded in 1946, was the destination for political prisoners from all over Spain, including those suffering from TB. As an institution it had functioned since 1943 as a tuberculosis sanatorium (if only in name), despite later converting to penitentiary use, and a number of 'healthy' inmates, kept in close confinement with other inmates, died due to being exposed to TB during their time in the institution.[161] This was also the case in the Sanatorium Penitentiary of Porta Coeli in the Province of Valencia, where there seems to have been a deliberate policy of not only isolating Republican prisoners with TB in camps, but also then leaving them to die untreated.[162]

A number of infirm prisoners who were captured in the port of Alicante at the end of the conflict were also imprisoned in this camp. Lluis Marcó i Dachs, an administrator for health and pharmaceuticals under the Republic, was sent to Port Coeli from Alicante but was able to recover from a pulmonary lesion caused by TB after his release from the camp.[163] Nevertheless, many thousands were to die in camps and hospitals across Spain due to the deplorable state that medical infrastructure had been left in by the loss of medical personnel, many of whom died in captivity, were executed, or were simply denied the right to practice.[164]

The conditions for Republican prisoners in Spanish hospitals and for the wounded and infirm in the prisons and camps after the fall of Catalunya may have in part been due to the disruption that an invading army brings in its wake, but throughout Spain these appalling conditions also resulted from the deliberate policies of the new dictatorship. The discourse firmly embedded in the Law of Political Responsibilities of 9 February 1939, was primarily predicated on punishing the losers, rather than healing the nation. The law made clear that restitution was only possible through the purging of the 'red disease' that gripped Republicans, and thus investing in the healing or even feeding of the vanquished was not high on the list of a new regime intent on cleansing Spain.[165] Subsequent legislation, including the Law for the Repression of Freemasonry and Communism and the tribunal set up to process and purge university staff, including academic medical personnel, only compounded this problem. It meant that alongside the lack of facilities or beds to treat the more seriously ill, there were simply not enough trained medical personnel to confront the immediate healthcare and medical problems faced and in most cases ignored by the new Francoist regime.[166] The flight of so many medical personnel into France, the distrust by the authorities of medical staff who remained, and the lack of resources with which to tackle a mounting medical crisis meant that high levels of care that had been frequently achieved in both the civilian and military field in Republican Spain during the conflict were no longer possible.[167]

Although in the sphere of military medicine, medical and surgical care had been broadly similar across both sides, Insurgent military concerns had been dominated with winning the war. Numerous doctors and other medical staff militarised during the conflict had not been replaced in the rear-guard or in the territories conquered by the Insurgents, and with martial law in place until 1948, this also affected the number of qualified medical staff available to treat the civilian population as many doctors were not immediately demobilised at the end of the conflict.[168] This was why those among the poor sections of society who had supported Franco were also adversely affected, as their poverty made it difficult for them to access limited medical facilities. Therefore, the immediate post-war crisis in health not only affected those who found themselves the target of the repressive policies of the regime, but also the population more widely. When medical services began to unravel it would be years before they could regain the reach that they had enjoyed during much of the Civil War in Republican areas, or indeed in the whole of Spain.

Across the Pyrenees

A witness to the unravelling of the Republican medical services at the end of the conflict, and to conditions in the concentration camps in France, was a young Lieutenant Practitioner, Francisco Urzaiz. Born in Melilla on 7 October 1919, he was studying medicine at university in Madrid when the war broke out. Initially he was drawn towards a combat role and joined the Republican Air force as a pilot in 1937. His stay there, however, was short-lived as he soon joined the Armed Forces, and after taking a short course in medicine and surgery in early summer 1938 was appointed as a Lieutenant Practitioner and posted to Hospital Train No. 6 on the Segre Front in Catalunya. Urzaiz was to serve as a medical practitioner in Catalunya for the remainder of the war. He took part in the Battle of the Ebro, the Catalan Campaign and the retreat to the French border and spent ten months in the internment camp at St Cypriens. He was later transferred to a French labour battalion where he ended up working as a medical practitioner. It was at this point that he worked in a forced labour battalion in German camps in France under the auspices of Organisation Todt, the body responsible for a large number of engineering projects in German-occupied territories.[169]

His participation as a medical practitioner in such diverse situations and the memories he related to the historian Ángeles Egido León, who, through an examination of the sources provides evidence that support his memories, proffers a rare glimpse of exile, incarceration and the work of a medical practitioner in a number of capacities as refugee and captive in Vichy France.[170]

Urzaiz states that during the evacuation of a hospital at Vilanova i Geltru during the retreat from Catalunya, he was informed that Regulares had entered and killed with bayonets patients confined to their beds, a charge that had been levelled against the North African troops on a number of occasions.[171] However, when the hospital train was later occupied during the closing days of the conflict in Catalunya, by either a company or a tabor of Regulares, he states that they were all treated well, despite being put under guard as prisoners on the train before being handed over to the French Military Health Authority. Urzaiz, concerned about his father whom he knew had been evacuated to Girona, managed to escape through the floor of the train. He made his way to Girona on foot, a difficult journey of sixty miles with planes bombing and strafing from the air the fleeing troops and refugees.

Urzaiz was able to find his father, a professional military man and veteran of several campaigns in the protectorate, who was able to present his son to the head of the evacuation services. Urzaiz was then assigned to Hospital Train No. 9 stationed at Llançà not far from the French border. Urzaiz noted of the train that it had the exact same layout as the Hospital Train No. 6, in which he had seen service during the Ebro Campaign. However, this time he noted that there was no abundance of materials but a shortage of time as there had been during the Battle of the Ebro; now there was time to spare to treat those on the train but virtually no materials, and in a nearby building wounded soldiers who could not be cared for on the train languished on piles of straw waiting to be evacuated to France.

The stay in Llançà was to be short-lived. With the unrelenting Insurgent advance, the train was ordered to make its way towards the frontier. It made its way to Cerbère laden with wounded and soldiers, both inside and out. It was here that Urzaiz again encountered his family who had been evacuated on a Republican army ministry train that had crossed over into France. Hospital Train No. 9 was commandeered by the French Military Health Service upon its arrival in Cerbère, who then used it to transport refugees to the internment camp of Saint-Cyprien, among them Urzaiz and his family.[172]

The confiscation of Republican medical vehicles and materials by the French authorities and the limited medical aid available to Republican refugees greatly exacerbated the poor health of the wounded and the infirm soldiers in the camps.[173] What is difficult to explain, however, is why, with

France alongside other European nations actively preparing for the forthcoming World War, the French Military Health Services did not do more to offer medical assistance.[174] Spanish civilian refugees did enjoy limited access to medical treatment, although the provision of this care varied widely, but medical treatment for the soldiers in internment camps in the first few weeks was almost entirely absent. If the military authorities had been allowed to treat the Republican wounded in the interest of national defence, it would have served as a valuable training exercise for the French Military Health Services. However, despite calls from both the Minister of the Interior and the Minister for Public Health for these facilities to be used to treat the Spanish wounded, Edouard Daladier, President of the Council of Ministers and Minister for War and National Defence, rejected their overtures on 15 March 1939.[175]

Care in France and in the French internment camps

The arrivals of hundreds of thousands of refugees in France in such a short space of time not only put huge stresses on the French authorities' ability to provide medical care for so many people, but the feeding of such a multitude also posed huge logistical problems. Many of these were slow to overcome and there were a number of deaths as a result.[176] Malnutrition and exposure to the cold winter conditions similar to those in internment camps across the border in nearby Spain further debilitated those already wounded or ill.[177] A relief worker reported on 9 February 1939 that 'sanitary arrangements were completely lacking' in the camps, and this problem was made worse by Spanish medical units making their way into France having their medical equipment and vehicles confiscated.[178]

French policy regarding the refugees came under criticism from a number of humanitarian aid agencies, and a number of internees who had letters smuggled out of the camp accused the French authorities of a deliberate policy of withholding care in order to encourage refugees to return to Spain.[179] For many this traumatic experience was exacerbated by the rough treatment they received at the hands of Senegalese guards.[180] Although there were those who acknowledged that their brutal treatment by the colonial troops resulted from 'orders to be rough with us, so as to make us tired and oblige us, more or less, to go with Franco', the predominant reaction was predicated upon the cultural stereotype of the savage Moor, a figure of hate for many Republicans.[181]

There were some hospitals that provided for the treatment of sick and wounded Republican soldiers such as the Hôpital Saint-Jean and the Hôpital Saint-Louis in Perpignan, a small hospital at Arles sur Tech and the hospital at Amélie-les-Bains, which also cared for children with air-raid injuries. Nevertheless, much suffering could have been avoided by directly employing Republican medical exiles.[182] However, the hospital ships *Maréchal Lyautey* and the *Asni*, moored at Port Vendres, and the *Providence* and *Patria* moored at Marseilles provided a total capacity of 4,410 beds, and it was on these ships that 6,000 Republican wounded soldiers were treated.[183] Conditions, however, were far from ideal with the hold and cargo spacing below deck on the *Maréchal Lyautey* holding 800 wounded in cramped conditions, and the *Asni* was described as having 800 wounded under treatment on a ship that only had a capacity of 600 beds.[184]

The hospital ships were made ready by order of the French Minister for Public Health, Marc Rucart, but their facilities varied.[185] However, with an estimated 30,000 sick and wounded in need of hospitalisation, the number of hospital beds on the ships were far from sufficient, and the death rate rose as a result. There were 200 deaths recorded at the hospital at Perpingnan for February 1939, but many deaths among the refugees not hospitalised were not recorded.[186] For a number of reasons the hospital ships also served as spaces for quarantine. There was a perceived need to isolate those seriously ill with contagious diseases so as to avoid epidemics, even though the majority of patients appear to have been surgical cases.[187] A visible response was also required as international criticism had been mounting of the French response to the refugee crisis. An additional reason, however, should also be considered. Those treated on the ships were soldiers and thus prisoners of war and therefore the ships were also places of confinement.[188]

Being confined on a ship was an added trauma for those under treatment, as some of the soldiers believed that the vessels they were on would ultimately take them to freedom. David Scott, a journalist for the *News Chronicle*, who visited the *Maréchal Lyautey* on 21 February 1939, noted the cramped conditions on board alongside an apparent air of confusion among some of the wounded. He was asked by a number of patients who brandished passports at him, 'What is this place?', 'What is this ship?' 'When will she sail?' 'Are we going to England? To America? To Mexico?' 'What is going to happen to us?' The reality of their situation was that they would soon be embroiled in another conflict where their experiences as victims would be further prolonged.[189]

Some of the wounded who did make it to the relative safety of France and were treated on the *Maréchal Lyautey* found themselves under the charge of inexperienced doctors and surgeons. Among the wounded who suffered as a result were a number of soldiers with complicated limb fractures who were subjected to unnecessary amputations, as at this stage the French Academy of Surgery rejected the closed plaster method beyond its perceived limited applicability on the battlefield.[190] However, deplorable conditions in the camps from where the men had recently come, combined with the lack of proper medical facilities, had led to the neglect of careful wound management, and a number of amputations were as a result of gangrene.[191]

Apart from the *Asni*, the hospital ships were only in operation for a month, with the *Asni* operational for 98 days. By the end of March, with conditions in the camps improving, the wounded, with the exception of a number under treatment on the *Asni*, were moved out of the ships and into the camps. This constituted a considerable saving for the medical authorities, as the ships were an additional financial strain during the height of the refugee crisis of early 1939.[192]

In the camps themselves, facilities were at first improvised on a makeshift basis. In St Cypriens on 17 February 1939, when construction of wooden barracks first began, seven interned Spanish doctors set up and ran an infirmary, which was described as sufficient to serve the needs of a small village but which was open to the elements on one side and had no medicines except for aspirin and bromide.[193] However, even this limited help proved to be the exception rather than the rule. The French authorities initially spurned offers of outside help, which included turning away Swedish Red Cross vans 'which had come to save the wounded'.[194] It was nearly three weeks after the opening of the camp at Argeles before more organised efforts were made for looking after the inmates. Nevertheless, a Spanish refugee and doctor, José Pujol, stated that the only external help that was allowed in the camp during this period were daily two-hour visits from a French doctor, which were clearly inadequate.[195]

It was not until the beginning of April 1939 that each camp had an infirmary/hospital, but these were wooden barracks with limited facilities, some even lacking floors and bunks. By the summer of 1939 conditions had improved, with the camps at Le Barcarès and Gurs receiving more favourable reports in June of 1939.[196] At the same time as the building of new barracks to house those interned in the camps advanced, Spanish doctors and medical practitioners were provided for the first time with basic kit bags with which to treat patients.[197]

Outside help was eventually permitted, and by August 1939 aid agencies that included the British organisation of the National Joint Committee for Spanish Relief, which helped Spanish organisations arrange transport for those seeking to get to Mexico, were active in the camps.[198] Nevertheless, the provision of outside medical aid was still limited and further complicated by the outbreak of WWII.

From the point of view of the French authorities, the main purpose of the camps in the Département des Pyrénées-Orientales were as prison camps for soldiers from the Republican Army. However, despite the majority of women and children being dispersed throughout France during the first opening of the frontier on 28 January 1939, there were thousands of women and children who came during the height of the flight of refugees into France, and there were a number of births in the camps with only limited facilities provided for a small number of birthing mothers in the hospital in Perpignan. It was not until December 1939 that better access to maternity services for women in the beach camps was established. Elisabeth Eidenbenz, a Swiss aid worker for the Service Civil International, an international non-governmental voluntary service organisation, was able to organise a small maternity hospital at Elna close to the camps. Here, between December 1939 and February 1944, 597 babies were born.[199]

The Maternity Hospital at Elna was run on a day-to-day basis by Eidenbenz. There were two to three nurses and a midwife on staff, and a doctor was available for difficult cases, although there were no surgical facilities for carrying out caesarean sections.[200] During the four years it was open, Eidenbenz also helped organise visas for many of the Spanish women who passed through its doors. From the end of 1941, Eidenbenz also helped a number of Jewish women from the Ribesaltes Internment Camp, who were patients at the hospital, by changing the names of the babies entered in the civil register so as to obscure the origins of their surnames. On other occasions, however, Eidenbenz was forced to hand over mothers and infants to the Gestapo who would have otherwise closed the hospital.[201]

The facilities and assistance offered by the staff at Elna offered hope to a few once it had opened its doors, however, neo-natal (new-born) and infant deaths in the camps remained particularly high.[202] During the first few weeks that the camps were in operation many infants died at birth or shortly thereafter, and infant mortality rates remained high throughout their operation due to the poor sanitary conditions and inadequate diet of those interned.[203]

The ex-health minister and anarchist Federica Montseny, whose second child had been born in Spain in November 1938, crossed into France at the end of January 1939, witnessing first-hand the extreme difficulties faced by the women and infants seeking refuge there. Herself a new mother, she was fortunate to find shelter from the wet winter conditions near the frontier when she took refuge in a barn full of refugees where she could breastfeed her daughter. However, she also recalls that outside the barn, a young mother clamoured to get in to escape the winter rain and shelter her baby. Such instances of exposure to the elements contributed significantly to the high infant mortality rates.

Being in possession of a diplomatic passport meant that Montseny enjoyed a certain freedom of movement in France. She sought out and found her infirm mother who had been taken by a Red Cross ambulance at the frontier to an improvised medical centre set up in a school. This was also the location where a number of new mothers making the difficult crossing into France were seeking medical treatment for their infants. After speaking with two Spanish volunteers at the centre, Dr Serrano and SantaMaría, an anarchist medical practitioner, Montseny was informed that, of the infants, 'the greater part would die' from exposure, and that all had pneumonia. She was also informed that some of the young infants could have been saved with proper hospitalisation, which, however, was not available.[204]

The women she saw were described as being in an abject state.[205] The additional strains put on malnourished nursing mothers exposed to the elements in the camps was all too frequently followed by the trauma of their infant's death, as they were less able to withstand exposure to disease and the harsh winter climate. This trauma was a legacy of many of the women who gave birth in the camps, and both in France and Spain the women who left the camps having lost infants due to the appalling conditions found there carried with them a burden of guilt that comes from losing an infant.

A common theme among the testimony of some of the mothers who gave birth at Elna was that, despite the comprehensive maternal and post-natal care they received during their on-average eight-week stay at the hospital, which included a much improved diet, was the feeling of still being incarcerated as they were not free to wander outside of the hospital. Some mothers also expressed feelings of guilt at receiving such comfort and caring concern when their own relatives in nearby camps were forced to endure the harsh conditions found there. Coupled with these feelings of guilt was the anxiety of exposing their own infants to such conditions upon their return to the camps.[206] Nevertheless the treatment for those fortunate to receive maternity cover at Elna was exemplary, and in stark contrast to the treatment of incarcerated mothers across the frontier in Spain.[207]

Infants imprisoned: The Prison for Nursing Mothers in Madrid

The outlook for maternal care within Spain was also bleak. Infant mortality rates, which prior to the war had been steadily declining, markedly increased. According to official figures contained in a report by the General Directorate of Health for 1901–1950, infant mortality sharply increased in the years 1939, 1940 and 1941 to levels not seen since 1923.[208] Nursing mothers in the camps in France were not separated from their infants, and this was also the case in Spanish prisons until 30 March 1940, when a new law established the right for women to keep their children with them in prison until the age of three.[209] However, as a result of this law, which was reinforced by further legislation for the protection of orphans in November 1940, thousands of children above the age of three were removed from their parents and placed in state and religious institutions.[210] Additionally, conditions experienced by infants and nursing mothers in Spain resulted in regimes that were both traumatic and cruel. The following case study of the Prison for Nursing Mothers in Madrid demonstrates how this resulted from an intentional policy on behalf of the Francoist authorities, who were influenced by Antonio Vallejo Nájera's ideas on eugenics.[211]

The widespread imprisonment of Republicans who had resisted the Insurgency or were suspected of dissident beliefs alien to the thinking of the new regime led to overcrowding in penal institutions throughout Spain, where official state figures from 1946 showed 280,000 prisoners in a penitentiary structure with only 20,000 places, resulting in 'disastrous humanitarian consequences'.[212] Women's prisons and camps were no exceptions. The trauma suffered by Republican women, predominantly 'political prisoners' in cramped unsanitary penal institutions, where punishments based upon army and church ideologies were the norm was made worse by the suffering and death of children among their midst.[213] For the mothers of children and the children themselves, a burden that they additionally bore as part of their experience of the Francoist penal universe were the 'positive eugenicist policies' of the new regime. These effectively punished the children for the perceived sins of their parents, first by imprisoning them with their mothers and then by removing and placing them in church and state institutions.[214] Although conditions in Spanish internment camps were similar to or worse than those encountered in France, there were nevertheless important differences in how they were run prior to the Nazi occupation of France.[215] What differentiated Spanish spaces of internment from their French counterparts was their use by the new regime as places where the defeated were subjected to 'a sustained and brutal attempt to reconfigure their consciousness and values'.[216] The Prison of Nursing Mothers of Madrid exemplified this approach. Set up in July 1940 to relieve the strain on the prison of Las Ventas, a model prison inaugurated in 1933 under the directorship of Victoria Kent, the first female Director of Prisons in Spanish history, it had been designed to hold less than 500 prisoners but at one stage accommodated more than 11,000.[217]

Ever since its opening in 1940, the ethos of the institution reflected the eugenicist principles of Antonio Vallejo Nájera.[218] His 'scientific' psychological tests carried out towards the end of the war on Republican prisoners demonstrated, in his view, that Republicans were not worthy of respect. He concluded that they had 'no moral feeling and had become brutal through their universal historical resentment, depriving them of all humanity'.[219] In relation to those he perceived as 'degenerate red militia women', he highlighted their propensity for violence, blood-thirstiness and necrophagia, and Nájera's views on what he perceived as the subhuman nature of Marxists and Republicans more generally, gave 'scientific' validation to the repressive measures imposed by the Francoist regime.[220]

The main author of a psychiatric study of women prisoners in Málaga, Nájera was also influential at an administrative level, helping to prepare prison functionaries through his involvement on prison boards and with the School of Penitentiary Studies in Madrid.[221] It was one such functionary, María Topete Fernández – a follower of his ideas, and an influential figure at the Prison for Nursing Mothers, ultimately becoming its director in 1945 – who instigated a regime that was particularly harsh.

Topete, whose own experience of 'traumatic' captivity by the Republicans served as validating credential for her loyalty to the regime, had served as a free volunteer at Las Ventas after August 1939. There she had enjoyed a semi-official role despite her voluntary status, which included the authority to sign the release documents of prisoners. Topete, whose interest more than anything centred on the interned children, moved to the new prison when it opened as a paid official of the Feminine Section of the Prison Corps. Although she was not named as director of the prison until later, her active influence throughout the prison was felt from day one.[222]

Central to Vallejo Nájera's ideology was the necessity of state intervention for the 'regeneration of the race'.[223] He believed that it was through the separation of children from the 'amoral environment' of their 'fanatical' parents, and the placing of infants and children in an enveloping sphere of 'catholic rightness' that society would be improved. It was this policy that Topete carried out to the letter.[224]

Although the law of 1940 stipulated that infants from the age of three were to be removed from prisons, it did not specify that before this age they should be separated from their mothers. However, Topete only allowed mothers one hour's access to their children each day, and it was during this time that the children were provided with their only meal, a thin gruel often containing insects. The rest of the time the infants were placed in cots in the courtyard regardless of the weather and many died of exposure, bronchitis and pneumonia due to the damp caused by the hospital's close proximity to the River Manzanares. Mothers were tortured and beaten when they tried to resist this separation from their infants. For the mothers serving jail terms that saw their children reach their third birthday in prison, having to face the trauma of seeing their children removed from the prison before reaching the age of four was made even worse for many by this separation being permanent.[225]

These deliberate acts of separation were common in prisons throughout Spain. María Aranzazu Vélez de Mendizabal ran a particularly brutal regime at the prison for women at Saturrarán in the Northern Spain and the segregationist policies of Vallejo Nájera were pursued equally vigorously here as they were at the women's prison in Madrid. One hundred women and fifty children also died of illness in the prison of Saturrarán, and this experience was replicated across Spain during the early years of Francoism.[226]

Among the oral testimony of female prisoners' accounts collected by Tomasa Cuevas, a former political prisoner and inmate of Las Ventas and other prisons, was the common theme of emotional stress suffered by the women witnessing the appalling conditions endured by children that resulted in debilitating illnesses and death. Although the trauma experienced was clearly more acutely felt by the children and mothers themselves, women who were witness to such cruelties were affected long-term by what they had seen and heard, and remembered the enforced separation of mothers from children as a traumatic event.[227]

The Prison for Nursing Mothers in Madrid was held up as an exemplary institution and was described by the propaganda of the Franco Regime as being the first of its kind in Europe. It was visited by a number of dignitaries, including a 'managed' visit for a British Labour MP who sang its praises, and María Topete herself was awarded several medals for her 'dedication and care'.[228] It was important as part of the consolidation of the power of the new regime to project the message that state institutions were functioning normally. An important part of this propagandist discourse was that the health of the nation was in good hands. Included in the new state's propaganda campaign for the 'sacred defence of the race', were initiatives that claimed that with the traditional role of the mother reaffirmed by the new regime, maternal and infant mortality were being reduced. However, despite the passing of the

Law of Maternal and Infant Health in June 1941, it was not until after 1943 that maternal and infant mortality rates began to decrease, and it was not until the latter part of the 1940s that rates began to significantly decrease with rationing only abandoned in 1952.[229]

The collective experience of women and children who were incarcerated in the prisons of the Franco Regime left a lasting mark upon the lives of those who passed through these institutions. The trauma experienced by the separation of mothers and infants was a burden that for many was borne in silence. It was not until the turn of the twenty-first century that the voices, mainly of the children, were heard for the first time when the Catalan public broadcaster Televisió de Catalunya commissioned and screened the documentary *Els nens perduts del franquisme* (*The Lost Children of Francoism*).[230] Some accounts by the women themselves had appeared much earlier in 1985, when Tomasa Cuevas published her two volumes on women's prisons, but it was the impact that this documentary was to have in a Spain where there was a growing movement to address the hidden traumas of Francoism, that highlighted how many skeletons, both literal and metaphorical, remained to be uncovered.[231]

The majority of the women and children who survived their imprisonment were denied the opportunity to articulate their suffering as a result of the 'pact of forgetting' that effectively silenced the remembrance of state-inflicted repression in the post-Franco era, with many of the women taking their untold traumas to their graves. For those survivors who contributed their difficult and traumatic stories to the documentary *Els nens perduts del franquisme*, which also explored the sexual abuse experienced by children in the prisons and institutions of the post-war Francoist regime, participating in this documentary not only made it possible for this story to reach a television audience, but also helped provide some limited restitution by airing long-silenced voices – a catharsis denied to the many whose silence accompanied them to their graves.

Conclusion

In April 1969, Manuel Cortes, a medical orderly during the Spanish Civil War and the last Republican mayor of Mijas, a small town west of Málaga, before its capture by the Insurgents in February 1937, emerged from hiding after spending thirty years hidden away in his own home. During the war, he had joined the exodus on the road to Almeria that accompanied the fall of Málaga and served as an orderly both at the front and in the rear-guard throughout the conflict. He returned home in the early hours of 17 April 1939 after being processed in the bullring of Valencia at the end of the war, where he was ordered to return to his own village to face judgement by the local authorities. Prepared to face a prison term of twelve years, it soon became evident that, if he gave himself up, he faced summary execution, and, therefore, with the help of his wife he went into hiding in a secret room in his house.[232] His emergence on 12 April 1969 followed an amnesty for 'offences' committed during the Civil War, that had been issued two weeks previously on 28 March.[233]

His long period in hiding was not as a result of any crimes he had committed, apart from being a non-combatant medical orderly during the Spanish Civil War. His previous post as mayor had not involved him in conflict or repressive measures against local right-wing elements, although he had been a vocal advocate of agrarian reform. Nevertheless, as an active Republican and a man of the left, and despite having helped save the lives of several rightists in his own village prior to the Insurgent takeover of the Province of Málaga, his life, like the many of thousands whose only crime was to have belonged to Republican organisations, was undoubtedly in danger.[234] His subsequent experience of captivity, supported by his wife and other family members, stood in stark contrast to the hundreds of thousands whose own experiences of captivity left them at the mercy of harsh repression where hunger and disease were used as weapons of oppression.

Although Cortes' journey back to his village had been in a cattle truck as far as Cordoba, before continuing his journey on a passenger train to Málaga, he was nevertheless able to make his way undetected to his village after directing a taxi driver to a false address a few miles from his home.[235] A few weeks after Cortes set out on his journey from Valencia, a cattle truck also left the overcrowded camp near Alicante set up to accommodate the prisoners captured when the city fell and where dysentery was rife. In each wagon there were thirty women and thirty children who were given a small ration of water and two sardines from a tin before embarking upon their journey under the hot May sun. By the time it had made its tortuous journey to Valencia, two children had died.[236]

Individuals as well as whole families were sent back to their homes in this manner after April 1939, and the deliberate cruelty inflicted upon the defeated formed part of the traumatic experience that framed their post-war experience, which was a result of the expressed desire of the Francoist regime to punish the defeated.[237] The suffering inflicted by the authorities on children, women and men of all ages whose allegiance to the regime was suspect was a deliberate policy that saw hundreds of thousands incarcerated, with 20,000 executions carried out in the immediate post-war period.[238] For the hundreds of thousands who fled to France, French indifference to their fate and a desire to empty the camps as quickly as possible likewise resulted in trauma and death. The conditions suffered by those in the camps in France echoed those in Spain. For those who stayed in France the experience of WWII would have lasting effects, but for those who returned to Spain the widespread net of Francoist oppression awaited. The purges, particularly those of medical personnel, were to have disastrous consequences for both private and public health, and it took years before healthcare within Spain began to offer anything close to universal cover for society's poor, sick and infirm. This deliberate policy of systematic persecution, the active traumatisation of the defeated of the Spanish Civil War, continued well into the 1950s.[239]

This legacy of trauma is still alive in Spain today and as part of the conclusion to this study this uneasy inheritance bequeathed to the heirs of the victims of Francoism will be addressed. The proclamation that the war had ended in 1939 heralded the start of a much longer one-sided conflict that saw the supporters of the Second Republic and their heirs punished for their opposition to Francoism. Manuel Cortes, whose daughter was only three years and eight months old when he went into hiding, was nevertheless able to see his child and his granddaughters grow up, something denied to the parents of at least 30,000 stolen children who grew up in state and religious institutions and who were 'fostered' by 'good catholic parents' loyal to Franco's regime.[240]

Notes

1 Preston, *Reaction, Revolution and Revenge*, p. 299; Graham, H., *The Spanish Republic at War 1936–1939* (Cambridge, 2002), p. 425.
2 Preston, *Reaction, Revolution and Revenge*, pp. 38, 299.
3 Arco Blanco, M. A. del, "'Morir de hambre': autarquía, escasez y enfermedad en la España del primer franquismo", *Pasado y memoria: Revista de historia contemporánea*, No. 5 (2006), pp. 241–258, pp. 241–242.
4 Rubio, *Emigración* (Vol. 1), pp. 116–118, 124.
5 Ibid., p. 124.
6 Ibid., pp. 362–368; Harana, L., "Los barcos-hospital franceses: Los otros barcos del exilio", in H. Buffery, F. Lough, E. Marcer, & A. M. Sánchez (eds.), *Spanish Republican Exile Geographies/Geografías del exilio republicano español* (Birmingham, 2012), pp. 35–46, p. 38; MRCUW: 15X/2/226/2, "Get Them Away: The Story of the French Concentration Camps" (London, 1941), issued by the International Brigade Wounded and Dependants' Aid Committee.
7 Beevor, *Battle for Spain*, p. 404.
8 Graham, *Spanish Civil War*, p. 111.
9 Rodrigo, J., "Internamiento y trabajo forzoso: los campos de concentración de Franco", *Hispania Nova. Revista de Historia Contemporánea*, No. 6 (2006), pp. 615–642, pp. 633–634; Preston, *Spanish Holocaust*, pp. 503–507.
10 Guerra, *La medicina en el exilio*, pp. 204–206.
11 Casanova, *Spanish Civil War*, p. 191; Guerra, F., *La medicina en el exilio*, pp. 337–340.
12 Rubio, *Emigración* (Vol. 1), pp. 340–1; Preston, *Spanish Holocaust*, p. 479.
13 Thomas, *Spanish Civil War*, pp. 858–884; Rubio, *Emigración* (Vol. 1), pp. 340–341.
14 Graham, *Spanish Republic at War*, p. 425; *ABC* (Sevilla), 02.04.1939, p. 7.
15 Ealham, C., & Richards, M., "History, Memory and the Spanish Civil War: Recent Perspectives", in C. Ealham & M. Richards, (eds.), *The Splintering of Spain: Cultural History and the Spanish Civil War, 1936–1939* (Cambridge, 2005), pp. 1–22., p. 9; Gálvez Biesca, S., "La 'memoria democrática' como conflicto", *Entelequia: revista interdisciplinar*, No. 7 (2008), pp. 1–52; Moradiellos, E., "Ni gesta heroica, ni locura trágica: nuevas perspectivas históricas sobre la guerra civil", *Ayer* (2003), pp. 11–39, pp. 37, 19, 30.
16 www.memoriahistorica.org.es and www.foroporlamemoria.es.

17 Ruiz-Vargas, J. M., "Trauma y memoria de la Guerra Civil y de la dictadura franquista", *Hispania Nova. Revista de Historia Contemporánea*, Vol. 6 (2006), pp. 299–336, pp. 323–324.
18 Fernández Paredes, T., "Transitional Justice in Democratization Processes: The Case of Spain from an International Point of View", *International Journal of Rule of Law, Transitional Justice And Human Rights*, Vol. 1(2010), pp. 120–136, p. 132.
19 Aguilar, The Timing and the Scope of Reparation, pp. 505–506.
20 *BOE*, No. 125, 04.05.1940, pp. 3048–3049.
21 *BOE*, No. 44, 13.02.1939, pp. 824–847; Preston, *Spanish Holocaust*, pp. 502–504.
22 Preston, *Spanish Holocaust*, pp. 506–510; Algarbani, *Y Jimena se vistió de negro*, pp. 159–166.
23 Preston, *Spanish Holocaust*, pp. xiii, xv, xix, 511.
24 Ruiz-Vargas, Trauma y memoria, p. 321.
25 Preston, *Spanish Holocaust*, pp. 514–515.
26 Ibid.; Quiroga, A., & Arco del, M. Á., (eds.), *Right-Wing Spain in the Civil War Era: Soldiers of God and Apostles of the Fatherland, 1914–45* (London, 2012), pp. 195–224, pp. 195–197.
27 Ibid., pp. 323–324; Preston, *Spanish Holocaust*, pp. xix, 510–515.
28 Graham, *Spanish Civil War*, pp. 129–131; Ruiz-Vargas, Trauma y memoria, p. 326.
29 "Vidas Robadas: El doctor Vela será el primer juzgado por el 'caso de los bebés robados', *El País*, 30.06.2016, online edition: http://politica.elpais.com/politica/2016/06/30/actualidad/1467280294_451438.html (last accessed: 10.08.2016).
30 Anderson, P., "In the Name of the Martyrs: Memory and Retribution in Francoist Southern Spain, 1936–1945", *Cultural and Social History*, Vol. 8, No. 3 (2011), pp. 355–370, p. 355.
31 Junquera, N., "La promesa que Rajoy se cumplió", *El País* (5.10.2013), online edition: http://politica.elpais.com/politica/2013/10/05/actualidad/1380997260_542677.html (last accessed: 24.07.2015).
32 Anderson, In the Name of the Martyrs, p. 355; Ferllini, R., "Human Rights Investigations in Spain", *Annals of Anthropological Practice*, Vol. 38, No. 1 (2014), pp. 65–80; Graham, *Spanish Civil War*, p. 141.
33 Junquera, La promesa que Rajoy se cumplió; Ealham & Richards, History, Memory and the Spanish Civil War, p. 9.
34 Ruiz-Vargas, Trauma y memoria, pp. 319–320.
35 Preston, *Spanish Holocaust*, pp. xii–xiii.
36 Rodrigo, J., "La guerra civil: 'memoria', 'olvido', 'recuperación' e 'instrumentación'", *Hispania Nova. Revista de Historia Contemporánea*, No. 6 (2006), pp. 385–410, pp. 397–398.
37 Richards, M., "From War Culture to Civil Society: Francoism, Social Change and Memories of the Spanish Civil War", *History and Memory*, Vol. 14, No. 1–2 (2002), Special Issue: Images of a Contested Past, pp. 93–120, pp. 103–104.
38 Ruiz-Vargas, Trauma y memoria, pp. 319–320.
39 Ibid., pp. 331, 333–335; Rodrigo, La guerra civil, pp. 385–410.
40 Abrams, L., *Oral History Theory* (Oxford, 2010), pp. 92–95.
41 Trueta, *Treatment of War Wounds*, p. 132.
42 Egido León, Á., *Francisco Urzaiz. Un Republicano en la Francia ocupada: Vivencias de la guerra y el exilio* (Madrid, 2000), pp. 139–149; Algarbani, *Y Jimena se vistio de negro*, pp. 120–125; Preston, *Reaction, Revolution and Revenge*, pp. 308–309.

43 Ealham & Richards, History, Memory and the Spanish Civil War, pp. 19–20; Ruiz-Vargas, Trauma y memoria, p. 333.
44 Ealham & Richards, History, Memory and the Spanish Civil War, p. 4.
45 Anderson, In the Name of the Martyrs, p. 356.
46 Rina Simón, C., "La construcción de los imaginarios franquistas y la religiosidad "popular", 1931–1945", *Pasado y Memoria: Revista de Historia Contemporánea*, No. 14 (2015), pp. 179–196, pp. 191–192.
47 Gadow, M. R., "Una imagen controvertida de la Semana Santa malagueña: el Cristo de los Mutilados", *Los crucificados, religiosidad, cofradías y arte: Actas del Simposium 3/6-IX-2010* (2010), pp. 213–224; *ABC* (Sevilla), 08.04.1939, p. 2.
48 Richards, M., "'Presenting arms to the Blessed Sacrament': Civil War and Semana Santa in the city of Malaga, 1936–1939", in C. Ealham & M. Richards (eds.), *The Splintering of Spain: Cultural History and the Spanish Civil War, 1936–1939* (Cambridge, 2005), pp. 196–222.
49 Rina Simón, La construcción de los imaginarios, pp. 191–192; Marín Gómez, I., *El laurel y la retama en la memoria: tiempo de posguerra en Murcia, 1939–1952* (Murcia, 2004), pp. 123–124; *ABC* (Sevilla), 08.04.1939, p. 2.
50 *ABC* (Sevilla), 08.04.1939, p. 2.
51 Ibid.
52 Gadow, Una imagen controvertida, pp. 217–218.
53 Rina Simón, La construcción de los imaginarios, pp. 191–192.
54 Richards, *After the Civil War*, pp. 64–65.
55 Richards, Presenting Arms, p. 199.
56 *BOE*, No. 540 (Suplemento), 14.04.1938, p. 4; *BOE*, No. 63, 13.03.1976, pp. 5209–5215, 'Ley 5/1976, de 11 de marzo, de Mutilados de Guerra por la Patria'.
57 Ibid.; Marín Gómez, *El laurel y la retama*, pp. 123–124.
58 Gadow, Una imagen controvertida, pp. 217–218; "Un Cristo mutilado protagoniza un polémico Vía Crucis 'profranquista' en Málaga", *Elplural.com*, available at: www.elplural.com/2015/04/04/un-cristo-mutilado-protagoniza-un-polemico-via-crucis-en-Málaga-que-muchos-tildan-de-profranquista/ (last accessed 15.01.2016).
59 Anderson, In the Name of the Martyrs, pp. 355–356; Un Cristo mutilado protagoniza un polémico Vía Crucis.
60 Ruiz-Vargas,Trauma y memoria, pp. 333
61 Ibid., pp. 330–34.
62 Thomas, *Spanish Civil War*, pp. 703–705.
63 Casanova, *Spanish Civil War*, p. 179; Bescós Torres, Sanidad Militar, 2ª Parte, p. 445. See Thomas, *Spanish Civil War*, p. 704.
64 Graham, *Spanish Civil War*, pp. 110–111.
65 Pagès i Blanch, *War and Revolution in Catalonia*, p. 157.
66 Rubio, *Emigración* (Vol. 1), p. 268.
67 Ibid., pp. 65–72, 268, 297–299; Martínez Vidal, À., "Metges catalans refugiats a França. Observació clínica i recerca científica als camps de concentració (1939 – 1942)", in R. Barrie, M. Camiade, & J. Font (directors), *Déplacements forcés et exils en Europe au XXe siècle: le corps et l'esprit: actes du 2eséminaire transfronterer* [*Desplaçaments forçosos i exilis a l'Europa del segle XX: el cos i l'esperit: actes del 2on seminari transfronterer*] (La Region Languedoc Rousillon, 2013), pp. 105–129, p. 105; CULA manuscript no. 3/233, 26–27 January 1939.
68 Rubio, *Emigración* (Vol. 1), pp. 309–312; Grande Covian, F., "Deficiencias vitamínicas en Madrid durante la guerra civil: una reminiscencia", in *Los médicos*

y la medicina en la Guerra Civil Española: Monografías Beecham (Madrid, 1986), pp. 61–67.

69 Rubio, *Emigración* (Vol. 1), pp. 312–314.

70 Egido León, *Francisco Urzaiz*, p. 142.

71 Vásquez León, *Un boomerang en Jimena de la Frontera*, pp. 150–153; Guerra, *La medicina en el exilio*, p. 191.

72 Preston, *Spanish Holocaust*, p. 479–480.

73 Guerra, *La medicina en el exilio*, p. 191.

74 Ibid.; Graham, *Spanish Republic at War*, pp. 422–423.

75 Rickett, R. M., "Refugees of the Spanish Civil War and Those They Left Behind: Personal Testimonies of Departure, Separation and Return Since 1936" (University of Manchester, 2015), p. 53; Guerra, *La medicina en el exilio*, p. 194.

76 Rubio, *Emigración* (Vol. 1), pp. 217–218.

77 MRCUW: 292/946/26/2, "Conference Internationale D'Aide aux Refugies Espagnols/International Emergency Conference for Spanish Refugees Paris, 15–16 Juillet 1939/Paris, 15-16th July 1939. Spanish Refugees in France: Census List", p. 3.

78 Ibid., p. 206; Guerra, *La medicina en el exilio*, pp. 537–693; Thomas, *Spanish Civil War*, pp. 894–897.

79 Thomas, *Spanish Civil War*, pp. 894–897.

80 Graham, *Spanish Civil War*, pp. 117–126.

81 Rubio, *Emigración* (Vol. 1), p. 129; *BOE*, No. 14.02.1939., pp. 856–859 (Ley de 10 de Febrero de 1939 fijando normas para la depuración de funcionarios públicos); Rubio, J., "Las cifras del exilio", *Historia 16* Vol. 30 (1978), pp. 19–32; Stein, L., *Beyond Death and Exile: The Spanish Republicans in France, 1939–1955* (London, 1979), p. 86. An estimated total of 684,000 refugees sought refuge in France between July 1936 and the end of March 1939. See Rubio, *Emigración* (Vol. 1), pp. 105–106.

82 Rubio, *Emigración* (Vol. 1), pp. 129, 344–349.

83 Rubio, *Emigración* (Vol. 3), pp. 129, 409; Hernández de Miguel, C., *Los últimos españoles de Mauthausen: La historia de nuestros deportados, sus verdugos y sus cómplices* (Barcelona, 2015), p. 23.

84 Marset Campos, P., Martínez Navarro, F., & Sáez Gómez, J. M., "La Salud Pública durante el franquismo", *Dynamis: Acta Hispanica ad Medicinae Scientiarumque. Historiam Illustrandam*, Vol. 15 (1995), pp. 211–250, p. 222.

85 Otero Carvajal, L. E., "La destrucción de la ciencia en España: Las consecuencias del triunfo militar de la España franquista", *Historia y Comunicación Social*, No. 6 (2001), pp. 149–186, p. 165.

86 Fernández Sabaté, *Nuestros fundadores*, p. vii.

87 Fraser, *Blood of Spain,* p. 482; Beevor, *Battle for Spain*, p. 324; Madariaga Fernández, Las Industrias de Guerra de Cataluña, pp. 778–783.

88 Thomas, *The Spanish Civil War*, pp. 844–848, 860.

89 Fraser, *Blood of Spain*, p. 482.

90 Casanova, *The Spanish Civil War*, p. 184.

91 Fraser, *Blood of Spain*, pp. 609, 773, 785, 786, 787, 848; Balcells, L., "Death is in the Air: Bombings in Catalonia, 1936–1939", *Revista Española de Investigaciones Sociológicas*, Vol. 136 (2011), pp. 25–48; The National Archives (TNA), Medical Research Council, FD 1/5372/C674261, Air Raid Precautions Department, Intelligence Branch, Medical Aspects of Air Raid Casualties in Barcelona

(701, 666/251), 25 March, 1939, p. 2; Aracil & Villarroya, *El país valencià sota les bombes*; Domènech, X., & Zenobi, L., *Quan plovien bombes* (Barcelona, 2007).

92 Beevor, *Battle for Spain*, pp. 332–333; Preston, *Spanish Holocaust*, pp. 177, 465.

93 Ibid.; Trueta, *Treatment of War Wounds*; Trueta, *El tractament de les fractures de Guerra* (Barcelona, 1938).

94 Trueta, *Treatment of War Wounds.*

95 Coller & Valk, The Delayed Closure of Contaminated Wounds, pp. 256–270; Moynahan, Treatment of War Wounds and Infected Fractures, p. 229; Winnett Orr, Treatment of War Wounds, p. 585; Ross & Hulbert, Treatment of 100 War Wounds and Burns; Broster, A Survey of War Surgery, pp. 273–275; Wilson, The Treatment of Compound Fractures, pp. 915–924; Ponseti Vives, History of Orthopaedic Surgery, pp. 59–64.

96 Trueta, The Organization of Hospital Services for Casualties, pp. 13–23.

97 Roig, A. F., "40 Años de puericultura en Reus" *Revista del Centre de Lectura de Reus*, No. 27 (1954), pp. 109–112, p. 111; TNA (FD1/5372, I.O. 65.), Medical Aspects of Air Raid Casualties in Barcelona, 25 March 1939, p. 3.

98 TNA (FD1/5372, I. O. 65), p. 3.

99 Ibid., pp. 1–5; TNA (FD1/5372, Annex A. to I. O. 65), "Opinions Formed from Actual Experience of Aerial Bombardment in Barcelona by Dr. J. Trueta Raspall, Head of the Catalan General Hospital, Chief Surgeon of the Passive Defence Service, Barcelona," 25 March, 1939, pp. 1–20.

100 Grayzel, S. R., "'A Promise of Terror to Come': Air Power and the Destruction of Cities in British Imagination and Experience, 1908–39", in S. Goebel & D. Keene (eds.), *Cities Into Battlefields: Metropolitan Scenarios, Experiences and Commemorations of Total War* (Farnham, 2011), pp. 47–62, pp. 60–61; Crome, L., Fisher, R. E. W., & Shirlaw, G. B., "Casualty Organisation in Air Raids", *The Lancet* (18.03.1939), pp. 655–658 (Len Crome had served as Chief Medical Officer, XV Spanish Army Corps, and G. B. Shirlaw as an MO in the Spanish Army); and Shirlaw, G. B., *Casualty: The Civil Defence Casualty Services* (London, 1940).

101 Fernández Sabaté, *Nuestros fundadores*, p. 151.

102 Preston, *Spanish Holocaust*, pp. 177, 465–466.

103 Hervás I Puyal, *La xarxa hospitalária*, p. 120; *Mi Revista*, 15.6.1937, pp. 9–10.

104 Ibid., p. 66. Jimeno Vidal had previously studied under the acclaimed Austrian surgeon Lorenz Böhler at the Unfallkrankenhaus in Vienna, a specialist orthopaedic centre. See Fernández Sabaté, *Nuestros fundadoress*, pp. 149–150.

105 Ibid., p. 120; Fernández Sabaté, *Nuestros fundadores*, p. 299.

106 Guerra, *La medicina en el exilio*, p. 369.

107 Hervás I Puyal, *La xarxa hospitalária*, p. 66; Fernández Sabaté, *Nuestros fundadores*, p. 299; Beevor, *Battle for Spain*, pp. 350–351.

108 Hervás I Puyal, *La xarxa hospitalária*, p. 123.

109 Massons, *Historia de la Sanidad Militar Española: Tomo II,* pp. 408–410.

110 Rubio, *Emigración* (Vol. 1), pp. 301, 306.

111 Coller & Valk, The Delayed Closure of Contaminated Wounds, pp. 267–270.

112 Ibid.; Böhler, L., *Técnica del tratamiento de las fracturas*, Traducción de F. Jimeno Vidal. Prólogo de Joaquín Trías Pujol (Barcelona, 1934). First published in 1932, *Técnica del tratamiento de las fracturas* quickly became an influential work, and was translated by Jimeno Vidal in 1934. See Fernández Sabaté, *Nuestros fundadores*, pp. 161–165.

113 Fernández Sabaté, *Nuestros fundadores*, pp. 53, 88–89.
114 Guerra, *La medicina en el exilio*, p. 214; *Gaceta de la República: Diario Oficial*, No. 3, 03.01.1937, p. 45; Fernández Sabaté, *Nuestros fundadores*, p. 53.
115 Guerra, *La medicina en el exilio*, pp. 126–127, 214.
116 Preston, *Reaction, Revolution and Revenge*, p. 294; Beevor, *Battle for Spain*, pp. 377–378.
117 Vinyes, R., Armengou, M., & Belis, R., *Los niños perdidos del franquismo: Un estremecedor documento que sale por primera vez a la luz* (Barcelona, 2002), p. 85; Preston, *Spanish Holocaust*, p. 465.
118 Preston, *Spanish Holocaust*, p. 465; Pàmies i Bertran, T., *Quan érem capitans: memòries d'aquella guerra* (Barcelona, 1974), pp. 149–150.
119 Preston, *Spanish Holocaust*, p. 465.
120 Fernández Sabaté, *Nuestros fundadores*, pp. 510–511; Luttikhuizen, F., "Professor Ignasi Ponseti i Vives (1914–2009)", *Contributions to Science* (2012), Vol. 7, No. 2, pp. 205–214.
121 Fernández Sabaté, *Nuestros fundadores*, p. 510.
122 Ibid.; Hervás I Puyal, *La xarxa hospitalària*, p. 163.
123 Fernández Sabaté, *Nuestros fundadores*, p. 510.
124 Wilson, F. M., *In the Margins of Chaos: Recollections of Relief Work in and between Three Wars* (London, 1944), pp. 222–229.
125 Fernández Sabaté, *Nuestros fundadores*, p. 510; Montseny, F., *Pasión y muerte de los españoles en Francia* (Toulouse, 1969), p.13.
126 Trueta, J., "The Treatment of War Fractures by the Closed Method: Section of Surgery", *Proceedings of the Royal Society of Medicine* Vol. 33, No. 1 (1939), pp. 65–74, pp. 71–72.
127 Fernández Sabaté, *Nuestros fundadores*, p. 153
128 Beevor, *Battle for Spain*, pp. 381–382; Guerra, *La medicina en el exilio*, p. 190.
129 Fernández Sabaté, *Nuestros fundadores*, p. 153; *ABC* (Sevilla), 19.03.1939, p. 15.
130 Guerra, *La medicina en el exilio*, p. 369; *ABC* (Sevilla), 19.03.1939, p. 15.
131 Guerra, *La medicina en el exilio*, p. 369.
132 CULA, manuscript no. 3/233: 26.01.1939; 3/233: 27.01.1939–16.01.1939.
133 Scott-Ellis, *The Chances of Death*, p. 2.
134 CULA, manuscript no. 3/233: 24.01.1939.
135 Ibid., 25.01.1939.
136 Ibid., 26.01.1939.
137 Ibid., 03.02.1939; Preston, *Spanish Holocaust*, p. 465.
138 Hernández Holgado, F., "La prisión militante. Las cárceles franquistas de mujeres de Barcelona y Madrid (1939–1945)" (Universidad Complutense de Madrid, 2011), pp. 78–9; *La Vanguardia*, 04.05.2004, p.7.
139 *La Vanguardia*, 23.05.2002, p. 7
140 Ibid.; Hernández Holgado, La prisión militante, pp. 79–80.
141 Hernández Holgado, La prisión militante, pp. 79–80.
142 Casanova, *The Spanish Civil War*, p. 187.
143 Anderson, P., *The Francoist Military Trials: Terror and Complicity, 1939–1945* (New York and Abingdon, 2010), pp. 74–77.
144 Hernández Holgado, La prisión militante, pp. 178–9.
145 Anderson, *The Francoist Military Trials*, pp. 75–77.
146 Hernández Holgado, La prisión militante, pp. 177–180, 119, 204–205.

147 Ibid.; Ruiz-Vargas, Trauma y memoria, pp. 248, 321; Junquera, N., "Necrológica: Trinidad Gallego, testigo del robo de niños", *El Pais* (12.11.2011), http://elpais.com/diario/2011/11/12/necrologicas/1321052401_850215.html (last accessed 18.10.15); Vinyes et al., *Los niños perdidos del franquismo*, pp. 121–133.

148 Ruiz-Berdún, D., & Gomis, A., "La depuración de las matronas de Madrid tras la Guerra Civil", *Dynamis* (2012), Vol. 32, No. 1, pp. 439–465, p. 444.

149 Ibid.; Guerra, *La medicina en el exilio*, p. 139; Algarbani, *Y Jimena se vistió de negro*, pp. 106–111.

150 Ibid.; Guerra, *La medicina en el exilio*, p. 196

151 Navarro Carballo, J. R., "Creación y desarrollo del Cuerpo de Damas Auxiliares de Sanidad Militar", *Medicina Militar* (1987), Vol. 43, No. 3, pp. 320–331, p. 325.

152 Mila Nolla, M, "La mujer en la guerra: Enfermeras", in *Los médicos y la medicina en la Guerra Civil Española: Monografías Beecham* (Madrid, 1986), p. 303; Massons, *Historia de la Sanidad Militar Española: Tomo II*, p. 520.

153 Serrallonga i Urquidi, El cuento de la regularización sanitaria, pp. 94–95.

154 Navarro Carballo, Creación y desarrollo del Cuerpo de Damas Auxiliares, p. 117; Preston, *Reaction, Revolution and Revenge*, pp. 308–312; Oliver Olmo, P., Dueñas Iturbe, O., & Solé I Barjal, Q., "El hospital militar de la calle Tallers de Barcelona: tratamiento y represión de los prisioneros trabajadores forzados (1939–1942): Military Hospital of Tallers Street, Barcelona: Treatment and Repression of Forced Prison Workers (1939–1942)", in J. C. Urda Lozano (ed.), *La prisión y las instituciones punitivas en la investigación histórica: The Prison and the Punitive Institutions at the Historical Research* (Cuenca, 2014), pp. 570–574.

155 Anderson, *The Francoist Military Trials*, p. 133; Arco Blanco, Morir de hambre, p. 253; Grande Covian, Deficiencias vitamínicas, pp. 61–67.

156 Jiménez Lucena, I., "El tifus exantemático de la posguerra española (1939–1943): el uso de una enfermedad colectiva en la legitimación del Nuevo estado", *Dynamis: Acta Hispanica ad Medicinae Scientiarumque. Historiam Illustrandam*, Vol. 14 (1994), pp. 185–198, p. 188.

157 Rodríguez Ocaña, E., "La intervención de la Fundación Rockefeller en la creación de la sanidad contemporánea en España", *Revista Española de Salud Pública*, Vol. 74 (2000), pp. 27–34.

158 Coni, *Medicine and Warfare*, p. 88; Anderson, *The Francoist Military Trials*, p. 133.

159 Anderson, *The Francoist Military Trials*, p. 133.

160 Preston, *Spanish Holocaust*, pp. 509–513.

161 Vega Sombría, S., & García Funes, J. C., "Lucha tras las rejas franquistas: La prisión central de mujeres de Segovia", *Studia Histórica: Historia contemporánea*, Vol. 29 (2012), pp. 281–314, pp. 285, 289–290.

162 Díaz-Balart, M. N., "La doma de los cuerpos y las conciencias, 1939–1941: El campo de concentración de Porta Coeli (Valencia)", *Hispania Nova: Revista de historia contemporánea*, No. 10 (2012), pp. 284–310, pp. 299–304.

163 Ibid., pp. 305–306.

164 Guerra, *La medicina en el exilio*, pp. 63–185.

165 *BOE*, No. 44, 13.02.1939, pp. 824–847.

166 Guerra, *La medicina en el exilio*, p. 81; Serrallonga i Urquidi, El cuento de la regularización sanitaria, p. 79

167 Serrallonga i Urquidi, El cuento de la regularización sanitaria, pp. 74, 94–96.
168 Ibid., pp. 78–79; Preston, P., *The Politics of Revenge: Fascism and the Military in 20th-Century Spain* (London, 2003), p. 130.
169 Egido León, *Francisco Urzaiz.*
170 Ibid., pp. 1–294.
171 Ibid., p. 129; Jackson, *For Us It Was Heaven*, p. 108; Preston, *Spanish Holocaust*, pp. 206–207. Perhaps the most infamous occasion on which this happened was when 'Moors killed the wounded in the Republican Hospital' in Toledo in September 1936, and where 'grenades were thrown in among two hundred screaming and helpless men', also killing the doctors and nurses. See Preston, *Spanish Holocaust*, pp. 336–337.
172 Egido León, *Francisco Urzaiz*, pp. 130–132.
173 MRCUW: 292/946/43/33, "Report to Spanish Medical Aid Committee by Miss Rosita Davson, Wednesday 15th February 1939", p. 4.
174 Rubio, *Emigración* (Vol. 1), pp. 298–299.
175 Ibid., p. 367, fn. 93.
176 Ibid., p. 311.
177 Monfort i Coll, A., "Los campos de concentración franquistas y su funcionamiento en Cataluña", in *Hispania. Revista Española de Historia*, Vol. 69, No. 231 (2009), pp. 147–178.
178 MRCUW, 292/946/18a/3, p. 5.
179 Coni, *Medicine and Warfare*, p. 214; & MRCUW, 292/946/18a/3, pp. 13–14.
180 Montseny, *Pasión y muerte*, pp. 25–65; Egido León, *Francisco Urzaiz*, p. 139; MRCUW, 292/946/18a/3, pp. 5–8.
181 Ibid.
182 Coni, *Medicine and Warfare,* p. 214; MRCUW, 292/946/18a/3, pp. 13–14, 3, 4, 15; Rubio, *Emigración* (Vol. 1), pp. 340–341.
183 Harana, Los barcos-hospital franceses, p. 46.
184 Ibid.; MRCUW, 292/946/18a/3, pp. 13–14.
185 Harana, Los barcos-hospital franceses, p. 39.
186 Rubio, *Emigración* (Vol. 1), pp. 313–314.
187 Harana, Los barcos-hospital franceses, p. 39; MRCUW, 292/946/18a/3, p. 17.
188 Harana, Los barcos-hospital franceses, p. 39.
189 MRCUW, 292/946/18a/3, p. 17.
190 Harana, Los barcos-hospital franceses, pp. 39–40.
191 Montseny, *Pasión y muerte*, p. 30.
192 Harana, Los barcos-hospital franceses, pp. 39, 46.
193 MRCUW, 292/946/18a/3, p. 5.
194 Wilson, *In the Margins of Chaos*, pp. 222–223.
195 Montseny, *Pasión y muerte*, p. 29.
196 Ibid., p. 30; Rubio, *Emigración* (Vol. 1), pp. 320–321; Wilson, *In the Margins of Chaos*; Montellà, A., *La maternidad de Elna: La historia de la mujer que salvo la vida de 597 niños* (Badalona, 2007), p. 52.
197 Montseny, *Pasión y muerte*, p. 30.
198 Wilson, *In the Margins of Chaos*, pp. 228–229.
199 Montellà, *La maternidad de Elna*, pp. 149–157.
200 Montellà, *La maternidad de Elna*; Llunch-Prats, J., "La maternidad de Elna: Una isla de paz en medio de infierno", *Migraciones y Exilios*, No. 13 (2012), pp. 111–122.

201 Montellà, *La maternidad de Elna*, pp. 66–67, 110.
202 Llunch-Prats, La maternidad de Elna, p. 111.
203 Ibid.; Montellà, La maternidad de Elna, p. 21.
204 Montseny, *Pasión y muerte*, pp. 16, 24–25, 30.
205 Ibid.
206 Montellà, *La maternidad de Elna*, pp. 73–86.
207 Vinyes et al., *Los niños perdidos*, pp. 121–132; Vinyes, R., *Irredentas: Las presas políticas y sus hijos en las cárceles franquistas* (Madrid, 2002), pp. 72–82.
208 Gimeno, A. S., & Fariñas, D. R., "La caída de la mortalidad en la infancia en la España interior, 1860–1960: Un análisis de las causas de muerte", *Cuadernos de historia contemporánea*, Vol. 24 (2002), pp. 151–188; Jiménez Lucena, El tifus exantemático de la posguerra española, p. 187
209 Capuano, C. F., & Carli, A. J., "Antonio Vallejo Nagera (1889–1960) y la eugenesia en la España Franquista: Cuando la ciencia fue el argumento para la apropiación de la descendencia", *Revista de bioética y derecho*, Vol. 26 (2012), pp. 3–12.
210 Ibid.
211 Ibid.; Vinyes et al., *Los niños perdidos*, pp. 24–28.
212 Ibid., p. 25; Bravo, G. G., "The Origins of the Francoist Penitentiary System, 1936–48", *International Journal of Iberian Studies*, Vol. 23, No. 1 (2010), pp. 5–21, p. 6.
213 Ibid.
214 Vinyes et al., *Los niños perdidos*, p. 121.
215 Graham, *Spanish Civil War*, p. 115–117; Rubio, *Emigración* (Vol. 1), pp. 321–334.
216 Graham, *Spanish Civil War*, p. 129.
217 Hernández Holgado, La prisión militante, pp. 37, 132, 225.
218 Vinyes, *Irredentas*, p. 72; Vinyes et al., *Los niños perdidos*, pp. 125–6.
219 Ruiz-Vargas, Trauma y memoria, p. 322.
220 Ibid.
221 Ibid.; Nadal, A., "Experiencias psíquicas sobre mujeres marxistas Malagueñas: Málaga 1939", *Baetica: Estudios de Arte, Geografía e Historia*, No. 10 (1987), pp. 365–383.
222 Vinyes et al., *Los niños perdidos*, pp. 121–133.
223 Capuano & Carli, Antonio Vallejo Nágera, pp. 10–12.
224 Ibid.; Vinyes et al., *Los niños perdidos*, pp. 125–126; Cuevas Gutiérrez, T., *Testimonios de mujeres en las cárceles franquistas* (Huesca, 2004), pp. 321–347.
225 Vinyes et al., *Los niños perdidos*, pp. 125–126; Cuevas Gutiérrez, *Testimonios de mujeres*, pp. 321–347.
226 Preston, *Spanish Holocaust*, p. 513
227 Cuevas Gutiérrez, T., *Cárcel de mujeres 1939–1945* (Barcelona, 1985).
228 Vinyes et al., *Los niños perdidos*, pp. 129–130.
229 Bernabéu Mestre, J., "Madres y enfermeras: Demografía y salud en la política poblacionista del primer franquismo, 1939–1950", *Revista de demografía histórica*, Vol. 20, No 1 (2002), pp. 123–144, pp. 126–127; Bernabéu Mestre, J., Caballero Pérez, P., Galiana Sánchez, M. E., & Nolasco Bonmatí, A., "Niveles de vida y salud en la España del primer franquismo: las desigualdades en la mortalidad infantil", *Revista de Demografía Histórica*, Vol. 24, No. 1 (2006), pp. 181–202; Arco Blanco, Morir de hambre, pp. 241–258.
230 Vinyes et al., *Los niños perdidos*, pp. 15–16.

231 Cuevas Gutiérrez, *Cárcel de Mujeres.*
232 Fraser, R., *In Hiding: The Ordeal of Manuel Cortes* (New York, 1972), pp. xii, 7.
233 Ibid., pp. 205–207.
234 Ibid., pp. 133–139.
235 Ibid., p. 7.
236 Vinyes et al., *Los niños perdidos*, pp. 23–24.
237 Preston, *Spanish Holocaust*, pp. 471–473.
238 Vinyes et al., *Los niños perdidos*, pp. 23–24; Preston, *Spanish Holocaust*, p. xii.
239 Preston, *Spanish Holocaust*, p. 507.
240 Ibid., pp. 7–15; Vinyes et al., *Los niños perdidos*; Junquera, Necrológica.

6 Conclusion

Opening graves – closing wounds

On 1 December 2012, in the newly restored cemetery of La Sauceda the remains of the twenty-eight skeletons uncovered earlier that year at the farm of El Marrufo (officially designated by the Junta de Andalucía as a Site of Historic Memory in March 2012) were finally accorded a proper burial after seventy-six years. In a symbolic act of public homage, the boxed remains were formally interred in funeral niches and each one sealed with a dedicated ceramic plaque.[1]

The cemetery's restoration had been made possible in large part due to the financial support of Miguel Rodríguez Domínguez, a Spanish businessman whose grandfather had been killed at El Marrufo.[2] Miguel Rodríguez was also the main financial contributor to the excavations at El Marrufo, as despite an apparent willingness by the Andalusian Parliament to promote an exploration of the region's Francoist past, broader financial support has largely been absent, with excavations and reburials mostly funded through local initiatives.[3]

In December 2013, La Sauceda was also designated by the Junta de Andalucía as a Site of Historic Memory, joining a growing list of sites across Andalucía dedicated to victims of the Francoist repression and the dictatorship and designed to publicly identify and preserve the locations where acts of repression took place.[4]

In February 2016, the Ley de Memoria Histórica y Democrática de Andalucía (Law of Historic and Democratic Memory of Andalucía) reached the Andalusian parliament without opposition.[5] The following year, on 28 March 2017, the Parliament of Andalucía approved, promulgated and ordered the publication of the new law, a law that reflected directives by the United Nations relating to historic memory and further strengthened the previous memory legislation passed by the parliament.[6] There was an attempt by the government in Madrid to rule the law unconstitutional shortly after its first passage through the Andalusian parliament. The ruling Popular Party opposed a clause that called for documentary material in state archives relating to democratic memory in Spain's southernmost region be transferred to the General Archive of Andalucía.[7] However, and possibly as a result of the contested vote for independence in Catalunya in November 2017, with the ruling party in Madrid perhaps more open to regional sensitivities, the Spanish Government suspended its opposition in December 2017, with the text of the law left unchanged, including the addenda that allows for further negotiation on the ultimate fate of these archives. Together, these statutes place Andalucía at the forefront of the movement in Spain to address the traumatic legacy of the Spanish Civil War, a legacy that effects both the diminishing numbers of elderly survivors and their forebears.[8]

This legacy of trauma, the diminishing but still present scars inflicted during a bloody conflict on both the body and the mind of so many in Spain, have led to a certain polarisation within Spanish society, where there are still conflicting discourses regarding whether it is best to leave the past and its dead undisturbed, or whether, through a direct engagement that allows for identification, reburial and commemoration of the victims of the Francoist repression, that closure can be achieved for those denied the right to properly remember their dead. This in effect answers the question of why the Spanish Civil War is still relevant today, in that at the heart of Spanish society a deep wound remains untreated; however, it does not explain the significance of the conflict within its own contemporary setting, or why a war that took place within the borders of a single nation has engendered a historiography of a similar size to that of WWII. Undoubtedly, the significance of the Spanish Civil War lies in its position at the crossroads of the clash between fascism and democracy in a Europe on the brink of all-out war. Through its international dimensions, the struggle between the Insurgents and the Government became one of the defining anti-fascist struggles of the twentieth century and thus the subject of extensive study.[9]

What also made it significant, however, were the genuine advances made in the medical care available to both combatants and civilians alike. New models of organisation were an important contributor in this regard, and the aim of this book has been to offer the first full study that examines the evolution, organisation and provision of medicine and surgery during the Spanish Civil War, on both sides. However, for Franco, punishing the defeated was at the centre of his agenda both during and after the Civil War, and the destruction of what the Republic had achieved in a number of fields – including health. Therefore the post-war traumatic legacy of Francoism is an essential part of this study.

The advances made have mostly been attributed to improvements within the medical services in the Republican Zone. This is largely due to the fact that among the early published works on the Spanish Civil War, a number of medical textbooks and memoirs were written by people who had served the Republic, and it was these texts that served as a starting point for later scholars.[10] Partly as a result of this, and apart from one or two notable figures, the role of the Spanish medical practitioner during the conflict has been largely overlooked, but changes in Spain on both sides of the divide were driven in the main by Spanish doctors, and an important part of this book has been an exploration of their contribution.

As has been argued throughout this study, the delivery of forward care in the opposing zones was notable for much that it had in common, although organisational models for the delivery of care did differ as a result of different ideological approaches. These ideological differences, reflecting diverse approaches towards medical care during war, were influential on the development of evolved models of healthcare, with anarchist and socialist discourses on the socialisation of medicine having a direct impact on planning in the Republican Zone. Furthermore, ideologically based discourses surrounding the provision of care could, at times, appear contradictory, making an examination of the propaganda surrounding medicine during the conflict such an important analytical tool, as different perspectives might favour one side over the other, but the broader details that they reveal contain reference to wider organisational and medical concerns, and are thus revealing on a number of levels.

The contradictory Crusade rhetoric at the heart of the Francoist myth of reconquest clearly demonstrate differences in approach. While phrasing the struggle as a religious crusade against the infidel 'reds', efforts were made to provide for the cultural and religious needs of those who would have been traditionally labelled as the infidel, i.e., those without faith; the 55,468 Muslim combatants fighting for the Insurgency who were wounded during the conflict. Between 75,000 to 85,000 Maghrebi soldiers saw action in Spain during the course of the Civil War, and the medical care they received, a story largely absent from the history of medicine of the conflict, reflected an approach that also catered for their religious as well as cultural needs. These paid recruits, fighting for a cause not their own in a foreign land, were not primarily professional soldiers, especially after the number of veterans was depleted in the opening campaigns, and were largely made up of civilians prepared to serve for regular pay.[11] However, despite the Crusades rhetoric constructed around a common religiosity in Insurgent propaganda, Spain's traditional enemy from across the Strait of Gibraltar were not only viewed with suspicion by the forces they were brought over to fight, but also by people more generally in the Insurgent Zone. Considerable resources were therefore put towards providing separate medical provision. Through exploring how surgical care was administered, and the efforts made by the Insurgents to meet the cultural needs of hospitalised Muslim combatants, this book provides the first in-depth analysis of medical care of the Moroccan wounded during the Spanish Civil War.

This examination of the surgical care of Franco's Muslim combatants also serves an additional purpose beyond telling a tale largely untold, in that it also addresses an imbalance in the historiography, where they are predominantly portrayed as, on the one hand, professional and exceptional fighters, but on the other as the savage 'Moors', who pillaged and raped their way across Spain, a view that still predominates within Spain to this day.[12] The fact that

Franco's colonial troops did engage in such activity is clearly acknowledged in this study. However, its detailed exploration of the medical care offered to these troops has also shed further light on their participation to offer a more nuanced understanding than that normally found in the literature – as the majority of those who did serve in Spain were subsistence farmers and herdsmen, rather than professional fighters – and is an area in need of further study.

Recent histories of medicine of the Spanish Civil War, especially studies written in English, have by and large concentrated on the role played by international volunteers in the provision of medical aid during the conflict. These accounts engage with a wide variety of sources in telling their tale, but their engagement with the historiography have tended to favour extra-national and international perspectives, with little analysis of the propagandist sources that this entails. This study, in attempting to more fully assess the Spanish medical contribution, first and foremost relies on the Spanish literature, in support of its central thesis. Nevertheless, it also engages closely with the literature that originates from outside of Spain as these are also first-hand accounts, and therefore the observations by Douglas Jolly MD provide supporting evidence on organisation, with the account by Peter Chalmers Mitchell throwing light on local anarchist-driven health initiatives in Málaga. It is the inclusion of such a diversity of materials that situates this study within a new historiographical trend with a much wider multidisciplinary approach; one that engages with local, regional and national studies in exploring both the Spanish Civil War in its contemporary context but also its longer-term consequences.

This engagement with a wide variety of Spanish material and data, from medical admission and discharge cards and other archival documentation, through to articles in the press and film, allows for a more complete analysis of how medical services were organised across Spain, thus allowing for an analysis of the effect different ideologies had on models of care. Thus, an examination of how medical care was organised, has not only revealed similarities between how care was delivered in the different zones, but it has also revealed the wider contribution made by anarchists to the development of health services within the Republican Zone. Understanding the anarchist contribution to healthcare provision, and the important role they played in promoting civil defence measures against the possible use of chemical weapons would not have been possible without a close engagement with propaganda. By examining contemporary state papers confirming appointments, newspaper articles and books, and accompanying photographic evidence, this study has been able to demonstrate more fully the role played by anarchist medical personnel in this regard.

The analysis of propaganda and debates surrounding the advances made in blood transfusion further demonstrate the importance of propagandistic materials as a historical source. The importance attached to these technical advances were not only strongly felt among the medical community who applied this knowledge in helping save lives in both in Spain and the World

War that was to follow, but was also part of a much wider cultural discourse. Different ideas and ideologies lay at the heart of this propaganda and this is nowhere more clearly expressed in the energetic popular front clenched fist to facilitate blood flow seen in *Transfusió de Sang* and *Heart of Spain*, as opposed to the passive and gendered flexing of the fingers for the same purpose in *Defenders of the Faith*. This study, by closely scrutinising film, imagery and text, is able to offer different interpretations surrounding the giving of blood than would normally be found, and this allows for the provision of this life-saving service to be assessed in its broader cultural context.

The impact that lies at the heart of much propaganda often concerns the visible scars of warfare, the shattered limbs and the bloodied faces, which form an important part of the visual legacy of war, and this is certainly true of a conflict that received international press attention.[13] However, it is the invisible traumas of war, the scars on the psyche that are perhaps one of war's most lasting legacies. The defeated of the Spanish Civil War were left in no doubt at the end of the conflict exactly whom Franco held responsible. As such, part of the Francoist projection of culpability was a powerful discourse that argued for a need for the purification of Spain, and the Franco Regime actively pursued a widespread policy of reprisal and punishment. This involved widespread political purges, with nearly half a million prisoners passing through Spanish prisons and concentration camps between 1939 and 1948. Elsewhere, processes of 're-education' and re-Catholicisation were imposed upon the defeated and were facilitated by repressive and retroactive laws that allowed for prosecution of Republicans for 'offences' dating back to October 1934.[14]

Historical rigour requires that the historian fully explore all avenues relating to the questions they ask of their sources. In addressing the painful legacy of the trauma of the defeated, those hidden wounds that remain obscured due to the lack of a national reconciliation that inhibited expression of that trauma and the healing that this can offer, also requires that the historian also deals with 'uncomfortable truths'. If this involves challenging those within Spanish society who seek to deny expression and historical identity to the inert and largely unidentified remains in burial pits and unmarked graves across Spain, then this is a task that needs taking on with consideration and thought. This study, by engaging with trauma and its continued relevance to the families and descendants, and through its interlocking alignment with national as well as regional and local perspectives in exploring this further, seeks to provide its own unique historical perspective that contributes towards this trauma being addressed, by an inclusive examination of the contribution made by Spanish medical professionals across Spain during the Spanish Civil War and its aftermath.

To this day, there remain in unmarked burial pits and mass graves across Spain the remains of more than 30,000 victims of Francoism. Successive national governments have failed to provide resources for the proper investigation of the numerous sites and – despite the passing of statute 52/2007, the Law of Historic Memory – have failed to attribute proper significance to the importance of confronting the traumas of the past. This, by and large, has been left to those few survivors still standing, and their children and grandchildren. Spain stands alone as the only democratic country in the world in which 'governmental bodies have failed to investigate their own extrajudicial killings', and old bones may lie still, but they do not lie quietly if their existence still has meaning to those connected through ties of family and kinship.

Andrés Rebolledo Barreno, president of the Association of the Relatives of Repressed Victims of Francoism in La Sauceda and El Marrufo, although he never met Andrés Barenno Perez, the grandfather executed and killed at El Marrufo, was able – at the side of his mother, Barenno Perez' daughter – to finally provide him with a proper burial, seventy-six years after his death. It is the daughter, eighty-three-year-old Juana Barreno Ruiz, who on his commemoration plaque in the newly restored Cemetery at La Sauceda is credited with having the constancy of rescuing his memory, a daughter who as an infant too young at the time to remember, witnessed the destruction of her village of La Sauceda. Notions of loss concerning her father would develop over time as the grief of close family members who remembered the event were denied expression beyond the confining walls of home, with the evolution of her own 'memories' of this life-changing moment denied expression for most of her adult life.[15]

Alongside the wounded veterans who had served the Republic and were denied pensions until after the death of Franco, the commemorative tiles that serve to identify those who can be named and those who cannot stand testimony to why a continued engagement with history of Spain's recent past involves not treating the Spanish Civil War as a conflict resolved, but as a battleground upon which lie lives still in the need of healing.

Notes

1 "Acuerdo de 27 de diciembre de 2013, del Consejo de Gobierno, por el que se declaran 34 Lugares de Memoria Histórica de Andalucía" (Accord of 27 December 2012 of the Council of Government by which thirty four places of Historic Memory are declared); available at: www.juntadeandalucia.es/boja/2014/26/1 (last accessed 02.02.2016); Lozano, A., "Memoria Histórica en el cementerio de La Sauceda: Los caídos del cortijo del Marrufo yacen en paz", *El Mundo*, 01.12.2012, available at: www.elmundo.es/elmundo/2012/12/01/Andalucía/1354366901.html (last accessed 12.03.2016).

2 *El Mundo*, 01.12.2012; *La Vanguardia*, 28.12.2003, p. 59.

3 *El Mundo*, 01.12.2012; Sígler, F., "Celebrado en el cementerio de la Sauceda el homenaje y entierro digno de víctimas exhumadas en el Marrufo", *Papeles de la Historia*, 2.12.2012, available at: www.papelesdehistoria.org/2012/12/02/celebrado-en-el-cementerio-de-la-sauceda-el-homenaje-y-entierro-digno-de-victimas-exhumadas-en-el-marrufo.html (last accessed 12.06.2016).

4 Ibid.

5 Limón, R., "El parlamento Andaluz tramita sin oposición la Ley de Memoria Histórica", *El País*, 10.02.2016, available at: http://politica.elpais.com/politica/2016/02/10/actualidad/1455127117_595274.html (last accessed 12.03.2016).
6 Ley 2/2017, de 28 de marzo, de Memoria Histórica y Democrática de Andalucía, available at: www.juntadeandalucia.es/boja/2017/63/1 (last accessed 20.01.2018).
7 Limón, El parlamento Andaluz tramita sin oposición la Ley de Memoria Histórica.
8 "Andalucía y Gobierno central firman la paz sobre la Ley de Memoria", *Publico*, 1.12.2017; Ley 2/2017, de 28 de marzo, p. 31.
9 Graham, *Spanish Civil War*, p. ix.
10 Jolly, *Field Surgery*; Trueta, *Treatment of War Wounds*; Mira, *Psychiatry in War*.
11 Balfour, *Deadly Embrace*, p. 312.
12 Martin Corrales, Maurofobia/islamafobia, pp. 39–51.
13 Riegel, O. W. "Press, Radio, and the Spanish Civil War", *The Public Opinion Quarterly*, Vol. 1, No. 1 (1937), pp. 131–136; Preston, P., *We Saw Spain Die: Foreign Correspondents in the Spanish Civil War* (London, 2008).
14 Rodrigo, Internamiento y trabajo forzoso, pp. 633–634; Preston, *Spanish Holocaust*, pp. 503–507.
15 León Moriche, *La Sauceda*.

Bibliography

Primary sources

Archives

Archivo Casa de la Memoria de La Sauceda
Archivo General Militar de Ávila
Biblioteca Nacional de España
Boletín Oficial del Estado
British Film Institute
British Library
British Library Sound Archive
Cardiff University Library Archive
Centro Documental de la Memoria Histórica
Filmoteca Catalunya
Filmoteca Española
Goyanes Family Archive
Imperial War Museum Sound Archive
Marx Memorial Library
Modern Records Centre University of Warwick
Wellcome Library Archives and Manuscripts

Contemporary newspapers and periodicals

AMI Periódico de la Ayuda Médica Extranjera (Barcelona)
ABC (Madrid)
ABC (Sevilla)
Caras y Caretas (Buenos Aires)
Crónica (Madrid)
El Compostelano (Santiago de Compostela)
Estampa (Madrid)
Heraldo de Aragón (Zaragoza)
Libertad (Cuenca)
Mi Revista (Barcelona)
Mundo Gráfico (Madrid)
El Pueblo Gallego (Vigo)
Solidaridad Obrera (Barcelona)
The Times (London)

La Vanguardia (Barcelona)
La Voz (Madrid)

Contemporary journals

British Medical Journal (BMJ)
Ejercito: Revista Ilustrada de las Armas y Servicios
Científica Médica
Crónica Médica
Lancet
Revista Sanidad de Guerra (5-1937 to 5-1938 Republican)
Revista Española de Medicina y Cirugía de Guerra (post May 1938 Insurgent)
Semana Medica Española
St. Bartholomew's Hospital Journal

Contemporary journal articles

Balmori, H., "Servicios sanitarios de antigás: Táctica y organización de estos Servicios en el ejército", *Revista Española de Medicina y Cirugía de Guerra*, Vol. 2, No. 5 (1939), pp. 49–63.

Bastos Ansart, M., "Conferencias y resumen de revistas", *Revista de Sanidad de Guerra*, Vol. 1, No. 1 (1937), pp. 27–33.

——— "Dos problemas de asistencia a los heridos en retaguardia", *Revista de Sanidad de Guerra*, No. 1 (1937), pp. 9–14.

——— "Sobre el pronóstico en las heridas de guerra del vientre", *Revista de Sanidad de Guerra*, Vol. 2 , No. 9 (1938), pp. 1–17.

——— "Varios 'standards' de cirugía de guerra", *Revista de Sanidad de Guerra*, Vol. 1, No. 5 (1937), pp. 173–181.

——— "Varios 'standards' de cirugía de guerra: 2. – Tratamiento de las heridas vasculares de los miembros", *Revista de Sanidad de Guerra*, Vol. 1, No. 7 (1937), pp. 257–266.

Broster, L. R., "A Survey of War Surgery", *BMJ*, Vol. 1, No. 4207 (1941), pp. 273–275.

Coller, F. A., & Valk, W. L., "The Delayed Closure of Contaminated Wounds: A Preliminary Report", *Annals of Surgery*, Vol. 112, No. 2 (1940), pp. 256–270.

Consell de Sanitat de Guerra, "Instruccions sobre defensa passiva de la població civil, per al cas d'atac amb gasos", *La Medicina Catalana*, Vol. 7, No. 39–40 (1936–1937), pp. 375–383.

Cuadrado, F., "Resultados inmediatos en heridas cráneo-cerebrales de guerra", *Revista Española de Medicina y Cirugía de Guerra*, Vol. 3, No. 3 (1940), pp. 203–220.

Dubash, J., Clegg, O., & Vaughan, J., "Changes Occurring in Blood Stored in Different Preservatives", *BMJ*, Vol. 2, No. 4162 (1940), pp. 482–484.

Durán-Jordà, F., "El Servicio de Transfusión de Sangre de Barcelona: Técnicas y utillaje", *Revista de Sanidad de Guerra*, Vol. 1, No. 8 (1937), pp. 307–321.

Ellis, R. W. B., "Blood Transfusion at the Front", *Proceedings of the Royal Society of Medicine*, Vol. 31, No. 6 (1938), pp. 684–686.

Gómez Durán, M., "Impresiones sobre cirugía en los hospitales de sangre en el frente", *Galicia Clínica*, Vol. 9, No. 5–6 (1937), pp. 89–140.

——— "Principios fundamentales en cirugía de guerra", *Revista Española de Medicina y Cirugía de Guerra*, Vol. 3, No. 2 (1939), pp. 2–35.

——— "Principios fundamentales en cirugía de guerra: Parte 2ª, hospitales de evacuación y especialidades", *Revista Española de Medicina y Cirugía de Guerra*, Vol. 3, No. 12 (1939), pp. 81–101.

——— "Puestos quirúrgicos avanzados", *Galicia Clínica*, Vol. 10, No. 3–4 (1938), pp. 37–48.

——— "Táctica terapéutica de urgencia en fracturas de guerra en el frente", *Galicia Clínica*, Vol. 11, No. 7 (1939).

González Romero, A., "Transfusión de sangre", *Boletín del Colegio Médico de Pontevedra* (1939), pp. 8–11.

Gordon-Taylor, S. R. A. G., & Hamilton, F. H., "Surgical Experience in the Spanish War", *BMJ*, Vol. 2, No. 4164 (1940), pp. 560–561.

Hernández Giménez, J., "La transfusión sanguínea en el ejército", *Ejército: Revista Ilustrada de las Armas y Servicios*, No. 67 (1945), pp. 13–20.

Lockwood, A. D., "Some Experiences in the Last War", *BMJ*, Vol.1, No. 4130 (1940), pp. 436–438.

Martín Santos, L., "Nuestro criterio en el tratamiento de los fracturados de guerra en la zona de vanguardia", *Medicina Española*, Vol. 1 (1938), pp. 653–681.

Molla, V. M., "Algunas consideraciones sobre cirugía en nuestros frentes de Guerra", Crónica Médica, Vol. 41 (1937), pp. 91–110.

Montserrat, S., "Gómez Ulla y su hospital quirúrgico de montaña", *Revista Española de Medicina y Cirugía de Guerra* Vol. 7, No. 2 (1945), pp. 600–604.

Moynahan, E. J., "Treatment of War Wounds and Infected Fractures", *BMJ*, Vol. 1, No. 4127 (1940), p. 229.

Oleo Herraiz, I., "Apostillas a los servicios de sanidad Militar en campaña", *Revista Española de Medicina y Cirugía de Guerra*, Vol. 2, No. 9 (1939), pp. 254–261.

Ross, J. A., & Hulbert, K. F., "Treatment of 100 War Wounds and Burns", *BMJ*, Vol. 1, No. 4190 (1941), pp. 618–621.

Ruiz Albéniz, V., *España en el Rif: estudios del indígena y del país, nuestra actuación de doce años, la guerra del veintiuno* (Madrid, 1921), p. 150.

Saxton, R. S., "The Madrid Blood Transfusion Institute", *The Lancet*, Vol. 230, No. 5949 (1937).

"Técnicas de actualidad: Defensa pasiva organizada", *Crónica Médica*, No. 110 (1937), pp. 47–79.

"Treatments of War Wounds and Fractures", *BMJ*, Vol. 2, No. 4108 (1939), p. 694.

Trueta, J., "The Organisation of Hospital Services for Casualties due to the Bombing of Cities, Based on Experience Gained in Barcelona – with Special Reference to the Classification of Casualties", *Proceedings of the Royal Society of Medicine*, Vol. 33, No. 13 (1939), pp. 13–23.

——— "The Treatment of War Fractures by the Closed Method: Section of Surgery", *Proceedings of the Royal Society of Medicine*, Vol. 33, No. 1 (1939), pp. 65–74.

Vaughan, J., "War Wounds and Air Raid Casualties: Blood Transfusion", *BMJ*, Vol. 1 (1939), pp. 933–936.

Welch, C. E., "War Wounds of the Abdomen", *New England Journal of Medicine*, Vol. 237, No. 5 (1947), pp. 156–162.

Wilson, P. D., "The Treatment of Compound Fractures Resulting from Enemy Action", *Annals of Surgery*, Vol. 113, No. 6 (1941), pp. 915–924.

Winnett Orr, H., "Treatment of War Wounds and Infected Fractures", *BMJ*, Vol 1, No. 4135 (1940), p. 585.

Contemporary printed sources/contemporary memoirs

Acier, M., *From Spanish Trenches: Recent Letters from Spain; Collected and Edited by M. Acier* (London, 1937).
Álvarez, A., "El Cuerpo de Sanidad Militar ha organizado un tren-hospital para los heridos del Frente", *Crónica* (01.11.1936).
——— "A Nation in Retreat", MRCUW: 292/946/18a/3.
Ayesta y Daguerre, L., "Mohamed Belkaid. El Morito Matarife", *El Compostelano* (27.04.1937), p. 1.
Barbiela, F. F., Bastos Ansart, M., & Ramon Otaola, J., *Manual de Sanidad Militar* (Valencia, 1938).
Bastos Ansart, M., *Algunos aspectos clínicos de las heridas por arma de fuego* (Barcelona, 1936).
Bethune, N., *The Crime on the Road Malaga – Almeria: Narrative with Graphic Documents Revealing Fascist Cruelty* (Spain, 1937).
——— *El crimen del camino Málaga-Almería: Relato con documentos gráficos reveladores de la crueldad fascista* (Spain, 1937).
——— *Le crime sur la route Malaga-Almeria: Narrative avec documents graphiques révélant la cruauté fasciste* (Spain, 1937).
Böhler, L., *Técnica del tratamiento de las fracturas*, Traducción de F. Jimeno Vidal. Prólogo de Joaquín Trías Pujol (Barcelona, 1934).
BOE, No. 540 (Suplemento), 14.04.1938, "Reglamento Provisional del Benemérito Cuerpo de Mutilado de Guerra por la Patria (Decreto de 5 de abril de 1938–11 Año Triunfal)", pp. 1–72.
BOE, No. 44, 13.02.1939, pp. 824–847.
BOE, 14.02.1939, "Ley de 10 de febrero de 1939 fijando normas para la depuración de funcionarios públicos", pp. 856–859.
BOE, No. 125, 04.05.1940, pp. 3048–9.
BOE, 17.10.1977, Ley 46/1977, de 15 de octubre, de Amnistía, pp. 22765–6.
BOE, 2.10.1936–27.02.1961.
Boletín Oficial de la Junta de Defensa Nacional de España (25.07.1936–2.10.1936).
Brenan, G., *The Spanish Labyrinth: An Account of the Social and Political Background of the Spanish Civil War* (Cambridge, 1943).
"Bulletin No. 5", MRCUW: 292/946/16a/47
Calvo García, "La ayuda sanitaria internacional a la República española (1936–1939)", *Sanidad Militar*, Vol. 50, No. 3 (1994), pp. 338–347.
Casares López, R., "La Farmacia Militar Española en la pasada guerra", *Discursos* (Madrid, 1940).
Chalmers Mitchell, P., *My House in Málaga* (London, 1938).
Colmegna, H., *Diario de un Médico Argentino en la Guerra de España 1936–1939* (Buenos Aires, 1941).
Conselleria de Sanitat i Assistència Social, *La Reforma Eugénica del Aborto*, Generalitat de Catalunya, Ediciones de la Consejería de Sanidad y Asistencia Social, Sección de Propaganda (Barcelona, 1937).
Cultura en el frente, No. 31, 18.10.1937.
Diario Oficial del Ministerio de Defensa Nacional, No. 296, Tomo 10 (Barcelona, 1937).
Donato, M., "Viaje en un tren hospital", *Estampa* (13.11.1937), pp. 4–5.

Durán-Jordà, F., *The Service of Blood Transfusion at the Front: Organisation-Apparatus by Frederic Duran-Jorda, Technical Chief of the Service, Director of Emergency Hospital No. 18* (Barcelona, 1937).

——— *El servei de transfusió de sang al front: Organització-utillatge* (Barcelona, 1937).

Duchess of Atholl, *Searchlight on Spain* (Harmondsworth, 1938).

Elósegui, C., "Editorial: El Instituto Español de Hematología y Hemoterapia", *Semana Medica Española*, Vol. 1, No. 3 (1942), pp. 231–241.

"Entrega de seis tiendas de campaña y veinticinco ambulancias al Ejército", *La Vanguardia* (09.07.1938), p. 4.

España, Servicio de Guerra Química, *Información del servicio de guerra química* (Madrid, 1938).

Esteva Villarasa, J., "La Química como arma bélica", *Mi Revista* (10.02.1938), pp. 39–41.

Gaceta de la República: Diario Oficial (10.11.1936–28.03.1939).

Gaceta de Madrid: Diario Oficial de la República (01.04.1934–08.11.1936).

"Get Them Away: The Story of the French Concentration Camps", MRCUW: 15X/2/226/2 (London, 1941).

Gollonet, M., & López, M., *Rojo y Azul en Granada (más datos por la historia de la guerra civil española), Ilustraciones fotográficas … cuarta edición* (Granada, 1937).

González, R., "Transfusión de sangre", *Boletín del Colegio Médico de Pontevedra* (31.12.1939), pp. 8–11.

Gómez Ulla, M., "Impresiones de una visita al frente francés de los Vosgos", *La Guerra y su preparación*, Vol. 5, No. 7 (1917), pp. 152–183.

——— "Una visita a las instalaciones sanitarias de los frentes francés e inglés", *La Guerra y su preparación*, Vol. 8, No. 1 (1920), pp. 207–235.

Goyanes Álvarez, V., "La transfusión de sangre en el Sector Centro", *Revista de Sanidad de Guerra*, Vol. 11, No. 12 (1938), pp. 159–176.

"Guerra química: Las dificultades para llegar a una prohibición de este terrible medio de lucha", *Caras y Caretas* (02.07.1938), pp. 12–13.

"Guerra química: Cómo deberá ser protegida la población civil contra el terrible peligro", *Caras y Caretas* (14.08.1937), pp. 12–13.

Guindal y Calderero, J. M., "Problemas de salubridad que ha planteado la guerra", Real Academia Nacional de Medicina, Instituto de España, *Anales de la Real Academia de Medicina* – 1943 (Madrid, 1944), pp. 503–538.

"Jefatura de Sanidad del Ejército de Tierra", *Cartilla sanitaria del combatiente* (Madrid, 1937).

Jolly, D. W., *Field Surgery in Total War* (London, 1940).

Koestler, A., *Spanish Testament* (London, 1937).

"La Cruz Roja y la guerra: La labor de los comités locales, los consultorios gratuitos, los puestos de socorro, las patrullas antigás", *Mundo Gráfico* (08.09.1937), p. 10.

"La estancia en Vigo del Visir del Majzen", in *El Pueblo Gallego*, (28.02.1937), p. 10.

"La guerra química", *Mundo Gráfico* (1937), p. 12.

"La guerra química II: Las dificultades para llegar a una prohibición de este terrible medio de lucha", *Mundo Gráfico* (26.05.1937), pp. 15–16.

"La guerra química III", *Mundo Gráfico* (02.06.1937), pp. 10–11.

Langdon-Davies, J., *Behind the Spanish Barricades* (London, 1938).

"La química como arma de guerra: Como era una nueva guerra?", *Mi Revista* (01.01.1938), pp. 58–60.

Laslet, A., "Report on the Health Mission in Spain: 28th December, 1936, to 15th January, 1937" (Geneva, 1937), MRCUW: 292.946.15b.11.
López Cotarelo, A., "Organización de los servicios sanitarios militares de vanguardia", in L. Girones, L. (ed.), *Cuestiones médico-quirúrgicas de guerra* (Castellón de la Plana, 1938), pp. 527–553.
Marín Gómez, I., *El laurel y la retama en la memoria: tiempo de posguerra en Murcia, 1939–1952* (Murcia, 2004).
McNeill-Ross, G., *The Epic of the Alcázar* (London, 1937).
"Medical Aid for Spain", MRCUW: 292/946/42/104.
Mira, E., *Psychiatry in War* (New York, 1943).
Morata Cantón, J., *Defensa de guerra tóxico química: En colaboración con otros compañeros y ed. por el "Sindicato Única de Sanidad"* (Madrid, 1937).
——— *Guerra química y bacteriológica* (Barcelona, 1938).
Nombela Gallardo, D., "El porqué de los hipertrofias cardiacas en la Guerra: Dirigidos a los Jefes de Cuerpo, División y Brigadas", *Libertad*, Vol. 1, No. 4 (1937), pp. 13–14.
——— "Nuestro Servicio Sanitario en la toma de Albarracín", *Libertad*, Vol. 1, No. 6 (1937), pp. 4–6.
Ortiz de Villajos, C. G., *Crónica de Granada en 1937, II Año Triunfal* (Granada, 1938).
Oteyza, L. D., *Abd-el-Krim y los prisioneros: una información periodística en el campo enemigo* (Madrid, 1925).
Parrilla Hermida, M., *Los gases de combate: Síntomas, tratamiento y protección* (La Coruña, 1936).
——— "Los gases de guerra", in L. Girones (ed.) *Cuestiones médico-quirúrgicas de guerra* (Castellón de la Plana, 1938), pp. 527–553.
Primo de Rivera, P., *4 Discursos de Pilar Primo de Rivera* (Madrid, 1939).
Reglamento para el servicio sanitario en campaña: Aprobado por real orden el 1º de Julio 1896 (Madrid, 1896).
"Report on International Conference for Medical Aid to Spain", MRCUW: 292/946/42/15.
"Reports Received from Mrs Leah Manning and Circulated to the Committee in Accordance with Resolution 10th August 1938", MRCUW: 292/946/42/16, p. 1.
Rico Belestá, F., "La Sanidad en Campaña" *Libertad*, Vol. 1, No. 5 (1937), p. 5.
——— "Servicio Sanitario en Campaña", *Libertad*, Vol. 1, No. 7 (1937), pp. 6–7.
Rodríguez Castelao, A. D., *Galicia Mártir: Estampas* (Madrid and Valencia, 1937)
Sarto, J. de, "Actividades de la Cruz Roja Española: El secretario general de esta magnífica institución, señor Morata, habla para los lectores de Crónica", *Crónica* (16.01. 1938), p. 3.
——— "Actividades de la Cruz Roja Española: Cómo se prepara a la población civil para su defensa contra la guerra química", *Crónica* (30.01.1938), p. 5.
Sim, *Estampas de la Revolución Española 19 Julio de 1936* (Barcelona, 1936).
"St. Pancras and Holborn Spain Week, 22–28 January, 1938 (Tuesday, 25th January. 8 p.m. Lantern Lecture by Dr. Janet Vaughan on the British Medical Unit in Spain)", MRCUW: 292/946/42/104, p. 1.
TNA, Medical Research Council, FD 1/5372/C674261, Air Raid Precautions Department. Intelligence Branch. *Medical Aspects of Air Raid Casualties in Barcelona* (701, 666/251), 25.03.1939.
TNA (FD1/5372, Annex A. to I. O. 65), *Opinions formed from actual experience of Aerial Bombardment in Barcelona by Dr. J. Trueta Raspall, Head of the Catalan General Hospital, Chief Surgeon of the Passive Defence Service, Barcelona*, 25.03.1939, pp. 1–20.

"The Treaty Between France and Spain Regarding Morocco", *The American Journal of International Law*, Vol. 7, No. 2 (1913), Supplement: Official Documents, pp. 81–99.
Trueta, J., *El tractament de les fractures de Guerra* (Barcelona, 1938).
——— *Treatment of War Wounds and Fractures: With Special Reference to the Closed Method as Used in the War in Spain* (London, 1940).
"Una Ambulancia Inglesa para el Frente", *La Vanguardia* (01.09.1936), p. 36.
"Una exposición de periódicos murales en Madrid", *Mundo Gráfico* (01.06.1938), pp. 1–2.
"Visita a un hospital: como se efectuá la transfusión de sangre en el frente", *La Vanguardia* (25.11.1936), pp. 2–3.
Viñuales Fariñas, M., "La ciencia al servicio de la barbarie: los horrores de la guerra aeroquímica", *Revista Blanca* (Barcelona, 1936).
Wilson, F. M., *In the Margins of Chaos: Recollections of Relief Work in and between Three Wars* (London, 1944).
Yudin, S., *La transfusion du sang de cadavre à l'homme* (Paris, 1933).

Film and documentary sources

Andrew Whitehead Interviews with Political Radicals, BLSA: C1377/47.
Blood Transfusion, Director: M. Nieter (United Kingdom, 1941).
Bethune, Director: Donald Brittain (National Film Board of Canada, 1964).
Norman Bethune: Spain and China, BLSA (Missing shelfmark) phonographic recording on vinyl (1976).
Blood Bank Service in Spain (Laya Films, 1937).
Defenders of the Faith, Director: Russell Palmer (US, 1938).
El Laberinto Marroquí, Director: Julio Sánchez Veiga (2007).
Els internat de la por, Directors: R. Vinyes, M. Armengou, & R. Belis (Televisió de Catalunya, 2015).
Heart of Spain, Director: Herbert Kline (Frontier Films, 1937).
La Sauceda, de la utopía al horror, Director: Juan Miguel León Moriche (Foro por la Memoria del Campo de Gibraltar/Asociación de Familiares de Represaliados por el Franquismo en La Sauceda y el Marrufo, 2013).
Las maestras de la República, Director: Pilar Pérez Solano (FETE-UGT, Transit Producciones, 2013).
Transfusió de Sang (Laya Films, 1937).
Victoire de la Vie, Directors: Henri Cartier Bresson and Herbert Kline (Centrale Sanitaire Internationale, 1937).

Secondary sources

Unpublished doctoral theses

Brasa Arias, B., "La Facultad de Farmacia de Santiago de Compostela (1900–1971)" (Universidad de Santiago de Compostela, 2011).
Hernández Holgado, F., "La prisión militante. Las cárceles franquistas de mujeres de Barcelona y Madrid (1939–1945)" (Universidad Complutense de Madrid, 2011).
Madariaga Fernández, F. J., "Las Industrias de Guerra de Cataluña durante la Guerra Civil" (Universitat Rovira i Virgili, Tarragona, 2003).

Rickett, R. M., "Refugees of the Spanish Civil War and Those They Left Behind: Personal Testimonies of Departure, Separation and Return Since 1936" (University of Manchester, 2015).

Books and articles (including participants' later memoirs)

Abrams, L., *Oral History Theory* (Oxford, 2010).

Aguirre González, J. V., *Al fin de la batalla, y muerto el combatiente … La Rioja 1936–1939* (Logroño, 2014).

Aguilar, P., "Agents of Memory: Spanish Civil War Veterans and Disabled Soldiers", in J. Winter & E. Sivan (eds.), *War and Remembrance in the Twentieth Century* (Cambridge, 1999), pp. 84–103.

——— "The Timing and the Scope of Reparation, Truth and Justice Measures: A Comparison of the Spanish, Argentinian and Chilean Cases", in K. Ambos, J. Large, & M. Wierda (eds.), *Building a Future on Peace and Justice: Studies on Transitional Justice, Conflict Resolution and Development: The Nuremberg Declaration on Peace and Justice* (Berlin, 2009), pp. 503–532.

Alexander, W., "Frontier Films, 1936–1941: The Aesthetics of Impact", *Cinema Journal*, Vol. 15, No. 1 (1975), pp. 16–28.

Alexi-Meskishvili, V., & Konstantinov, I. E., "Sergei S. Yudin: An Untold Story", *Surgery*, Vol. 139, No. 1 (2006), pp. 115–122.

Algarbani, J. M., *Y Jimena se vistió de negro: II República, Guerra Civil y posguerra en Jimena de la Frontera* (Cádiz, 2011).

Allen, T., Allen, J., & Gordon, S., *The Scalpel, the Sword: The Story of Doctor Norman Bethune* (Toronto, 2009).

Al Tuma, A., "The Participation of Moorish Troops in the Spanish Civil War (1936–1939): Military Value, Motivations, and Religious Aspects", *War and Society*, Vol. 30, No. 2 (2011), pp. 91–107.

Ametlla, C., *Catalunya: Paradís perdut. La guerra civil i la revolució anarco*-comunista (Barcelona, 1984).

Amo García, A., & Ibáñez Ferradas, M. L. (eds.), *Catálogo general del cine de la Guerra Civil/edición a cargo de Alfonso del Amo García; con la colaboración de M. Luisa Ibáñez Ferradas* (Madrid, 1996).

"Andalucía y Gobierno central firman la paz sobre la Ley de Memoria", *Publico* (1.12.2017).

Anderson, P., *The Francoist Military Trials: Terror and Complicity, 1939–1945* (New York and Abingdon, 2010).

——— "In the Name of the Martyrs: Memory and Retribution in Francoist Southern Spain, 1936–1945", *Cultural and Social History*, Vol. 8, No. 3 (2011), pp. 355–370.

——— *Friend or Foe? Occupation, Collaboration and Selective Violence in the Spanish Civil War* (Brighton, 2016).

Aracil, R., & Villarroya, J., *El país valencià sota les bombes, 1936–1939* (Valencia, 2010).

Arco Blanco, M. A. del, "'Morir de hambre': autarquía, escasez y enfermedad en la España del primer franquismo", *Pasado y memoria: Revista de historia contemporánea*, No. 5 (2006), pp. 241–258.

Armstrong, K., *Islam: A Short History* (New York, 2002).

Asbridge, T., *The Crusades: The Authoritative History of the War for the Holy Land* (New York, 2010).

Ávila Álvarez, A (ed.), *Todos los nombres. Base de datos sobre la represión franquista en Andalucía accesible a través de internet* (Sevilla, 2007).

Azzuz Hakim, M. I., *La actitud de los moros ante el alzamiento, Marruecos 1936* (Málaga, 1997).

Balcells, L., "Death is in the Air: Bombings in Catalonia, 1936–1939", *Revista Española de Investigaciones Sociológicas*, Vol. 136 (2011), pp. 25–48.

Balfour, S., *Deadly Embrace: Morocco and the Road to the Spanish Civil War* (Oxford, 2002).

Barona, J. L., & Bernabéu Mestre, J. (eds.), *Ciencia y sanidad en la Valencia capital de la República* (Valencia, 2007).

Barona, J. L., & Perdiguero-Gil, E., "Health and the War: Changing Schemes and Health Conditions During the Spanish Civil War", *Dynamis*, Vol. 28 (2008), pp. 103–126.

Bastos Ansart, M., *De las guerras coloniales a la guerra civil: memorias de un cirujano* (Barcelona, 1969).

Beevor, A., *The Spanish Civil War* (London, 1982).

——— *The Battle for Spain: The Spanish Civil War 1936–1939* (London, 2006).

Beneito Lloris, A., *El hospital Sueco-Noruego de Alcoi durante la Guerra Civil Española* (Alcoi, 2004).

——— "El Dr Manuel Bastos, profesor y militar represaliado", in J. L. Barona (ed.), *El exilio científico Republicano* (Valencia, 2010), pp. 315–333.

Benjelloun, A., "La participación de los mercenarios marroquíes en la Guerra Civil Española", *Revista Internacional de Sociología*, Vol. 46, No. 4 (1988), pp. 527–541.

Bentley, B. P. E., *A Companion to Spanish Cinema* (Woodbridge, 2008).

Bernabéu Mestre, J., "El papel de la Escuela Nacional de Sanidad en el desarrollo de la salud publica en España, 1924–1934", *Revista de Sanidad e Higiene Pública*, Vol. 68 (1998), pp. 65–89.

——— "La utopía reformadora de la Segunda República: la labor de Marcelino Pascua al frente de la Dirección General de Sanidad, 1931–1933", in *Revista Española de Salud Pública*, Vol. 74 (2000), pp. 1–13.

——— "Madres y enfermeras: Demografía y salud en la política poblacionista del primer franquismo, 1939–1950", *Revista de demografía histórica*, Vol. 20, No 1 (2002), pp. 123–144.

Bernabéu Mestre, J., Caballero Pérez, P., Galiana Sánchez, M. E., & Nolasco Bonmatí, A., "Niveles de vida y salud en la España del primer franquismo: las desigualdades en la mortalidad infantil", *Revista de demografía Histórica*, Vol. 24, No. 1 (2006), pp. 181–202.

Bernecker, W. L., *Colectividades y Revolución Social: El Anarquismo en la Guerra Civil Española, 1936–1939* (Barcelona, 1982).

Bescós Torres J., "Las enfermeras en la guerra de España (1936–1939)", *Revista Historia Militar*, Vol. 53 (1982), pp. 97–143.

——— "La Sanidad Militar en la guerra de España (1936–1939). 1ª Parte – La Sanidad en el Ejército Republicano", *Medicina Militar*, Vol. 43, No. 1 (1987), pp. 88–100.

——— "La Sanidad Militar en la Guerra de España (1936–1939), 2ª Parte – La Sanidad en el Ejército Nacional", *Medicina Militar*, Vol. 43, No. 4 (1987), pp. 434–447.

Bjerström, C. H., *Josep Renau and the Politics of Culture in Republican Spain, 1931–1939: Re-imagining the Nation* (Brighton, 2015).

Blanco Rodríguez, J. A., "La Historiografía de la guerra civil española", in S. Gálvez (ed.), *Dossier generaciones y memoria de la represión franquista: un balance de los movimientos por la memoria en Hispania Nova. Revista de Historia Contemporánea*, No. 7 (2007), pp. 741–775.

Blond Álvarez Del Manzano, C., "El Protectorado. Firma del convenio hispano-francés y Guerra del Rif 1912–1927", *Revista de Historia Militar*, Vol. 2 (2012), pp. 103–135.

Boyd Haycock, D., *I Am Spain: The Spanish Civil War through the Eyes of the Britons and Americans Who Saw it Happen* (London, 2013).

Brasa Arias, B., & Landín Pérez, M., "El trabajo de las mujeres voluntarias en el laboratorio de Farmacia Militar de Santiago de Compostela (1936–1939)", *Sanidad Militar*, Vol. 67, No. 1 (2011), pp. 177–192.

Bravo, G. G., "The Origins of the Francoist Penitentiary System, 1936–48", *International Journal of Iberian Studies*, Vol. 23, No. 1 (2010), pp. 5–21.

Broggi, M., *Memòries d'un cirurgià (1908–1945)*, Vol. 1 (Barcelona, 2001).

Browne, J. S., "Anaesthesia and the Spanish Civil War: The Delivery of Anaesthetic Care in a Divided Spain", *History of Anaesthesia Society Proceedings* Vol. 46 (2013), pp. 74–80.

——— "History of Anaesthesia: Anaesthetics and the Spanish Civil War: The Start of Specialisation", *European Journal of Anaesthesiology*, Vol. 31, No. 2 (2014), pp. 65–67.

Burleigh, M., *Sacred Causes: The Clash of Religion and Politics, from the Great War to the War on Terror* (London, 2006).

Burón, L., "Hospital de sangre de retaguardia: Actuación de un médico durante la guerra civil española. 1936–1939", *Los médicos y la medicina en la Guerra Civil Española: Monografías Beecham* (Madrid, 1986), pp. 245–258.

Cabañas González, J., *La Bañeza 1936. La vorágine de julio. Golpe y represión en la comarca Bañezana*, Vol. 1 (León, 2010).

Calvocoressi, P., & Wint, G., *Total War: Causes and Courses of the Second World War* (London, 1972).

Campo Rizo, J. M., "El Mediterráneo, campo de batalla de la Guerra Civil Española: la intervención naval Italiana. Una primera aproximación documental", *Cuadernos de Historia Contemporánea*, Vol. 19, No. 55 (1997), pp. 55–87.

Campos, M. L., "La historiografía española y la internacionalización de la Guerra Civil (1936–1939): un estado de la cuestión", *Ab Initio*, No. 5 (2012), pp. 59–79.

Capuano, C. F., & Carli, A. J., "Antonio Vallejo Nagera (1889–1960) y la eugenesia en la España Franquista": Cuando la ciencia fue el argumento para la apropiación de la descendencia", *Revista de bioética y derecho*, Vol. 26 (2012), pp. 3–12.

Carr, E. H., *The Comintern and the Spanish Civil War* (New York, 1984).

Carr, R., *Spain 1808–1975*, 2nd edn. (Oxford, 1982).

Carrie, L. E. S., & Simpson, P. J., *Understanding Anaesthesia* (London, 1982).

Carrol, P. N., *The Odyssey of the Abraham Lincoln Brigade: Americans in the Spanish Civil War* (Stanford, 1994).

Casals Meseguer, X., "Franco 'El Africano'", *Journal of Spanish Cultural Studies*, Vol. 7, No. 3 (2006), pp. 207–224.

Casanova, J., A Short History of the Spanish Civil War (New York, 2013)

Cayón García, F., & Muñoz Rubio, M., "Transportes y comunicaciones", in P. Martín Aceña & E. Martínez Ruiz (eds.), *La economía de la guerra civil* (Madrid, 2006), pp. 229–272.

Cenarro, Á., *La sonrisa de Falange: Auxilio Social en la guerra civil y la posguerra* (Barcelona, 2006).

Conde Lopez, M., "Médicos Exiliados (1492–1939)", in *Los médicos y la medicina en la Guerra Civil Española: Monografías Beecham* (Madrid, 1986), pp. 311–334.
Coni, N., *Medicine and Warfare: Spain, 1936–1939* (Abingdon, 2008).
Corse, E., *A Battle for Neutral Europe: British Cultural Propaganda during the Second World War* (London, 2013).
Cortada, J. W., *Modern Warfare in Spain: American Military Observations on the Spanish Civil War, 1936–1939* (Washington, DC, 2012).
Crawford, D., "Morocco's Invisible Imazighen", *The Journal of North African Studies*, Vol. 7, No. 1 (2002), pp. 53–70.
Crusells, M., "El Cine durante la Guerra Civil Española 1936–1939", *Comunicación y Sociedad*, Vol. 11, No. 2 (1998), pp. 123–152.
Cuevas Gutiérrez, T., *Cárcel de Mujeres 1939–1945* (Barcelona, 1985).
——— *Testimonio de mujeres en las cárceles franquistas* (Huesca, 2004).
Cull, N. J., Culbert, D., & Welch, D., *Propaganda and Mass Persuasion: A Historical Encyclopaedia 1500 to the Present* (Santa Barbara, 2003).
Davies, A., "The First Radio War: Broadcasting in the Spanish Civil War, 1936–1939", *Historical Journal of Film, Radio and Television*, Vol. 19, No. 4 (1999), pp. 473–513.
Derby, M., *Petals and Bullets: Dorothy Morris, New Zealand Nurse in the Spanish Civil War* (Brighton, 2015).
Díaz-Balart, M. N., "La doma de los cuerpos y las conciencias, 1939–1941: El campo de concentración de Porta Coeli (Valencia)", *Hispania Nova: Revista de historia contemporánea*, No. 10 (2012), pp. 284–310.
Díaz-Plaja, F., *La vida cotidiana en la España de la Guerra Civil* (Madrid, 1994).
Doll, R., "Vaughan, Dame Janet Maria (1899–1993)", in *Oxford Dictionary of National Biography* (Oxford, 2004).
Domènech, X., & Zenobi, L., *Quan plovien bombes* (Barcelona, 2007).
Domínguez Pérez, A., *El verano que trajo un largo invierno: La represión político-social durante el primer franquismo en Cádiz, 1936–1945*, Vol. 1 (Cádiz, 2004).
Ealham, C., "'Myths' and the Spanish Civil War: Some Old, Some Exploded, Some Clearly Borrowed and Some Almost 'Blue'", *Journal of Contemporary History*, Vol. 42, No. 2 (2007), pp. 365–376.
Ealham, C., & Richards, M., "History, Memory and the Spanish Civil War: Recent Perspectives", in C. Ealham & M. Richards, (eds.), *The Splintering of Spain: Cultural History and the Spanish Civil War, 1936–1939* (Cambridge, 2005), pp. 1–22.
Egido León, A., *Francisco Urzaiz. Un Republicano en la Francia ocupada. Vivencias de la guerra y el exilio* (Madrid, 2000).
Espuelas Barroso, S., "La evolución del gasto social público en España, 1850–2005", *Estudios de Historia Económica*, Vol. 63 (2013), pp. 1–122.
Estellés Salarich, J., "La sanidad del ejército Repúblicano del centro", in *Los médicos y la medicina en la Guerra Civil Española: Monografías Beecham* (Madrid, 1986), pp. 37–60.
Ferllini, R., "Human Rights Investigations in Spain", *Annals of Anthropological Practice*, Vol. 38, No. 1 (2014), pp. 65–80.
Fernández Paredes, T., "Transitional Justice in Democratization Processes: The Case of Spain from an International Point of View", *International Journal of Rule of Law, Transitional Justice And Human Rights*, Vol. 1 (2010), pp. 120–136.
Fernández Sabaté, A., *Nuestros fundadores y maestros en 1935 y 1947: Sociedad Española de Cirugía y Traumatología* (Madrid, 2013).

Ferrer Córdoba, P., "La sanidad en la marina republicana", in *Los médicos y la medicina en la Guerra Civil Española: Monografías Beecham* (Madrid, 1986), pp. 127–138.

Fleming, S., "Spanish Morocco and the Alzamiento Nacional, 1936–1939: The Military, Economic and Political Mobilisation of a Protectorate", *Journal of Contemporary History*, Vol. 18, No. 1 (1983), pp. 27–42.

Fletcher, R. A., *Moorish Spain* (London, 1992).

Franco Grande, A., Álvarez Escudero, J., & Cortés Laiño, J., *Historia de la anestesia en España: 1847–1940* (Madrid, 2005).

Franco Grande, A., Cortes, J., Alvarez, J., & Diz, J. C., "The Development of Blood Transfusion: The Contributions of Norman Bethune in the Spanish Civil War (1936–1939)", *Canadian Journal of Anaesthesia*, Vol. 43, No. 10 (1996), pp. 1076–1078.

Franco Grande, A., Diz, J. C., Aneiros, F. J., Cortés, J., & Alvarez, J., "The 'Servicio Hispano-Canadiense de Transfusión de Sangre' in the Spanish Civil War (1936–1939)", *Bulletin of Anaesthesia History*, Vol. 17, No. 2 (1998), pp. 14–16.

Fraser, R., *In Hiding: The Ordeal of Manuel Cortes* (New York, 1972).

——— *Blood of Spain: An Oral History of the Spanish Civil War* (London, 1979).

Frutos Herranz, M. de, *Hospitales en Burgos durante la Guerra Civil, 1936–1939* (Burgos, 2009).

Fundación Pablo Iglesias, *Carteles de la Guerra* (Madrid, 2008).

Fyrth, J., *The Signal Was Spain: The Aid Spain Movement in Britain, 1936–1939* (London, 1986).

Fyrth, J., & Alexander, S. (eds.), *Women's Voices from the Spanish Civil War* (London, 1991).

Gadow, M. R., "Una imagen controvertida de la Semana Santa malagueña: el Cristo de los Mutilados", *Los crucificados, religiosidad, cofradías y arte: Actas del Simposium 3/6-IX-2010* (2010), pp. 213–224.

Gálvez Biesca, S., "La 'memoria democrática' como conflicto", *Entelequia: revista interdisciplinar*, No. 7 (2008), pp. 1–52.

Garate Córdoba, J. M., "Las tropas de África en la Guerra Civil Española", *Revista de Historia Militar*, No. 70 (1991), pp. 9–66.

García Bravo, L. A., *Un valle de belleza y dolor: La tragedia de la Sauceda* (Ubrique, 2014).

García Cruz, J. F., "Las fuerzas militares nativas procedentes del Protectorado de Marruecos. Transcendencia política de su aplicación en las operaciones militares durante la Guerra Civil española", *Hispania Nova. Revista de Historia Contemporánea*, No. 2 (2001–2002), pp. 1–23.

García Ferrandis, X., "La asistencia sanitaria en la provincia de Valencia durante la Guerra Civil Española (1936–1939)", *Llull*, Vol. 34, No. 73 (2011), pp. 13–38.

——— "Anarcosindicalismo y sanidad en la retaguardia y en el frente: Los casos de Valencia y de la Columna de Hierro en la Guerra Civil Española (1936–1937)", *Asclepio*, Vol. 66, No. 2 (2012), pp. 63–76.

——— "La cobertura sanitaria de un ejército en retirada: la actuación de un Capitán Médico durante la Batalla del Maestrazgo (abril-julio de 1938)", *Sanidad Militar*, Vol. 68, No. 3 (2012), pp. 189–194.

——— *L'assistència sanitària A la ciutat de València durant la Guerra Civil* (Valencia, 2015).

García Ferrandis, X., & Munayco Sánchez, A. J., "La asistencia sanitaria en el frente de Teruel durante la primera campaña republicana (agosto de 1936-febrero de 1937)", *Sanidad Militar*, Vol. 66, No. 4 (2010), pp. 245–249.

Gasch-Tomás, J. L., "Spanish Empire: Vol. 2. From 1580", in J. M. MacKenzie (ed.), *The Encyclopedia of Empire* (Hoboken, 2015).

Giangrande, P. L. F., "The History of Blood Transfusion", *British Journal of Haematology*, Vol. 110, No. 4 (2000), pp. 758–767.

Gimeno, A. S., & Fariñas, D. R., "La caída de la mortalidad en la infancia en la España interior, 1860–1960: Un análisis de las causas de muerte", *Cuadernos de historia contemporánea*, Vol. 24 (2002), pp. 151–188.

Gómez Teruel, J. M., *La hospitalización militar en Sevilla a través de los tiempos* (Sevilla, 2006).

González Calleja, F., Cobo Romero, F., Martínez Rus, A., & Sanchez Pérez, F., *La Segunda República Española* (Barcelona, 2015).

González Canomanuel, M. A., "El comienzo del transporte aéreo sanitario en España. De la campaña del norte de África (1909–1927) al Servicio de búsqueda y salvamento (1955)", *Sanidad Militar*, Vol. 69, No. 4 (2013), pp. 276–282.

González Fernandez, A., *Fundamentos antropolóxicos da obra de Castelao* (Santiago de Compostela, 1999).

Goya y de Lucientes, F., *Los desastres de la guerra: Colección de ochenta láminas inventadas y grabadas al agua fuerte por Don Francisco Goya* (Madrid, 1863).

Gracia Rivas, M., "La sanidad de la armada en la Zona Nacional durante la guerra de 1936–1939", in *Los médicos y la medicina en la Guerra Civil Española: Monografías Beecham* (Madrid, 1986), pp. 103–126.

Graham, H., *The Spanish Republic at War 1936–1939* (Cambridge, 2002).

——— *The Spanish Civil War: A Very Short Introduction* (Oxford, 2005).

Grande Covian, F., "Deficiencias vitamínicas en Madrid durante la guerra civil: una reminiscencia", in *Los médicos y la medicina en la Guerra Civil Española: Monografías Beecham* (Madrid, 1986), pp. 61–67.

Grayzel, S. R., "'A Promise of Terror to Come': Air Power and the Destruction of Cities in British Imagination and Experience, 1908–39", in S. Goebel & D. Keene (eds.), *Cities Into Battlefields: Metropolitan Scenarios, Experiences and Commemorations of Total War* (Farnham, 2011), pp. 47–62.

Guerra, F., *La medicina en el exilio republicano* (Madrid, 2003).

Guijo Mauri, J. M., & Pecero Espín, J. C., *Estado de las investigaciones antropológicas en el cortijo de el Marrufo: Fundamentos científicos de inhumaciones clandestinas y episodios de violencia* (Jimena de la Frontera, 2012).

Gurriarán, R., *Fernando Alsina E O Seu: Diario de Guerra* (Santiago de Compostela, 2015).

Hannant, L., *The Politics of Passion: Norman Bethune's Writing and Art* (Toronto, 1998).

——— "'My God, Are They Sending Women?': Three Canadian Women in the Spanish Civil War, 1936–1939", *Journal of the Canadian Historical Association/Revue de la Société historique du Canada*, Vol. 15, No. 1 (2004), pp. 153–176.

Harana, L., "Los barcos-hospital franceses: Los otros barcos del exilio", in H. Buffery, F. Lough, E. Marcer, & A. M. Sánchez (eds.), *Spanish Republican Exile Geographies/Geografías del exilio republicano español* (Birmingham, 2012), pp. 35–46.

Harrison, M., *The Medical War: British Military Medicine in the First World War* (Oxford, 2010).

Hastings, M., *The Real Band of Brothers: First-Hand Accounts from the Last British Survivors of the Spanish Civil War* (London, 2009).

Hernández de Miguel, C., *Los últimos españoles de Mauthausen: La historia de nuestros deportados, sus verdugos y sus cómplices* (Barcelona, 2015).

Herraiz Muñoz, M., "Aplicación y avances en el tratamiento de los heridos en la Guerra civil Española", in *Los médicos y la medicina en la Guerra Civil Española: Monografías Beecham* (Madrid, 1986), pp. 279–290.

Herranz-Loncán, A., "Infrastructure Investment and Spanish Economic Growth, 1850–1935", *Explorations in Economic History*, Vol. 44, No. 3 (2007), pp. 452–468.

Herrera, A., & Las Mulas, M. de, "In Memoriam Fidel Pages Mirave (1886–1923) on the 75th Anniversary of the Publication of Anesthesia Metamerica", *Revista Española de Anestesiología y Reanimación*, Vol. 43, No. 2 (1996), pp. 59–66.

Hervás I Puyal, C., *La xarxa hospitalária a Catalunya durant la Guerra Civil 1936–1939* (Manresa, 2014).

Huertas, R., "Política sanitaria: De la dictadura de Primo de Rivera a la IIª República", *Revista Española Salud Publica*, Vol. 74 (2000), pp. 35–43.

International Boundary Study, No. 84 (Revised), July 1, 1970, Algeria – Western (Spanish) Sahara Boundary.

Jackson, A., *British Women and the Spanish Civil War* (London and New York, 2002).

——— *Beyond the Battlefield: Testimony, Memory and Remembrance of a Cave Hospital in the Spanish Civil War* (Abersychan, 2005).

——— *'For Us It Was Heaven'. The Passion, Grief and Fortitude of Patience Darton: From the Spanish Civil War to Mao's China* (Brighton, 2012).

Jackson, M., *The Oxford Handbook of the History of Medicine* (Oxford, 2001).

Jiménez Lucena, I., "El tifus exantemático de la posguerra española (1939–1943): el uso de una enfermedad colectiva en la legitimación del Nuevo estado", *Dynamis: Acta Hispánica ad Medicinae Scientiarumque. Historiam Illustrandam*, Vol. 14 (1994), pp. 185–198.

Junquera, N., "La promesa que Rajoy se cumplió", *El País* (5.10.2013).

——— "Necrológica: Trinidad Gallego, testigo del robo de niños", *El País* (12.11.2011).

Keene, J., *The Last Mile to Huesca: An Australian Nurse in the Spanish Civil War* (Sydney, 1998).

Klein, H. G., Spahn, D. R., & Carson, J. L., "Transfusion Medicine 1: Red Blood Cell Transfusion in Clinical Practice", *The Lancet*, Vol. 370 (04.08.2007), pp. 415–426.

La Porte, P., "Civil Military Relations in the Spanish Protectorate in Morocco: The Road to the Spanish Civil War, 1912–1936", *Armed Forces and Society*, Vol. 30, No. 2 (2004), pp. 203–226.

Larraz Andía, P., *Entre el frente y la retaguardia. la sanidad en la guerra civil: el hospital "Alfonso Carlos", Pamplona 1936–1939* (Madrid, 2004).

Larraz, P., & Barrola, C., "'Los pies de Teruel': Asistencia y tratamiento de las heridas por congelación en los hospitales navarros durante la guerra civil", *Anales de Sistema Sanitario de Navarra*, Vol. 28, No. 2 (2005), pp. 197–212.

Leal, J. M. "El Stanbrook: un barco mítico en la memoria de los exiliados republicanos", *Pasado y memoria: Revista de historia contemporánea*, Vol. 4 (2005), pp. 65–82.

Ledesma, J. L., "Enemigos seculares: La violencia anticlerical (1936–1939)", in J. de la Cueva & F. Montero (eds.), *Izquierda obrera y religión en España (1900–1939)* (Alcalá de Henares, 2012), pp. 219–244.

Lethbridge, D., *Norman Bethune in Spain: Commitment, Crisis, and Conspiracy* (Brighton, 2013).

Leval, G., *Collectives in the Spanish Revolution* (London, 1975).

Ley 2/2017, de 28 de marzo, de Memoria Histórica y Democrática de Andalucía.

Limón, R., "El parlamento Andaluz tramita sin oposición la Ley de Memoria Histórica", *El País* (10.02.2016).

Llunch-Prats, J., "La maternidad de Elna: Una isla de paz en medio de infierno", *Migraciones y Exilios*, No. 13 (2012), pp. 111–122.

Lozano, A., "Memoria Histórica en el cementerio de La Sauceda: Los caídos del cortijo del Marrufo yacen en paz", *El Mundo* (01.12.2012).

Lozano, M., & Cid, J., "Pioneers and Pathfinders; Frederic Durán-Jordà: A Transfusion Medicine Pioneer", *Transfusions Medicine Reviews*, Vol. 21, No. 1 (2007), pp. 75–81.

Llavona, R., & Bandrés, J., "Psicología y anarquismo en la Guerra Civil Española: La Obra de Félix Martí Ibañez", *Psicothema* Vol. 10, No. 3 (1998), pp. 669–678.

Lloret Pastor, J., "La depuración de científicos tras la guerra civil", in J. Luis Barona, (ed.), *Ciencia, salud pública y exilio (España, 1875–1939)* (Valencia, 2003), pp. 131–168.

Luttikhuizen, F., "Professor Ignasi Ponseti i Vives (1914–2009)", in *Contributions to Science*, Vol. 7, No. 2 (2012), pp. 205–214.

MacKay, R., "History on the Line; The Good Fight and Good History: the Spanish Civil War", *History Workshop Journal*, Vol. 70, No. 1 (2010), pp. 199–206.

Madariaga, M. R. de, *Los moros que trajo Franco: La intervención de tropas coloniales en la Guerra Civil Española* (Barcelona, 2002).

Mangini, S., *Memories of Resistance: Women's Voices from the Spanish Civil War* (New Haven, 1995).

Márquez, C. J., *Cómo se ha escrito la Guerra Civil* (Madrid, 2006).

Marset Campos, P., Martínez Navarro, F., & Sáez Gómez, J. M., "La Salud Pública durante el franquismo", *Dynamis: Acta Hispánica ad Medicinae Scientiarumque. Historiam Illustrandam*, Vol. 15 (1995), pp. 211–250.

Martí Boscà, J. V., "Algunos hombres buenos: Francisco Trigo Domínguez", *Revista de Salud Ambiental*, Vol. 14, No. 2 (2014), pp. 151–157.

——— "Federica Montseny y Pedro Vallina", *Revista de Salud Ambiental* Vol. 13, No. 1 (2013), pp. 95–102.

Martin Corrales, E., "Maurofobia/islamafobia y maurofilia/islamofilia en la España del siglo XXI", *Revista CIDOB d'Afers Internacionals*, No. 66–67 (2004), pp. 39–51.

Martín Rodríguez, M., "La industria azucarera española 1914–1936", *Revista de Historia Económica*, Vol. 5, No. 2 (1987), pp. 301–324.

Martin Sierra, F., "Hospital quirúrgico de montaña 'Gómez Ulla'", *Medicina Militar*, Vol. 56, No. 2 (2000), pp. 117–121.

Martinez Alonso, E., *Adventures of a Doctor* (London, 1962).

Martínez Antonio, F. J., "Entre la diplomacia médica y la política sanitaria: Médicos militares en el Protectorado Español en Marruecos (1906–1927)", *Revista de Historia Militar*, Vol. 2 (2012), pp. 203–242.

Martínez Vallina, P., *Mis Memorias* (Córdoba, 2000).

Martínez Vidal, À., "Metges catalans refugiats a França. Observació clínica i recerca científica als camps de concentració (1939–1942)", in R. Barrie, M. Camiade, & J. Font (directors), *Déplacements forcés et exils en Europe au XXe siècle: le corps et l'esprit: actes du 2eséminaire transfronterer* [*Desplaçaments forçosos i exilis a l'Europa del segle XX: el cos i l'esperit: actes del 2on seminari transfronterer*] (La Region Languedoc Rousillon, 2013), pp. 105–129.

Massons, J. M., *Historia de la Sanidad Militar Española: Tomo II* (Barcelona, 1994).

——— "L'Obra de Frederic Duran I Jorda Viscuda Per Mi", *Revista de la Reial Academia de Medicina de Catalunya*, No. 21 (2006), pp. 52–55.

Mateos Royo, J. A., "All the Town is a Stage: Civic Ceremonies and Religious Festivities in Spain During the Golden Age", *Urban History*, Vol. 26, No. 2 (1998), pp. 165–189.

Matthews, J., "'The Vanguard of Sacrifice'? Political Commissars in the Republican Popular Army during the Spanish Civil War, 1936–1939", *War in History*, Vol. 21, No. 1 (2014), pp. 82–101.

Medhurst, K., "The Coming of the Spanish Civil War: Reform, Reaction and Revolution in the Second Republic 1931–1936. (Book Review)", *International Affairs (Royal Institute of International Affairs 1944-)*, Vol. 55, No. 3 (1979), pp. 473–474.

"Memory of the World: Lost Memory – Libraries and Archives destroyed in the Twentieth Century", prepared for UNESCO on behalf of IFLA by Hans van der Hoeven and on behalf of ICA by Joan van Albada (Paris, 1996).

Merroun, M. E., *Las tropas marroquíes en la Guerra Civil española, 1936–1939* (Madrid, 2003).

Mesa, J. L. D., *Los moros de la Guerra Civil española* (Madrid, 2004).

Mila Nolla, M., "La mujer en la guerra: Enfermeras", in *Los médicos y la medicina en la Guerra Civil Española: Monografías Beecham* (Madrid, 1986), pp. 301–308.

Ministerio de la Defensa, *Historia militar de la Guerra Civil en Madrid: Fuentes primarías* (Madrid, 2014).

Monfort i Coll, A., "Los campos de concentración franquistas y su funcionamiento en Cataluña", *Hispania. Revista Española de Historia*, Vol. 69, No. 231 (2009), pp. 147–178.

Molero-Mesa, J., "'Salud, actuación y actividad'. La Organización Sanitaria Obrera de la CNT y la colectivización de los servicios médico-sanitarios en la Guerra Civil Española", in R. Campos, A. González, M. I. Porras, & L. Montiel (eds.), *XVI Congreso de la Sociedad Española de Historia de la Medicina. Medicina y poder político* (Madrid, 2014), pp. 103–107.

Montellà, A., *La maternidad de Elna: La historia de la mujer que salvo la vida de 597 niños* (Badalona, 2007).

Montseny, F., *Pasión y muerte de los españoles en Francia* (Toulouse, 1969).

——— "Mi experiencia en el Ministerio de Sanidad y Asistencia Social", in J. L. Barona & J. Bernabéu Mestre (eds.), *Ciencia y sanidad en la Valencia capital de la República* (Valencia, 2007), pp. 119–125.

Moradiellos, E., "Ni gesta heroica, ni locura trágica: nuevas perspectivas históricas sobre la guerra civil", *Ayer* (2003), pp. 11–39.

Moral Torres, J., "El 'método español' en el tratamiento de heridas de Guerra", in *Los médicos y la medicina en la Guerra Civil Española* (Madrid, 1986), pp. 157–166.

Moran Cifuentes, B., "Equipo quirúrgico de Traumatología", in *Los médicos y la medicina en la Guerra Civil Española: Monografías Beecham* (Madrid, 1986), pp. 167–176.

Moreno Cantano, A. C., "Proyección propagandística de la España franquista en Norteamérica (1936–1945)", *Hispania Nova: Revista de Historia Contemporánea*, No. 9 (2009), pp. 93–118.

Moreno Fernández-Caparrós, L. A., *Historia de la veterinaria militar española: organización de la veterinaria militar durante la Guerra Civil española, 1936–1939* (Madrid, 2013).

Nadal, A., "Experiencias psíquicas sobre mujeres marxistas Malagueñas: Málaga 1939", *Baetica: Estudios de Arte, Geografía e Historia*, No. 10 (1987), pp. 365–383.

Navarro Carballo, J. R., "Creación y desarrollo del Cuerpo de Damas Auxiliares de Sanidad Militar", *Medicina Militar*, Vol. 43, No. 3 (1987), pp. 320–331.

——— *Frederic Duran i Jorda: Un hito de la historia de la transfusión sanguínea* (Madrid, 2006).

Navarro Suay, R., & Plaza Torres, J. F., "1925: Cuando volvimos a ser grandes ... el apoyo sanitario en el desembarco de Alhucemas", *Sanidad Militar*, Vol. 68, No. 4 (2012), pp. 247–256.

——— "Una 'hazaña prácticamente desconocida': la participación de médicos militares españoles en la Primera Guerra Mundial", *Sanidad Militar*, Vol. 70, No. 1 (2014), pp. 51–57.

Oliver Olmo, P., Dueñas Iturbe, O., & Solé I Barjal, Q., "El hospital militar de la calle Tallers de Barcelona: tratamiento y represión de los prisioneros trabajadores forzados (1939–1942): Military Hospital of Tallers Street, Barcelona: Treatment and Repression of Forced Prison Workers (1939–1942)", in J. C. Urda Lozano (ed.), *La prisión y las instituciones punitivas en la investigación histórica: The Prison and the Punitive Institutions at the Historical Research* (Cuenca, 2014), pp. 557–578.

Orledge, R., *Charles Koechlin (1867–1950): His Life and Works* (Luxemburg, 1981).

Otero Carvajal, L. E., "La destrucción de la ciencia en España: Las consecuencias del triunfo militar de la España franquista", *Historia y Comunicación Social*, No. 6 (2001), pp. 149–186.

Overy, R., "Saving Civilization: British Public Opinion and the Coming of War in 1939", in D. Welch & J. Fox (eds.), *Justifying War: Propaganda, Politics and the Modern Age* (Basingstoke, 2012).

Pagès i Blanch, P., *War and Revolution in Catalonia, 1936–1939*, translated by Patrick L. Gallagher (Boston, 2013).

Palfreeman, L., *¡Salud! British Volunteers in the Republican Medical Service during the Spanish Civil War, 1936–1939* (Brighton, 2012).

——— *Aristocrats, Adventurers and Ambulances: British Medical Units in the Spanish Civil War* (Brighton, 2014).

——— *Spain Bleeds: The Development of Battlefield Blood Transfusion during the Civil War* (Brighton, 2015).

Paulino Pérez, J., "La sanidad del arma de aviación Republicana", in *Los médicos y la medicina en la Guerra Civil Española: Monografías Beecham* (Madrid, 1986), pp. 231–236.

Payne, S. G., *The Franco Regime, 1936–1975* (London, 1987).

——— "Historiography on the Spanish Republic and Civil War", *The Journal of Modern History*, Vol. 60, No. 3 (1988), pp. 540–556.

Pelis, K., "Taking Credit: The Canadian Army Medical Corps and the British Conversion to Blood Transfusion in WWI", *Journal of the History of Medicine and Allied Sciences*, Vol. 56, No. 3 (2001), pp. 238–277.

Pérez Ribelles, V., "La sanidad del aire en Zona Nacional durante la Guerra Civil Española", in *Los médicos y la medicina en la Guerra Civil Española: Monografías Beecham* (Madrid, 1986), pp. 203–210.

Picardo Castellón, M., "Experiencia personal en un hospital quirúrgico de primera línea durante nuestra Guerra Civil", in *Los médicos y la medicina en la Guerra Civil Española: Monografías Beecham* (Madrid, 1986), pp. 177–202.

Pita, R., *Armas Químicas: La Ciencia en Manos de Mal* (Madrid, 2008).

Ponseti Vives, I., "History of Orthopaedic Surgery", *The Iowa Orthopaedic Journal* (1991), pp. 59–64.

——— "Treatment of Congenital Club Foot", *The Journal of Bone and Joint Surgery* Vol. 74, No. 3 (1992), pp. 448–454.

Preston, P., *The Coming of the Spanish Civil War: Reform, Reaction, and Revolution in the Second Republic, 1931–1936* (London, 1978).

——— "The Historiography of the Spanish Civil War", in *People's History and Socialist Theory*, History Workshop Series (London, 1981).

——— *Franco: A Biography* (London, 1993).

——— *A Concise History of the Spanish Civil War* (London, 1996).

——— *Doves of War: Four Women of Spain* (London, 2002).

——— *The Politics of Revenge: Fascism and the Military in 20th-Century Spain* (London, 2003).

——— *The Spanish Civil War: Reaction, Revolution, and Revenge*, revised and expanded edition (London, 2006).

——— "Two Doctors and One Cause: Len Crome and Reginald Saxton in the International Brigades", *International Journal of Iberian Studies*, Vol. 19, No. 1 (2006), pp. 5–24.

——— *We Saw Spain Die: Foreign Correspondents in the Spanish Civil War* (London, 2008).

——— *The Spanish Holocaust: Inquisition and Extermination in Twentieth-Century Spain* (London, 2012).

Pretus. G., *La ayuda humanitaria en la Guerra Civil española, 1936–1939* (Granada, 2015).

Puyal, C. H., & Mur, M. C., "Notas históricas sobre el hospital de sangre número 18 de Barcelona (1936–1939)", *Gimbernat: Revista Catalana d'història de la medicina i de la ciencia*, Vol. 27 (1997), pp. 173–184.

Quiroga, A., & Arco del, M. Á. (eds.), *Right-Wing Spain in the Civil War Era: Soldiers of God and Apostles of the Fatherland, 1914–45* (London, 2012).

Ramiro Rivera, Dr., Presidente de la Organización Médico Colegial, "Epilogo: Soldados de la ciencia, el humanismo y la libertad", in *Los Médicos y la Medicina en la Guerra Civil Española: Monografías Beecham* (Madrid, 1986), pp. 347–350.

Renshaw, L., *Exhuming Loss: Memory, Materiality and Mass Graves of the Spanish Civil War* (Walnut Creek, 2011).

Requena Gallego, M., & Sepúlveda Losa, R. M. (eds.), *La sanidad en las Brigadas Internacionales* (Cuenca, 2006).

Ribeiro de Meneses, F., "Popularizing Africanism: The Career of Víctor Ruiz Albéniz, El Tebib Arrumi", *Journal of Iberian and Latin Studies*, Vol. 11, No. 1 (2005), pp. 39–63.

Riegel, O. W., "Press, Radio, and the Spanish Civil War", *The Public Opinion Quarterly*, Vol. 1, No. 1 (1937), pp. 131–136.

Rina Simón, C., "La construcción de los imaginarios franquistas y la religiosidad 'popular', 1931–1945", *Pasado y Memoria: Revista de Historia Contemporánea*, No. 14 (2015), pp. 179–196.

Richards, M., "From War Culture to Civil Society: Francoism, Social Change and Memories of the Spanish Civil War", *History and Memory*, Vol. 14, No. 1–2 (2002), Special Issue: Images of a Contested Past, pp. 93–120.

——— "'Presenting Arms to the Blessed Sacrament': Civil War and Semana Santa in the City of Malaga, 1936–1939", in C. Ealham & M. Richards (eds.), *The Splintering of Spain: Cultural History and the Spanish Civil War, 1936–1939* (Cambridge, 2005), pp. 196–222.

——— *After the Civil War: Making Memory and Re-Making Spain since 1936* (Cambridge, 2013).

Rodrigo, A., *Doctor Trueta: Héroe anonimo de dos guerras* (Barcelona, 1977).

Rodrigo, J., "La guerra civil: 'memoria', 'olvido', 'recuperación' e 'instrumentación'", *Hispania Nova. Revista de Historia Contemporánea*, No. 6 (2006), pp. 385–410.

——— "Internamiento y trabajo forzoso: Los campos de concentración de Franco", *Hispania Nova. Revista de Historia Contemporánea*, No. 6 (2006), pp. 615–642.

Rodríguez Ocaña, E., "La intervención de la Fundación Rockefeller en la creación de la sanidad contemporánea en España", *Revista Española de Salud Pública*, Vol. 74 (2000), pp. 27–34.

Rodríguez Padilla, E., *Mujeres de Almería condenadas a muerte o reclusión perpetua tras la Guerra Civil 1939–1945* (Almería, 2014).

Roig, A. F., "40 Años de puericultura en Reus", *Revista del Centre de Lectura de Reus*, No. 27 (1954), pp. 109–112.

Rojo Fernández, V., "Algunos aspectos durante la operaciones de Teruel", in *Los médicos y la medicina en la Guerra Civil Española: Monografías Beecham* (Madrid, 1986), pp. 139–156.

Romero Romero, F., *Alcalá del Valle. República, Guerra Civil y represión 1931–1946* (Cádiz, 2009).

Rubio, J., *La emigración de la guerra civil de 1936–1939: Historia del éxodo que se produce con el fin de la II República española* (Madrid, 1977).

——— "Las cifras del exilio", *Historia 16*, Vol. 30 (1978), 19–32.

Ruiz-Berdún D., & Gomis, A., "La depuración de las matronas de Madrid tras la Guerra Civil", *Dynamis*, Vol. 32, No. 1 (2012), pp. 439–465.

Ruiz-Vargas, J. M., "Trauma y memoria de la Guerra Civil y de la dictadura franquista", *Hispania Nova. Revista de Historia Contemporánea*, Vol. 6 (2006), pp. 299–336.

Said, E., *Orientalism: Western Conceptions of the Orient* (London, 1978).

Sánchez-Biosca, V., *Cine y Guerra Civil Española: Del mito a la memoria* (Madrid, 2006).

Sánchez Ruano, F., *Islam y Guerra Civil Española: Moros con Franco y con la República* (Madrid, 2004).

Scott-Ellis, P., *The Chances of Death: A Diary of the Spanish Civil War*, edited by Raymond Carr (Norwich, 1995).

——— The Diary of Pip Scott-Ellis (Cardiff University Library Archive (CULA): manuscript no. 3/233).

Schmidt, U., *Medical Films, Ethics, and Euthanasia in Nazi Germany: The History of Medical Research and Teaching Films of the Reich Office for Educational Films – Reich Institute for Films in Science and Education, 1933–1945* (Husum, 2002).

——— *Secret Science: A Century of Poison Warfare and Human Experiments* (Oxford, 2015).

Schneider, W. H., "Blood Transfusion Between the Wars", *Journal of the History of Medicine and Allied Sciences*, Vol. 58, No. 2 (2003), pp. 187–224.
Serrallonga i Urquidi, J., "El cuento de la regularización sanitaria y asistencial en el régimen franquista: Una primera etapa convulsa, 1936–1944", *Historia social*, No. 59 (2007), pp. 77–98.
Shepard, D. A. E., & Levesque, A. (eds.), *Norman Bethune: His Times and His Legacy* (Ottawa, 1982).
Shumacker, H. B., *Leo Eloesser, MD: Eulogy for a Free Spirit* (New York, 1982).
Sotomayor Blásquez, C. T., "El moro traidor, el moro engañado: variantes del estereotípico en el Romancero republicano", *Anaquel de Estudios Árabes*, Vol. 15 (2005), pp. 233–249.
Sígler, F., "Celebrado en el cementerio de la Sauceda el homenaje y entierro digno de víctimas exhumadas en el Marrufo", *Papeles de la Historia* (2012).
Stein, L., *Beyond Death and Exile: The Spanish Republicans in France, 1939–1955* (London, 1979).
Stewart, R., & Majada, J., *Bethune en España* (Madrid, 2009).
Stewart, R., & Stewart, S., *Phoenix: The Life of Norman Bethune* (Montreal, 2011).
Swan, H., "S. S. Yudin: A Study in Frustration", *Surgery*, Vol. 58, No. 3 (1965), pp. 572–585.
Thackrah, J. R., *Routledge Companion to Military Conflict Since 1945* (Oxford, 2009).
Thomas, H., *The Spanish Civil War*, revised edition (Toronto, 2001).
Torre Fernández, J. M., *Gómez Ulla, Hospital Militar Central, cien años de historia,* (Madrid, 1996).
Trueta, J., *Trueta: Surgeon in War and Peace: The Memoirs of Josep Trueta, M.D., F.R.C.S., D.Sc.* Translated by Meli and Michael Strubell (London, 1980).
Tse Tung, M. [Zedong, M.], *Quotations from Chairman Mao Tse Tung*, trans. W. Barnstone (San Francisco, 1972).
Unzueta Merino, M. C., Hervás Puyal. C., & Villar Landeira. J, "Robert R. Macintosh y España: una relación fecunda", *Revista Española de Anestesiología y Reanimación*, Vol. 48, No. 1 (2001), pp. 21–28.
Valls, R., et al., *Infermeres catalanes a la Guerra Civil espanyola* (Barcelona, 2008).
Van de Ven, H., "Introduction to Part 1", in R. Chickering, D. Showalter, & H. Van de Ven (eds.), *The Cambridge History of War Volume IV: War and the Modern World* (Cambridge, 2012), pp. 9–15.
Vásquez León, A., *Un boomerang en Jimena de la Frontera: Guerra, huida y exilio de una niña campogibraltareña* (Algeciras, 1998).
Vega Sombría, S., & García Funes, J. C., "Lucha tras las rejas franquistas: La prisión central de mujeres de Segovia", *Studia Histórica. Historia contemporánea*, Vol. 29 (2012) pp. 281–314.
Vincent, M., "The Keys of the Kingdom: Religious Violence in the Spanish Civil War, July–August 1936", in C. Ealham & M. Richards (eds.), *The Splintering of Spain: Cultural History and the Spanish Civil War, 1936–1939* (Cambridge, 2005), pp. 68–92.
Vinyes, R., *Irredentas: Las presas políticas y sus hijos en las cárceles franquistas* (Madrid, 2002).
Vinyes, R., Armengou, M., & Belis, R., *Los niños perdidos del franquismo: Un estremecedor documento que sale por primera vez a la luz* (Barcelona, 2002).
Zelizer, B, "Why Memory's Work on Journalism Does Not Reflect Journalism's Work on Memory", *Memory Studies*, Vol. 1, No 1 (2008), pp. 79–87.

Zubelzu, L. S., "Obra Quirúrgica de Fermín Palma García", *Seminario Medico*, No. 38 (1979), pp. 59–78.
Zumel, M. F., "Cirugía de guerra", in *Los médicos y la medicina en la Guerra Civil Española: Monografías Beecham* (Madrid, 1986), pp. 69–92.

Electronic sources

www.bbc.co.uk/history/british/britain_wwtwo/orwell_01.shtml
https://commons.wikimedia.org/wiki/Los_desastres_de_la_guerra
www.elplural.com
www.foroporlamemoria.es
www.fpabloiglesias.es
www.juntadeandalucia.es
www.ibms.org/go/nm:history-blood-transfusion
www.memoriaHistórica.org.es
www.oxforddnb.com
www.papelesdehistoria.org/2012/12/02/celebrado-en-el-cementerio-de-la-sauceda-el-homenaje-y-entierro-digno-de-victimas-exhumadas-en-el-marrufo.html
www.todoslosnombres.org

Modern newspapers

ABC
El Mundo
El País
La Vanguardia
Publico
The Independent

Index

Note: Page numbers in *italics* refer to images.